Acclaim for the writing of Niall McLaren, M.D.

"Not only does Dr. Niall McLaren point out the various shortcomings of the established views of psychology/psychiatry, and of some other scientific disciplines, but he also proposes the most cogent model of mind that does not violate fundamental scientific laws and is also compatible with the norms of common sense and logic. He has endangered the foundations of contemporary mainstream psychiatry while, at the same time, creating a rescue channel."
—Ernest Dempsey, editor of *Recovering the Self Journal*

"This book is a *tour de force*. It demonstrates a tremendous amount of erudition, intelligence and application in the writer. It advances an interesting and plausible mechanism for many forms of human distress. It is an important work that deserves to take its place among the classics in books about psychiatry."
—Robert Rich, PhD, AnxietyAndDepression-Help.com

"I found Niall McLaren's book to be an incredibly well-written and thought-provoking. It is not, by any means, easy reading. It is also not for someone who doesn't have some form of background in understanding the various psychological theories and mental health conditions. I think that this would make an excellent textbook for a graduate class that allows students to question the theories that we already have."
—Paige Lovitt for *Reader Views*

"It is impossible to do justice to this ambitious, erudite, and intrepid attempt to dictate to psychiatry a new, 'scientifically-correct' model theory. The author offers a devastating critique of the shortcomings and pretensions of psychiatry, not least its all-pervasive, jargon-camouflaged nescience.
—Sam Vaknin, PhD, author *Malignant Self Love: Narcissism Revisited*

"McLaren's book has been thirty years in the making and is obviously well researched and thought-out. The author makes very strong, intelligent arguments that, I believe, will have a large impact on the future of psychiatry. McLaren's book would make an excellent read for a psychiatry student or for those already in the field."

—Kam Aures for *Rebecca's Reads*

"This is an academic book about psychiatric methods. As a psychology graduate as well as a user of the various services, I find this a fascinating subject. It's not for a beginner, but for someone who has some experience of the mental health services, it's interesting and thought-provoking. We need to get over the stigma attached to mental health and see it on the same level as physical health issues. It's not a new theory, but more of an overview of what has gone before and where the future direction of psychiatry should lead."

—Josie Henley-Einion, author of *Silence*

"Ultimately, McLaren says that any theory of the mind has to provide a rational explanation of mental disorder. He boldly speaks his mind throughout the book, backing up his points with multiple examples, and he is not afraid to cry "Humbug!" when necessary. McLaren has been practicing psychiatry since 1977 in Australia. His discussion of his own education and the shortcomings of the education system he went through as well as weaknesses in current psychiatric practices demonstrate that psychiatry has many more steps to take before it is a completely effective science. This work may well lead to a new understanding of mental illness in future years as younger psychiatrists read his book and follow his example in rejecting the ineffective theories he derides."

—Tyler R. Tichelaar, PhD, author of *The Gothic Wanderer*

"This is a paradigm-challenging work, to say the very least, and McLaren's views require a person who has a vested interest in these subjects to confront their own resistance to challenge. It's worthwhile, because McLaren's book is affirmative concerning something which many people may have found lacking in modern psychology, and psychiatry: namely, a psyche.

With the technological revolutions occurring in the past century-and-a-half, it seems every scientist wanted to find a way to reduce the psyche to a physical property, or some combination of physical properties, or completely deny its existence (behaviorism). While this has certainly been in vogue, and has yielded many useful results in terms of understanding neurobiology and its connection to moods and perception, it has not been successful in penetrating an understanding of 'the Self', or the psyche. Some will say this is because the self/psyche doesn't exist, but is only a fiction that appears to the individual: still, this is just a reduction to absurdity- what is the person who perceives the self, but indeed the self?"

—Kevin Brady, *Clear Objectives*

The Mind-Body Problem Explained:

The Biocognitive Model for Psychiatry

Niall McLaren, M.D.

An application of the philosophy of science to psychiatry

Future Psychiatry Press

Distributed by: Ingram Book Group (USA/CAN), Bertram's Books (UK)

Library of Congress Cataloging-in-Publication Data

McLaren, Niall, 1947-
  The mind-body problem explained : the biocognitive model for psychiatry / Niall McLaren.
      p. ; cm.
  Includes bibliographical references and index.
  ISBN 978-1-61599-171-6 (hardcover : alk. paper) -- ISBN 978-1-61599-170-9 (pbk. : alk. paper) -- ISBN 978-1-61599-172-3 (ebook)
  I. Title.
  [DNLM: 1. Cognition. 2. Psychiatry--methods. 3. Models, Psychological. 4. Psychological Theory. WM 100]

  616.89--dc23
                          2012028891

Future Psychiatry Press is an imprint of
Loving Healing Press
5145 Pontiac Trail
Ann Arbor, MI 48105
USA

http://www.LovingHealing.com or
info@LovingHealing.com
Fax +1 734 663 6861

To my long-suffering family.

"Behind it all is surely an idea so simple, so beautiful, that when we grasp it—in a decade, a century, or a millennium—we will all say to each other, how could it have been otherwise? How could we have been so stupid?"

—John A Wheeler

Contents

Table of Figures

Introduction:
Psychiatry and the Biocognitive Model of Mind

> "Every great and deep difficulty bears in itself its own solution. It forces us to change our thinking in order to find it."
>
> —Niels Bohr

The purpose of this book is to start to fill in the details of the model of mind outlined in my previous monographs [1,2,3]. For want of a better term, I named it the 'biocognitive model of mind,' unaware that somebody else had a prior claim to the word [4]. Fortunately, that hasn't been a problem as we are of similar philosophical inclinations, and two heads are surely better than one.

This model says that the mind is an informational space generated by the brain by means of principles and processes that, these days, are universally applied throughout industry, commerce, at home and at play—in fact, everything we do these days seems to depend on these principles. There is nothing new about any of them as they have been transforming society throughout my lifetime, and before. However, there is no guarantee that what works in a laboratory or in a laptop or mobile phone has anything to do with the human mind. While it may even be the case that the principles behind a desktop computer apply perfectly to animal "minds," we can't ever assume that they apply to human mental function, which seems to reach so much further in its scope.

It's possible that this particular debate may never be resolved because, if the brain does function like an ordinary computer, it's not clear that we can ever know the codes by which it operates. At this stage, I don't think that's a problem. All I am doing is setting out the case for a new model of mind based on the notion that the mind emerges from the brain in its normal function as a switching device of almost incomprehensible complexity and power.

The first consequence of this is that we have to take the mind seriously and stop trying to devise theories of mind or behavior that start with the idea that we can never know anything about it, or that science can't deal with it, or that it is inherently antiscientific, or all the other arguments that have been raised against this type of project. The mind exists, it is a reality, it arises from the brain by principles that are neither mysterious nor magical, and it then acts upon the universe by non-magical means to produce changes that we choose by an act of willpower [5]. In essence, this project is about giving a formal, rational basis to most of what ordinary people have always understood of minds—the Folk Psychology concept of mind, to use Wilhelm Wundt's apt term.

Of course, this puts the project on the other side of the fence from all serious theories of mind or psychology developed in the twentieth century. They all started with the notion that the idea of mind was too silly or too abstruse or irrational or whatever for scientists to talk about, even in their sleep. The American psychologist, John B. Watson, who played a major part in initiating the behaviorist movement, said in about 1916 that he wanted his students to be as ignorant of questions of mind as engineering students. He achieved that particular goal but I don't think the world, or several generations of psychologists, were any the better for it—or that they will thank him. The philosopher Daniel Dennett is scathing about the concept of a dualist mind and never misses an opportunity to hammer mentalist theories as magical gibberish and "green slime" nonsense. He is aware that his own theory, functionalism, is counter-intuitive but that doesn't worry him as he believes the correct theory of mind has to be counter-intuitive as we have tried all the intuitive ones and they went nowhere.

It is ironic, then, that Dennett's own theory is based in his intuitive rejection of dualism at the age of eighteen. If the correct theory of mind turns out to be dualist, which I believe is the case, then he will be able to say he got something right: his own intuitive antidualist reaction, way back then, was wrong. There is no reason to believe that dualism implies magic at all.

The second point I like to make about theories of mind is that if they don't immediately generate a theory of mental disorder, they aren't worth the paper they are written on. Any valid theory of mind must be able to predict how and why the mind will begin to malfunction. The only theory of mind that makes any attempt to do this is the theory I will be talking about here, the bio-cognitive theory of mind for psychiatry. The rest don't even offer a starting point. Unfortunately, they have left the field wide open for psychiatry to embrace the notion that, whatever the mind is, mental disorder is nothing more than a biological disease of the brain. I also believe that notion, called biological reductionism, is completely wrong and is causing huge damage to mentally-troubled people, as well as needlessly costing the taxpayer a large and ever-increasing fortune.

This book follows the same format I have used in the past, mainly because this is what they call "a work in progress." It is technical, because I think it has to be. I'm not writing for popularity (that's lucky, as I'm not getting much, especially in psychiatric circles) but I try to write so that non-psychiatrists can read it. The theory has to be comprehensible to educated non-medical people; if I can't convince them, then I will end up in the same hole as the psycho-analysts who only ever convinced people who wanted to be convinced. I see my job as convincing all the people who still believe that science can't come to grips with the mind just because it is magical.

Each chapter in the book tackles a particular problem and treats it at depth. In this book, I am largely relying on my three previous books and my other publications, so I won't be giving a lot of references. Any new material will be referenced but that's all. The first part (Chapters 1-7) develops the principles behind the notion of the mind as a natural phenomenon that emerges predictably from a specialized switching device. There are gaps, of course, but that is to be expected. My goal is to make sure there are no conceptual gaps in the chain of explanation from brain to mind and back again. There is no magic, no miracles, no smoke or mirrors or whipping the real problem off the table and leaving a pseudo-problem to be resolved with a fanfare. Unfortunately, this process becomes a bit tedious because I have to raise and then deal with one objection after another so it is sometimes difficult to keep track of the main theme.

The second part is more interesting because the new model is tested against a number of existing theories to see if it can give an account of the observations that led to the theories. This leads to a discussion on the concept of human nature and the relationship between our more primitive drives and instincts and our capacity for abstract thinking and reasoning. I also include in this section criticisms of some other ideas, mainly the notion that mental disorder is a myth, ably marketed these past fifty years by the late Thomas Szasz. My case is that Szasz (who also decided he knew everything there is to know about minds as a teenager) is completely wrong: his approach fails to take into account the notion that mental disorders are primary dysfunctions in the informational state known as the mind. Despite anything Thomas Szasz has said, mental disorder is a reality. I also review the latest developments in the apparently endless progress of biological psychiatry from A to B and back to A again, driven only by technology and financed at stupefying cost by taxpayers who have no idea what is being done on their behalf. I will show that this research is all wrong: mental disorder is a reality but it will never be explained by looking down a microscope.

Part III develops some of the ideas using clinical material, the main emphasis being to show how the notion of biological reductionism inevitably leads to gross misunderstandings of the nature of mental disorder, and ends up causing more damage than it could hope to solve. I had hoped to talk more about how I treat mental disorder as a primary disorder of mind (i.e. psycho-therapy) but I ran out of space so that may have to wait for another book. The case histories point to serious misdiagnosis and mismanagement as the norm in psychiatry. I have always argued that this arises just because psychiatry doesn't have a formal, articulated model of mental disorder to guide its practice, its teaching and its research. While this remains the case, orthodox psychiatry will continue to chase after fads, ably encouraged and misled by academics pushing their own agendas and drug companies on the lookout for new marketing opportunities.

I mentioned style. Some readers have said they find the style in the earlier books pedestrian, pedantic and pugnacious. I really don't know how to prove a lot of people wrong when they don't want to believe it, unless I take an opposing point of view (pugnacious), sort out exactly what they are saying (pedantic) and then wearily go through each of their points and every consequence of each of their points (pedestrian) without coming across as pedestrian, pedantic and pugnacious. My problem is that if I don't take a strongly opposed point of view, orthodox psychiatry will ignore anything critical and everything novel, as they have resolutely done for decades, just because that is their only way of dealing with criticism: shut it out, make sure it doesn't get an airing. In particular, they are determined to make sure that medical students and trainees (residents) don't get to hear of any arguments against their own position. Yes, their behavior is completely against the spirit of science as a process of free, open inquiry but that's how they play the game. That means I have no alternative but to play it by their rules, only better. For twenty-five years, I knocked politely at the doors of the psychiatric establishment, only to realize that they took courtesy as a sign of weakness, and put extra locks on the door. Now I kick at the doors. If nothing else, it makes me feel better.

The title of this book may cause some concern but the precedent was set nearly twenty years ago by Dennett himself, with his *Consciousness Explained.* Right at the end, he said:

> "I haven't replaced a metaphorical theory, the Cartesian Theater, with a *non*-metaphorical ("literal, scientific") theory. All I have done, really, is to replace one family of metaphors and images with another.... It's just a war of metaphors, you say – but... metaphors are the tools of thought... Look what we have built with our tools. Could you have imagined it without them?"

That is, he hadn't explained anything at all. In this work, my goal is to get rid of all metaphors and replace them with formal, proven working models to assemble a concept of mind that does not rely on legerdemain to bridge conceptual gaps. Whether I have succeeded or not rests with the readers.

So that's it. As I said, I don't give a lot of references in this book as everything depends on the case developed in my earlier works. At this stage, if my argument doesn't stand on its own feet, unsupported by libraries of references, then it isn't convincing.

Enjoy.

Part I:
The Irreducible
Mentality of Mind

"Everything should be made as simple as possible, but not simpler."
—Albert Einstein

<table>
<tr>
<td>1</td>
<td>

The Irreducible
Mentality of Mind

</td>
</tr>
</table>

"If the creator had a purpose in endowing us with a neck, he surely meant us to stick it out."

—Arthur Koestler

1.1 Introduction

The astounding success of modern science depends on reductionism, the concept that the properties or behavior of a higher-order entity can be fully explained in terms of the properties or behavior of the lower-order entities of which it is composed. As an intellectual program, it lies at the core of our efforts to see the universe as a rational or rule-abiding place whose laws we can discover by pursuing a rational or rule-governed program. We can call this approach 'naturalism,' to contrast it with the ancient idea of a supernatural element above and beyond the natural or material world which we mortals can approach only by intuition or supplication, if at all. To a very large extent, the history of western science has been the history of reducing what was once seen as mysterious or beyond comprehension to matters of mechanics and chemistry.

In attempting to explain human behavior, the ancient model was the intuitive: each of us has a resident supernatural soul or spirit that does the hard work of separating us from the beasts of the field. The notion of an inner self was formalized by the French polymath, Rene Descartes, who concluded that, while the body is a machine of essentially the same order of nature as that of all other animals, the soul is both real and utterly different. That is, he saw the universe as having a dual nature, consisting of the natural or material world, which obeys the laws of physics (although he didn't use that term), and a supernatural world, which does not. This, of course, leads to an insuperable problem: if the soul is of a non-material nature, how can it interact with the material body to produce observable behavior? How can some untouchable thing touch us? For several centuries after Descartes, nobody worried greatly about this as most people accepted that it just did: after all, that is what supernatural means. There was enough work for scientists to do without offending religious sensibilities by tackling a mind-body problem which seemed to have no beginning.

However, from about the middle of the nineteenth century, it was becoming increasingly obvious that something was very wrong. Either the universe was a natural, rule-governed sort of place, or it wasn't. Political programs, such as Marxism and anarchism, began to challenge the idea of a benevolent deity, while the onward rush of materialist science seemed to overcome every challenge in its path. More to the point, the concept of a causally effective soul or spirit started to appear incongruous, if not downright silly: science was based on hard evidence, but if there was no conceivable evidence for a soul, then how could science deal with it? By the turn of the century, there was open rebellion. The American psychologist, John B. Watson, proclaimed that all talk of a mind tethered psychology to a nonsensical standard. What was needed, he said, was a science of behavior in which students of psychology knew as much about the mind as students of physics—essentially, nothing [1, Chap. 2].

In fairly short order, the notion that there could and should be a formal science of human mentality took control. There were three possible forms, a mechanistic model of mentation, as in Freud's psychoanalytic notion of mind; the behaviorist approach, which regarded all talk of minds as gibberish; or the concept that reductionist science would explain the mind just as it was explaining everything else. By the 1950s and 60s, the intellectual world had more or less stabilized in these three approaches. Neuroscientists and physicians accepted that the phenomena of mind would eventually be explained *in toto* by the principles and methods of reductionist laboratory science. Psychologists had their behaviorism, and psychiatrists had both of those plus psychoanalysis, as the fancy took them. Philosophers, the smallest but most durable group of theorists of mind, were moving to a hard-nosed materialism, doing everything they could to distance themselves from the insurmountable difficulties of dualism.

By the 1980s, however, the world was changing fast. First psychoanalysis, then behaviorism, fell by the wayside as 'non-science.' Psychiatrists rushed to embrace reductionist biologism, psychologists fell hungrily upon a semantically-modified mentalism (relabeled 'cognitivism'), while philosophers discovered a middle road called functionalism. That, roughly, is the position today, so we need to look a little more closely at what these terms mean.

1.2 Failed Theories

The term 'cognitive psychology' can be misleading as, in practice, it has two distinct meanings. The first, and more restricted, meaning applies to the investigative or laboratory discipline which is part of the broader field of cognitive sciences. Cognitive sciences means roughly the intersection of the neurosciences, psychology, philosophy, linguistics and computer sciences. Ulrich Neisser defined cognition as referring to all the processes by which the sensory input is transformed, reduced, elaborated, stored, recovered and used. This includes not only the obvious mental events of which we are aware, but also the many brain processes underlying knowing and awareness that are not open to introspection. Cognitive research examines mental processes such as sensory perception, memory, motor processing, judgment and many other complex events, often using laboratory animals rather than humans. There is no conceptual boundary between this and ordinary neurophysiology as researchers in each field approach the same general topic from different but complementary directions. Cognitive psychologists and other neuroscientists freely borrow techniques and concepts from each other.

When cognitive psychology is used in the context of treating mental disorders, it is normally in the loose sense of what is now known as Cognitive-Behavioral Therapy (CBT). Overlooking the fact that cognitivism and behaviorism are mutually contradictory, and that a therapy without a model is just a technology (or even an art), not a scientific theory, CBT uses techniques of moral suasion in a more focused sense than in the days of 'moral therapy.' It sees the human as a mind in a body, where the mind is causally effective, but it has no formal theory of mind and definitely no theory of mind-body interaction. The techniques have limited efficacy and are relatively harmless but the lack of a model of mind leads to a major problem: the absence of a demarcation criterion between the therapy and quackery. As Skinner noted in 1974 [2], the problem is that simple cognitivism is not a theory at all. It simply attributes to an 'inner person' that which requires explanation. Thus, we have the bizarre spectacle of psychologists trained in the scientific method indulging in all sorts of non-scientific practices, such as aura therapy, rebirthing, massage, prayer, macrovitamin therapy, QEEG and anything else that takes their fancy. The reason they can do this is because there is nothing in their theory that says they can't. At the same time, many psychologists are now claiming that, by virtue of their training in areas of mind, they should be granted the right to prescribe psychoactive drugs. In general, this is not a good combination. Governments should resist steadfastly the drive to mate Kirlian photography with depot antipsychotics.

Unlike psychology, psychiatry has not had to change horses in mid-stream, merely to let two of them go while everybody crowded on the last. Worldwide, since early in the nineteenth century, there has been a very strong tradition of what is now known as biological psychiatry. In about 1867, this was summarized by the British psychiatrist, Henry Maudsley, in his famous dictum "mental disease is brain disease" (also attributed to Benjamin Rush, of the US). This means that all cases of mental disorder are simply cases of neurological disorder in which the symptoms are manifest as psychological dysfunction rather than, say, as paralysis or speech defects. It must never be forgotten that, despite all the publicity it generated, the foray into psycho-analysis was a very small show indeed. In every country, at all times in the past several hundred years, the vast majority of people with any sort of mental disorder received "treatment," where treatment meant something like what ordinary medical practitioners do to people with ordinary physical illnesses, or what vets do to horses. Until about fifty years ago, this meant incarceration and isolation (like people with infectious diseases) and a wide range of more or less brutal physical "treatments." A brief but shocking history of some of the physical methods used to control the mentally disturbed is available in Whitaker's *Mad in America* [3].

The concept that mental disorder is, at base, a form of brain disturbance, has a powerful appeal to people trained in the tradition of reductionist science, meaning all medical practitioners. Western physical medicine is a compelling argument for the notion that, if you want to know why something isn't working properly, you need only look at its component parts and the answer will thrust itself at you. All physicians are trained in anatomy, physiology and biochemistry, while therapeutics consists of understanding how particular chemicals change the biochemical status of the body. It is thus a small step to the view that, since the mind is a function of the brain, a full understanding of the brain is both necessary and sufficient for a full understanding of all disorders of the mind. In one sentence, that is the credo of biological psychiatry which, since the collapse of psychoanalysis and behaviorism, has more or less had the field of psychiatry to itself. The social pressures that have contributed to biological psychiatry's spectacular success in taking control of the profession are another issue; what counts here is that psychiatrists needed a scientific stance, and biology is the strongest, or even the only, candidate they know.

It has been said of psychiatrists that they studied medicine but don't practice it, and practice psychology, which they never studied. Intellectually, turning from psychologism to biologism represents a conceptual retreat, from either the arcane mysteries of psychoanalysis or a borrowed science of behaviorism, to the certainty of reductionist biology. Psychiatrists no longer study or practice psychotherapy; they say they are conventional physicians of the mind, diagnosing chemical imbalances of the brain, either by ordinary interview alone or supported by laboratory tests, and treating them with a range of drugs which are finely targeted on the specific disorders they find. Since the human genome project, it has become commonplace for psychiatrists to talk in terms of genes for mental disorder. The profession as a whole has no doubt that, in the near future, there will be massive "breakthroughs" allowing the development of drugs to treat mental disorders diagnosed wholly by chemical analysis. Psychoanalysis will give way to genome analysis so that, after generations in the wilderness, psychiatry will take its rightful place among the rest of the medical specialties.

For ordinary psychiatrists, the new biologism in psychiatry represents a return to intellectual certainty and safety. It is not so much a retreat as a reorientation of limited resources: psychiatry must be based in science; the only science we have is reductionism; therefore, psychiatry must be biological, as Samuel Guze proved to his satisfaction [4]. In addition, this strategic shift will make the training of tomorrow's psychiatrists easier as they will no longer be required to learn a completely new language (ego, libido, Thanatos and all that) nor will they need to distract themselves with patients' problems of living. If depression is a chemical imbalance of the brain, then losing his job and his wife must be coincidental, so the depressed patient can therefore see psychologists and social workers about his bit of "collateral damage."

1.3 Theories of Mind

The world of philosophy is never quite so clear as fields that claim to be scientific. Philosophers are the 'forward scouts,' you could say, ranging far and wide in their enquiries, finding the paths for the technicians plodding in the rear. Early in the last century, there was general agreement that the soul was a non-starter. By the 1950s, philosophers had rushed ahead of the psychologists. The behaviorist idea of a science of mind without a mind was not yielding the benefits claimed for it [5], so the drive was to provide an account of mind that did not set up a mind-body problem. To this end, some philosophers adopted the leitmotiv of science, reductionism. Mind, they averred, was material at base. There are many different options by which this claim can be realized, and all of them have been explored at some stage or other. All of them have failed, too. The notion that the mind is identical with the brain, or can be reduced to brain, or will be explained away by the march of science, etc., in all its permutations and combinations, has gone nowhere (this means, of course, that of all the people professing an interest in matters of mind, only psychiatrists still stick to biological reductionism, but that's another question).

As the dust of philosophical battle has cleared, one group of theories remains in more or less robust shape. This is the group known as functionalist theories of mind, of which the best known is the work of Daniel Dennett, so this will suffice as the exemplar of a modern theory of mind. Dennett's approach to the question of mind has three bases: dualism is false; the mind is biological; and the mind is a virtual machine generated by the brain. The following quotes, largely taken from Chap. 9 of [1], will demonstrate how he approaches these points:

(i). "...YES," he says, "My theory is a theory of consciousness" [6, p281; all emphasis in quotes is in the original]. Note that he uses the terms mind and consciousness more or less interchangeably, which is possibly tendentious as the set of conscious events is a subset of the universal set of mental events. That is, some mental events are not conscious, but this is not central to his case.

(ii). It is a materialist theory: "The prevailing wisdom... is materialism: there is only one sort of stuff, namely matter—the physical stuff of physics, chemistry, and physiology—and the mind is somehow nothing but a physical phenomenon... We can (in principle!) account for every mental phenomenon using the same physical principles, laws and raw materials that suffice to explain radioactivity, continental drift, photosynthesis..." [6, p33]. "Somehow, the brain must be the mind..." (p41). See also his *Intentional Stance*: "I declare my starting point to be the objective, materialistic, third-person world of the physical sciences" [7, p5].

(iii). Consciousness is all sorts of things, but mostly it is about computation and information [6, pp43-65].

(iv). When consciousness is not about computation, the extra bits can be explained away: "...we will try to remove the motivation for believing in these (special, subjective) properties (of our internal discriminative states)... by finding alternative explanations for the phenomena that seem to demand them" [6, p373].

(v). Dualism always means substance dualism, which violates the laws of physics [6, pp33-35]; therefore dualism is bad: "There is the lurking suspicion that the most attractive feature of mind stuff is its promise of being so mysterious that it keeps science at bay forever. This fundamentally anti-scientific stance of dualism is, to my mind, its most disqualifying feature, and is the reason why in this book I adopt the apparently dogmatic rule that dualism is to be avoided at all costs... given the way dualism wallows in mystery, accepting dualism is giving up (as in 'then a miracle occurs')" [6, pp37-38]. "...'adopting' dualism is really just accepting defeat without admitting it" [6, p41]. By this, he means that accepting dualism automatically means giving up on the quest for a rational explanation of mind. He does not compromise on this point.

(vi). Descartes' model, the 'Cartesian Theatre,' is bad, because wherever there is a Cartesian Theatre, there is a hidden observer, and wherever there is a hidden observer, there is dualism, but dualism means ectoplasm where ectoplasm is antiscientific.

(vii). Selves are good because they are abstractions [6, p368] which can be explained in terms of the same processes which result in snails' shells, beavers' dams and bower birds' bowers. While these natural features are interesting, "...the strangest and most wonderful constructions in the whole animal world are the amazing, intricate..." selves spun out of the brain of the primate, *Homo sapiens*. In constructing a self, a child no more knows what it is doing than do snails making their shells [6, p416]; therefore, the two processes are biological;

(viii). Selves, however, do not imply a Cartesian Theatre: "This idea of 'mechanical' interpretation in the brain is the central insight of any materialistic theory of the mind, but (it denies the idea that) there has to be someone in there... to witness the events... Witnesses need raw materials on which to base their judgments. These 'sense data' or... 'phenomenal properties of experience,' are props without which a Witness makes no sense" [6, p322]. Hidden observers need phenomenal properties, therefore getting rid of the phenomenal properties gets rid of the hidden observer. Selves do not rely on phenomenal properties because, despite appearances, consciousness isn't really about phenomenal properties anyway;

(ix) Materialism gets rid of phenomenal properties; therefore materialism gets rid of hidden observers; therefore materialism dispenses with Cartesian dualism which is "hopelessly wrong" (p106); therefore a materialist Self can do no wrong, even if it is immortal [6, pp368, 430];

(x) Dennett's materialist theory explains consciousness without doing anything naughty because it explains computation without leaving any loose bits called phenomenal experiences, which nobody would want to include in a sensible theory of consciousness anyway because they're far too difficult: "The phenomena of human consciousness have been explained... in terms of the operations of a 'virtual machine,' a sort of evolved (and evolving) computer program that shapes the activities of the brain" [6, p431]. "...when language came into existence, it brought into existence the kind of mind that can transform itself on a moment's notice into a somewhat different virtual machine, taking on new projects, following new rules, adopting new policies.

We are transformers. That's what a mind is, as contrasted with a mere brain, the control system of a chameleonic transformer, a virtual machine for making more virtual machines" [8, p250-51].

The rest of this paper will consider these claims in detail: dualism is false; the mind is biological; and the mind is a virtual machine generated by the brain. I will argue that the first two are simply wrong, while the last is a flat contradiction of his basic, antidualist stance. My case is that any attempt to reduce the mind to the biological brain will inevitably fail because it is based in a profound misunderstanding of the concept of "biological." In order to do this, it will be necessary to look more closely at the question of what we might mean when we say that the processes of mind are of the same nature as the processes of biology. We will then consider the concept of machine-based computation and ask whether it is of the same order of nature as the processes of "radioactivity, continental drift, photosynthesis..," not to mention snail shells, beaver dams and bird nests.

1.4 The Case Against Dualism

This will be brief. Dennett leaves absolutely no doubt about his position. He sees dualism as a hopelessly myth-ridden bit of prescientific nonsense that could only appeal to starry-eyed dreamers. His hostility goes back to his first year in college, when he read Descartes' *Meditations* and was "...hooked on the mind-body problem" [6, first line of preface]. However, the classic Cartesian formulation bothered him greatly: "How on earth," the 18yr old freshman Dennett asked, "could my thoughts and feelings fit in the same world with the nerve cells and molecules that made up my brain?" Intuitively, he understood that the only conceivable way the Cartesian approach could survive was by a small miracle connecting the two realms, but miracles are irrational, so Cartesian dualism must also be irrational. He has not modified his views one iota in the ensuing half century. To him, dualism *means* magical, non-scientific and all other scornful expressions he can throw at it. To accuse somebody of being a dualist is just an insult. I believe he is wrong, as there is nothing in the term 'dualism' that implies, means, requires or depends upon the concept of magic or mysterious substances.

The definition of dualism is just what the word suggests: twofold. "The crux of dualism is an apparently unbridgeable gap between two incommensurable orders of being that must be reconciled if we (wish to justify) our assumption that there is a comprehensible universe..." (Watson, in [9], p210). That is all there is to it: we start with the overwhelming impression that the universe consists of two utterly separate parts, each of which seems to require nothing more than itself to exist, but, if we wish to make sense of what we observe, we must find a way of showing that they do, in fact, relate by rational means. This means that the formal definition of 'dualism' deliberately and explicitly requires a rational account of mind-body interaction, which means it deliberately and explicitly eschews magic. So why does the word make Dennett tremble with outrage? Clearly, he is convinced that dualism has only one meaning: Cartesian substance dualism, meaning magic. In this respect, I suggest he still holds to the unmodified notions he absorbed during his first year at college in 1960, when the harsh world view of reductionist science reigned triumphant. That is the sort of mistake an 18 year old novice is likely to make in his first few days in the world of philosophy. Perhaps he should have paid more attention to the Sage of Minnesota, Garrison Keillor: "At fourteen, you're no skeptic but a true believer starting with belief in yourself as a natural phenomenon never before seen on this earth and therefore incomprehensible to all others" (Lake Wobegon Days; from my recollection, it is still largely true at 18yrs old).

It is quite clear that Dennett has constructed his theory of functionalism on the single misperception that any hint of dualism in the formulation necessarily implies an observer, which has to be of a different substance. However, I have argued that this is the wrong error implicit in the dualist case: the problem for naïve dualism is not substance dualism but an infinite regress. That is, as Skinner described decades ago, if we postulate a little man or spirit inside the head to acquit the human functions, then the risk is that we will have to invent a littler man inside the little man to acquit his functions, *ad infinitum*. However, if we prevent the infinite regress at the outset, there is no reason to believe we cannot devise a non-magical or rational dualism. By this means, we may be able to bridge the "...apparently unbridgeable gap between two incommensurable orders of being that must be reconciled (and thereby we can justify) our assumption that there is a comprehensible universe..." I believe we can indeed prevent the infinite regress, so Dennett's case against dualism collapses. Ironically, his own work shows how to bridge the gap, by breaking down each and every function to be explained to its atomic elements until each step is so simple that it could be performed by a mindless automaton, such as a neuron. A non-magical dualism is definitely possible in theory, so Dennett's carefully crafted monism is based on a straw man.

1.5 The Mind as a Tool

We need to look at this in some detail as Dennett's case is vague at a number of points where it requires the utmost precision. He starts boldly enough: "I declare my starting point to be the objective, materialistic, third-person world of the physical sciences" [8, p5]. But what does this mean? In the documentary *The Singularity is Now*, which examines the work of Ray Kurzweil, the AI researcher Ben Goertzel makes the important point that he doesn't know if the next person has the same inner experience as he does, but he has to act as though they do. It then follows that, if he assumes they also have a private inner world, he must explain his own inner experience (the point is that if Goertzel thinks his own private experiences are unique, meaning he is some kind of freak, he doesn't really have to explain it; but if he thinks he isn't a freak, then he has set himself the huge task of explaining private experience). However, Dennett explicitly doesn't assume that. His declared starting position is "the objective, materialistic, third-person world of the physical sciences." As far as I know, there is nothing in that particular world that would qualify as a "subjective, immaterial, first-person world of a mental science."

Thus, from the outset, he has defined the subjective experience of being a sentient creature out of his search. In this sense, he is very like Skinner, who did much the same thing, when he remembered [1, Chap. 2]. Of course, Dennett is perfectly within his rights to try to build a theory of mental life out of third-person, physical-type building blocks, but he can't object when somebody doesn't agree with his choice of starting positions. For myself, I feel a duty to attempt to explain not just the observable behavior of humans, rats and worms, but also the compelling sense of there being something important "in here." It is important to remember Alfred Ayer's acerbic critique of behaviorism: "To be a behaviorist is to pretend to be anaesthetized from the neck up." Similarly, to claim that everything human can be explained in terms of "the objective, materialistic, third-person world of the physical sciences" is to pretend to be a zombie, that there is nothing "in here" that can be observed, even if by the one person, and therefore nothing worth bothering with.

In fact, Dennett's starting position is a matter of taste. He finds the idea of a mental life counter-intuitive. That is his personal choice, and his right, but I don't agree, and he has never shown any hint of an argument that would convince me that I am wrong. *De gustibus, non est disputandam.* In matters of taste, there can be no argument.

In case there is any doubt, he eggs his pudding: "...there is only one sort of stuff, namely matter—the physical stuff of physics, chemistry, and physiology—and the mind is somehow nothing but a physical phenomenon... the same physical principles, laws and raw materials that suffice to explain radioactivity, continental drift, photosynthesis..." This, all will agree, is a brave claim because it could lead in unexpected directions. For example, if minds can be explained by the same processes as photosynthesis in leaves, then it won't be long before somebody is claiming that leaves must have minds. For myself, I don't worry about that because I believe the claim is wrong, so blatantly and patently wrong that only a person who doesn't actually know very much about "...radioactivity, continental drift, photosynthesis..." snail shells, beaver dams and bird nests would ever bother making it. Dennett, however, is being consistent because, if he claims that the laws of physics will explain minds completely, then he can't claim any other properties for minds other than the purely physical.

So what is the mechanism by which a physical thing like the brain can generate symphonies and nuclear weapons? His answer is: "Somehow, the brain must be the mind" [6, p41]. This is important: everything hangs on that one word "somehow." Oddly enough, the philosopher who despises the pseudo-explanation "and so a miracle occurs" [6, p38] is quite taken by "somehow," as in "...the mind is somehow nothing but a physical phenomenon..." Clearly, he expects science to ride to the rescue, meaning "let's not worry about the finer details." This is not good policy as the devil lies in the details. Does he mean "the brain must be the mind," as in mind-brain identity theory; or mind can be reduced to brain, as in explaining mind away; or does he mean the brain "somehow" generates the mind? In fact, he means the latter, as his quote on virtual machines shows: "That's what a mind is, as contrasted with a mere brain ...a virtual machine for making more virtual machines."

I will come back to this point but, first, we should ask what it means to say that a machine such as the brain is governed wholly and solely by the same principles as govern leaves, kidneys, car engines and earthquakes. To begin with, we need to consider the difference between a tool and a machine. A tool is an implement or instrument that is used purely for its physical capacity to perform a task that humans cannot. It may be harder than a fist (such as a hammer or club), or sharper and tougher than finger nails (a knife), or able to exert more force, such as a lever, or reach further (a rope) or hold more (a jug). It may amplify a movement (a casting rod), provide more heat (a fire) or block the wind (clothes and blankets) and so on. A tool performs its task using only the direct physical properties of its constituents (such as metal or glass) or its shape to achieve something a human could do if he had time or hard enough hands. A worker using tools relies on their physical properties and nothing else. He must design them to do the job he wants done, and they can do only that job. A crowbar cannot float, a block of ice cannot cook a meal, a knife cannot hold water, and so on. Conceptually, tools place few demands on the intellect: they are made of ordinary physical materials and their performances remain wholly within the "...objective, materialistic, third-person world of the physical sciences," "...using the same physical principles, laws and raw materials that suffice to explain radioactivity, continental drift, photo-synthesis..." There is nothing magic about tools, so we can move on.

Machines are different, but they also remain within the material realm. A machine does more than a tool in that it uses energy to transform something. It may just change physical properties using a specific input of energy (cutting or bending steel) or, more commonly, it transforms chemicals to achieve an output that is thermodynamically highly unlikely. A good example of a simple machine is a wind or water mill. These collect one form of kinetic energy (moving air, moving water) and, by a system of levers and wheels, redirect it into another form of kinetic energy (usually rotary motion) in a different medium that can then be put to work. A further development is seen in the generators in a hydropower installation, where the kinetic energy of moving water is converted to electrical energy.

All machines, regardless of their complexity, work by the same principles. There is a physical structure and an energy input. By virtue of the precise physical arrangement of the machine, the energy is channeled in very tightly controlled directions, even if it involves temperatures and pressures that may not be seen outside volcanoes, which allows the machine to perform work. Everything fits together; the precise pathways of energy input, transformation and output are designed and manufactured to remarkable tolerances otherwise the machine would not do its job—and perhaps may even level a few cities in the process. An X-ray machine, a jet aircraft, a gas hot water system, a genome sequencer, every machine we use is built according to our understanding of the laws of the physical realm. In each machine, there is a direct causal chain of physicochemical events connecting every step of the process from initiation to completion, and we understand all of this in very great detail. There cannot be a break in the matter-energy pathways or the machine will fail. A single leak in a gasket of a diesel engine results in breakdown as the pressures in the cylinders drop too low to cause the temperature to reach ignition point. In diesel engines, and in biological machines such as leaves or kidneys, there is no magic involved.

If we look at the processes of photosynthesis, which we now know in great detail, it is possible to show precisely how the plant's genome produces the necessary enzymes—and no others—and how these are able to capture light energy and use it to build the complex chemicals that form the basis of plant growth. By processes which, in thermodynamic terms, are vanishingly unlikely, the energy and chemical inputs are passed along immensely complicated physicochemical structures to give just one output from the myriad possibilities. Every input photon and every input hydrogen ion (proton) can be followed through the process, showing exactly where each element is passed along the chemical chain, how it is joined to its neighbors in just such a form and no other, and how the final products are assembled from simpler components until a new plant cell is assembled and the plant becomes ever so slightly larger.

An error at any stage will quickly cause the superbly balanced processes of photosynthesis to begin to break down. It may be an enzymic error, or perhaps the sun is too hot or a viral invader is using one of the enzymes or a heavy metal is blocking another, the possibilities are endless, but the point is that the response to any interference is predictable. Given the exact physicochemical mechanism of the leaf, the outcome of any error can be understood wholly in terms of the laws of the physical universe. There is nothing magic in it: no *élan vital*, no pixie dust, no nymphs, universal spirits or telekinesis, nothing but matter and energy chugging mindlessly along paths that have emerged from evolution, all the while operating strictly according to the laws that govern their interaction. Instead of magic, there is an infinite series of one-to-one relationships, point-to-point equations joining every atom with every erg, dyne, calorie, photon and electron in the system (for those of you who don't remember ergs, dynes and calories, they were very small). These relationships are not just approximately true or roughly correct, they are true to the nth degree. There is no room for error. The corollary is that, if your tomatoes start to rot under the blossom scar, you know something has affected them physically (lack of calcium). You do not imagine your neighbor has placed a hex on them.

The same is true of organs such as the heart, the kidney and the eye. It is also true of any machine that humans can make, from a mousetrap (stored kinetic energy) to a space probe heading to its destination billions of kilometers from Earth. Everything about each of these examples, every tiny part or aspect without exception, is under the precise control of "...the same physical principles (and) laws... that suffice to explain radioactivity, continental drift, photosynthesis..." If there is any imbalance of *any* sort in the equations, it will accumulate until, slowly or suddenly, the imbalances will overcome the structural integrity of the machine and it will either grind wearily to a halt or explode in a ball of flame (for a good example of accumulating pressures, have another look at the videos of the Fukushima plant exploding). That is the nature of physical machines. Given their matter-energy relationships, it could not be otherwise. A nuclear power plant cannot suddenly start producing eggs, a kidney cannot start singing, a leaf cannot produce gold bars, so on and so forth. Because the universe is a rational place, machines can only do what they can do according to the laws of this "rational place," and nothing else. Anything else would be magic.

We can now move to Dennett's broader claim: "...there is only one sort of stuff, namely matter—the physical stuff of physics, chemistry, and physiology—and the mind is somehow nothing but a physical phenomenon... the same physical principles, laws and raw materials that suffice to explain radioactivity, continental drift, photosynthesis..." We need to look at this claim in some detail: "...there is only one sort of stuff, namely matter..." (He means matter-energy, but that is a minor quibble). It is certainly the case that, throughout human history and even today, the great majority of people who have ever lived were or are comfortable with the idea that there is actually more to the universe than mere matter and energy. Given their daily personal experience of being something different from what they imagine rocks to be, of being more than just zombies, they assume that the universe has at least two sorts or orders of being. That is, they inhabit what they believe to be a dualist universe. For the record, that is exactly how I grew up but, having been trained and immersed in the western materialist viewpoint for over fifty years, I now think we were wrong: that way lies intellectual chaos. I do not believe that the folk notion of dualism can give us the rational world we desire. But I also believe that you, my readers, are more than just a clever "objective, materialistic, third-person" machine, and I would like you to believe that is equally true of me.

Rightly or wrongly, I believe that, from the time you wake each day, to your dreams at night, your experience of being yourself is much the same as what I experience. As a physician, I deal every day with people with chronic pain. I do not, for example, believe that people with back pain are just "work shy" (to quote the experts at the American Pain Association). I believe that, when they complain of pain, they are having some kind of intensely discomforting inner experience, one with which I am personally over-familiar. I believe their inner experience is real in the context that they are real or complete humans (not just mannequins), in the same context that tells us it is not nice to test napalm on living chimps or to sell children for sexual purposes. Having said that, I do not believe that chimps have a resident soul or spirit composed of a second, supernatural order of being but, crucially, I also do not believe, as Dennett does, that that exhausts the possibilities. He says: "the mind is somehow nothing but a physical phenomenon... Somehow, the brain must be the mind," as though that is the end of the matter, but I don't think it is. I do not believe that the principles that explain a nuclear power station, or a leaf, or a mousetrap, are sufficient to explain the observable behavior of a human or the private experience of being a human or a chimp. There is more to humans (and chimps, dolphins, dogs and possibly rats but not eggs, cabbages, yeast or pork), more to us minded creatures than just the "...physical principles, laws and raw materials that suffice to explain radioactivity, continental drift, photosynthesis..."

Having said that, I now have to prove my case. Dennett's is actually the null hypothesis, so he has the easier job. He can announce to his classes: "There is nothing more to the universe than boring physics, so run along to your science classes where you will learn everything you need to know about humans." As it stands, I don't think physics and chemistry will tell us anything interesting about the human condition but I also don't think I can convince him that a full explanation requires something more. In the rest of this paper, I will propose a "something more" that can conceivably account for our experience of being more than dumb rocks on legs (and can justify our repugnance for cruelty to animals and sexual exploitation of children) but which does not invoke a supernatural realm to complete the explanatory chain. But first, we will have to digress a little through some of the laws of physics and special examples of when they don't apply.

1.6 The Mind as a Dumb Machine.

Just on 350 years ago, the comfortable world of the ancients was turned on its head by a most peculiar and even objectionable bachelor living in the little town near the bridge on the River Cam, deep in rural England. Working essentially alone, Isaac Newton challenged the received wisdom regarding the concept of motion as it had been set down by Aristotle and others nearly two thousand years before. To medieval scholars, motion was a very complex issue, riven by arcane mysteries such as goals, natural planes and orbits and so on, and certainly not helped by the notion that the world is the centre of the universe. Granted, some things make sense from that point of view, but a lot of other things don't; even planets don't stick to their prescribed motions. Newton's achievement (among many others) was to strip the supernatural accretions from what he saw as a blessedly simple concept, the idea that a moving object will continue on its path unless and until something changes it. From this, he was able to describe in purely mathematical form a set of equations that would predict where a moving object would be at a certain time. Motion was no longer a matter of supernatural teleology, but was just dumb physics (although the word had a different meaning then).

This is a very important and, in fact, a revolutionary concept. Metaphorically speaking, he reached into the morass of spiritualism, charlatanism and tomfoolery and extracted the vitals of the concept of motion as a rule-governed *natural* event (the ancients never thought it wasn't rule-governed; they just thought the rules were supernatural). As a result of Newton's labors, the world changed in ways we can no longer understand. His ideas were so penetrating and so powerful in their reach that spacecraft launched to travel billions of kilometers to their destinations are still guided by the principles he enunciated by candlelight. As an aside, the monkish Newton was a difficult and abrasive personality who spent much of his time pursuing alchemy and endless bitter vendettas with anybody, such as Leibniz, who crossed him. If he were alive today, working in a modern university, he would be diagnosed as having bipolar disorder and put on large doses of powerful psychotropic drugs, and perhaps given ECT (shock treatment), which would mean no more penetrating insights derived from staying up all night to pursue a dream. As I said, that's an aside.

Not two hundred years later, the world began to change again. Everybody is familiar with the Darwinian revolution but something even more powerful was already under way. Just as Newton (and others, of course) had pruned motion to its bare essentials as a set of equations with no content, so a series of highly original thinkers did the same thing to the way we view energy. Starting in the mid-eighteenth century, tinkerers and engineers such as Watt, Ampère and Faraday started the process of showing that energy was just another natural event. Increasingly, the hugely profitable supernatural embroidery such as life forces, *élan vital*, spiritual energy, telekinesis, poltergeists, divine interventions and the like were shown to be unnecessary. Nobody ever proved they didn't exist (that's actually not possible) but, using systems such as the Maxwell equations, energy became part of the natural world, ordered by strict relationships that could be understood with great precision in mathematical form.

As this revolution in physics accelerated during the latter part of the nineteenth century, the mystical element of the universe was shoved aside. In the twentieth century, of course, it transformed the universe as we understand it. Thanks to the work of such penetrating minds as Einstein, Schrödinger, Heisenberg, Bohr and so many others, we can never go back to pre-atomic thinking, whatever that was. Energy, actually matter-energy, is a fundamental component of the physical universe as we see it. There is nothing magic about how energy is released by nuclear fusion deep in the sun, how it travels through an ether-less space to the earth, and is then absorbed by chloroplasts and converted into the chemical energy which we either eat directly, as vegetables and grains, or indirectly, as eggs and meat. All of this is now part of our *Weltanschauung* or world-view, part of the process by which magical motion and supernatural energy were converted into standing in a crowded, smelly train while it lurches through the dreary suburbs on a rainy Tuesday morning. We have gone from a dark and threatening Tolkienesque world of infinite possibility to being stuck in a traffic jam, as yesterday's miracle becomes today's must-have mod con (and promptly breaks down). Once again, there was nothing magic about the transition. It was "simply" a matter of showing how the concept of the universe as a comprehensible, rule-governed place extended to areas which, previously, had seemed so extraordinary that we had to invoke magic to account for it.

The third part of this demystifying process was launched in the late 1930s by two young men who had not yet met. One was the British mathematician, Alan Turing, who published a paper of frightening complexity relating to the notion of reducing intelligence to machine-like steps. In 1937, an unknown student submitted what is now regarded as the most influential and widely-quoted masters thesis in history. Claude Shannon was born in 1916, in a lakeside town in Michigan which, even today, boasts only about 6,000 souls (Gaylord, where he went to school, had just 3,681 determined residents in 2000 and dropping). At the age of twenty, he graduated from the University of Michigan with two degrees, mathematics and electrical engineering, so we can assume he didn't spend a lot of time drinking at football matches. In his thesis, *A Symbolic Analysis of Relay and Switching Circuits*, by showing that information was just another commodity that obeyed ordinary laws that could be rendered in mathematical form, he helped lay the basis of the third great scientific triumph over the forces of the supernatural. Instead of thinking of information as something mystical that came from heaven with trumpet blasts, or arrived from "the other side" via poets and playwrights, or from the racial unconscious or other such nonsense, Shannon established the fundamentals of the concept of information as something that could be pumped through pipes like water, or sprayed across screens like confetti, or bundled and sold like pumpkins. My case is that the concepts outlined by these highly original thinkers can form the basis of a theory of mind (and mind-body interaction) for psychiatry. Needless to say, such a theory then has to generate a theory of mental disorder.

1.7 Defining Information

Clearly, the whole of this depends utterly on a convincing definition of information and a plausible account of how so insubstantial a concept could translate into the reality of human life. If I can't show how we can cast the concept of information in real terms, then my attempt at a theory of mind amounts to just another "Just So" story in the long, sorry history of psychology and psychiatry. Unfortunately, if anybody has ever defined information in a clear, non-circular way, I have yet to see it. Yes, we all know what information is, so why bother defining it? Well, the answer is that the concepts we all think we understand perfectly are just the ones to trip us up at a crucial point in the debate. At least part of the difficulty arises because our sense of selfhood is itself generated in an informational space. How then can we define information when it is the basis of our existence as mentally-capable beings? It is the ultimate recursive quandary, forcing us to reflect back on ourselves in such a manner as to doubt our personal reality. We will come back to this point later.

In the meantime, we can try this definition: *Information is an assessment of some aspect of the universe by an entity with an emergent capacity to represent the physical universe in a symbolic calculus.* Information is not a thing; it is the rule-governed process of mapping one system onto another but the catch is that only an entity with the emergent capacity we are trying to define can apprehend it (it takes one to know one, you could say, because entities without the capacity can't know anything). In brief, information is what we information users gather and use in our daily lives, about ourselves and the world we live in. That, as I am sure you will agree, is nicely circular but it will do for the time being. As we continue to explore the concept of mind as an informational space, refinements to this definition will emerge (sic) ostensively.

One thing is immediately clear: information describes, or is about, the physical universe, but it is not of the physical universe (the physical universe has no capacity to describe itself in a symbolic calculus). It represents another realm, another order of nature governed by rules which are conceptually distinct from and incompatible with those governing the physical realm. That is, I am defining a dualist universe, one in which the "mere atoms" of the physical world (including energy) stand distinct from and opposed to the symbols with which we information users represent those atoms. The physical world therefore precedes the symbolic, logically and as a matter of empirical necessity: there can be no symbols unless there is a medium on which to inscribe them. The imprint of the symbol in the medium is physical but the functional significance of the symbol is most definitely not physical: it exists in its own right as an element of an informational state that can be apprehended only by another informational state. A brick does not know that a newspaper contains information. There is always a disjunction between the medium and the message it expresses, such that the message is not identical with or reducible to the medium. One element of the medium can express many messages, and any message can be expressed in many different media. The message is more than the medium but, as long as they coincide at just one point, communication can take place.

If we define the mind as an emergent informational system in a "space" generated by the brain, one which is totally dependent on healthy brain function for its existence but which can act back upon the brain to achieve ends that would not otherwise occur, then we are defining a classic dualist system of mind and brain. It is, however, a natural dualist system, one which arises predictably from the particular architecture of the brain as a switching mechanism capable of representing the physical universe as symbols in a semantic realm or context [10]. The problem with any dualist system is to show how the parts relate to each other, and to define a mechanism for their interaction. By defining the mind as nothing more than an informational system, and bearing in mind that the body traffics in information all day, every day, then it should be clear that there is no logical impediment to mind-body interaction at the level of transfers of information. It is now only a matter of showing how the flow of data in the body, from exteroreceptors to the Central Nervous System (CNS) and back to effector organs, is organized at the molecular level. This, as should become quite clear, is conceptually not difficult but the first step is to show how, using proven concepts of informational systems, the mind is organized in such a way as to be open to inputs from the body, and what it can do with them. In simple terms, how can we decompose what we know of ourselves as mentally-capable beings to satisfy the requirements of some predefined theory of information? The answer, as will become clear, is that this is a relatively simple task as long as it is approached from the correct point of view. If not, it is intractable. As the mind-body problem has been until now.

1.8 Conclusion: A Non-Mentalist Mentalism

Can machines think? The essential preliminary to this question is: Can humans think? What do we mean by 'thinking'? As Chalmers has argued [10], the human mind divides readily in two parts, the experiential and the knowledge-based. The experiential mind is the feeling, sensing part while all the knowledge and decisions on which daily life is based are contained in the knowing or informational state. The two parts of mind stand in a direct, ordered relationship with each other but each is the product of prior events, arising from or supervening upon more primitive brain events.

The world of experience is vivid, private and ineffable: I can never explain to you what I feel or sense, but hope that you can understand from your own, comparable experiences. The world of knowledge is different. It is silent, in that I do not know how I know anything or how I make my decisions, they simply arrive and I act upon them. It is communicable, by language, and therefore becomes public knowledge. The great bulk of activity in this aspect of mind is very fast and takes place beyond introspection. I don't know how I reach my decisions, just the same as I don't know how my fingers reach for the keys on my keyboard. I speak, without knowing how I choose the words or why I arrange them in just this order. You hear my speech and, without knowing how, you decompose this constant stream of syllables into individual words, from which you build meaningful sentences. Amazingly, even if you don't remember a single word of the grammar you learned at school, you can even tell when I have made a mistake. All of this is done "for" us but we accept without question that we are doing it ourselves.

In order to make sense of these daily observations, we need to show how complex mental events can be understood in terms of less complex causes. That is, can we give a simple, non-mentalist account of these complex, mental events? I believe the answer is Yes, we can, but first, we need to reconsider some of the most profoundly influential events of the twentieth century.

Emergent Logic and Antimonism

"A new idea comes suddenly and in a rather intuitive way. But intuition is nothing but the outcome of earlier intellectual experience."

—Albert Einstein (1949)

2.1 Introduction

Seventy-five years ago, a young British mathematician, Alan Turing, asked: Can we devise a machine to do what we think is unique to humans? His goal was to give a non-mentalist explanation for quintessentially mental events. Can we, he wondered, find a mechanical way of computing complex decisions that doesn't involve human interference at any stage? His answer, detailed in a paper of numbing complexity, was, *Yes, we most certainly can* [1]. Any question can be broken down into a series of lesser questions, and each of these can be further decomposed into sub-questions, on and on until all we have is a very long series of questions that are so elementary that a machine can answer them. The mechanism he proposed has become the basis of all modern computing, although it required contributions from two other seminal thinkers before it became a physical reality (it is of interest that, in this profoundly influential paper, the author cited a mere five references).

As the basis of his "mechanical intelligence," Turing proposed a machine composed of just a few parts. There was an input-output tape, a read-write head, a memory store, an executive unit and a control. The tape was divided into squares, or cells, that could hold only one of two tokens, either 0 or 1, yes or no, on or off, etc. As the tape clicked forward, the mechanism scanned what was written in each cell and conveyed this to the executive unit, which checked with the memory and then decided what to do. It could either leave the token as it was, or erase it and write the other. Having done this, the machine then clicked on to the next cell on its list. That's all. The detail he provided was mathematical and said nothing about the engineering problems involved in building a mechanical computer. For example, in discussing the control mechanism, he said: "We have mentioned that the 'book of rules' supplied to the (human) computer is replaced in the machine by a part of the store. It is then called the 'table of instructions.' It is the duty of the control to see that these instructions are obeyed correctly and in the right order. The control is so constructed that this necessarily happens." Turing had no background in engineering and, in 1936, he probably had a physical mechanism in mind but, as it was written, it was little more than magical thinking. There were no details, just this vague promise that, "Oh, yes, the control will check that, don't worry about the details."

Turing understood that the first version of his computing machine would be built with a fixed memory, meaning it could only work on a single type of problem. In order to adapt it to dealing with other classes of problems, the memory would have to be physically taken apart and put back together in a different form or rewired, as we would now say. He called this a 'discrete state machine,' as it could only function in one state or another. However, he then took a huge conceptual leap. If a machine could be given a big enough memory, and its instructions were fed into it via the input tape, then it would be free of its inherent design constraints and would be able to calculate any known mathematical problem. He called this a 'universal computing machine,' now generally known as a Turing Machine. There was, however, a problem, because his universal computer worked at a pedestrian pace governed by its need to consider just one cell at a time. There would therefore be many problems for which it would not provide an answer in reasonable time, even, he intimated, within the lifetime of its operators. Clearly, something better was needed, especially as war was looming.

2.2 Electronic Logic

During World War II, there were desperate needs for prodigious feats of calculation in two areas. The first was the demand for massive computational power as the Allies strove to decipher the German military codes. The second was in the field of fire control, especially of anti-aircraft guns capable of tracking and intercepting the fast and agile fighter planes that dominated the skies. When the first mechanical computing machines were built, they were very expensive to build and run, slow and unreliable. Computation had to be lifted to another level, and that level was firstly electrical, then electronic. Working with telephone engineers, Turing's elegantly simple concepts were central to the construction of the first British electrical computers, which he called the 'Bombe' (probably following a Polish invention used to work on the German codes). This used cascades of computation, with arrays of analytic devices connected such that the output of one subunit became the input of the next. It seems most likely that Turing and his wider group understood the next level of complexity, in which the output of one part of the array becomes not just the data for the next level, but actually issues new instructions to it or, as we would now say, programs it. By this means, a finite machine with physical limitations on its calculating ability could, with time, generate essentially an infinite output. That is, it could mimic one of the most characteristic of human features, the ability to say or do something completely novel, day after day.

At about the same time, developments in switching mechanisms meant that machine-based computation no longer meant just mathematical computations. With suitable engineering, they became logic machines, capable of deciding much broader questions. The concepts behind this step were developed by an even younger man than Turing. Claude Shannon was just twenty-one when he submitted his thesis [2]. As part of his mathematics program, he had attended a course in logic, which included a section on Boolean algebra. Later, when he looked at switching devices used in long-distance telephony, he realized that the switches were actually functioning as small, Boolean logic machines.

So what is a Boolean switch? To answer that, we have to go back to the early part of the nineteenth century, to an ordained minister and mathematics teacher working in what was then the isolation of Cork, in Ireland. George Boole (1815-64) was a self-taught mathematician who developed the notion of a dual-valued algebra. At the age of twenty-four, without having attended university, he was appointed to the foundation chair of mathematics at Queens College, Cork, purely on the strength of his published work. His goal was to render logic in algebraic form, thus making it incorrigible. Logic, he understood, is a dual-valued calculus, where the only two values are true and false. If these are given numerical values, of 0 and 1, then the semantic operations of logic can be rewritten using the arithmetical operators of + (addition) and x (multiplication). In this approach, logic became formulaic, meaning it moved from being the plaything of the idle educated, to a branch of what we would now call science. Boole's life is another astounding example of how an outsider can turn an established field upside down just by seeing it from a different point of view. As was Claude Shannon's.

Shannon's paper [2] has been called the most famous master's thesis in history. It consists of 69 loosely typed pages (the first page contains a mere 172 words; very few have more) and the bibliography contains just six references. With precious little introduction, he tips the reader into a world where the mechanisms of electrical switches in series and in parallels are performing the same operations as a person using the dual-valued logic of a Boolean algebra. He presents very little in the way of actual argument: in the main, he offers his material as self-evident—which, with the helpful clarity of hindsight, it is. But at the time, it must have been shocking: mere machines, made of switches found lying on any engineer's workbench, could emulate the highest reaches of human thought.

What did this rather diffident young man see that had eluded his teachers? It isn't clear from this paper, or from any of his equally famous works, just what he saw but it seems likely that he simply had the flash of insight that, despite their differences, switching and logical operations were, at their core, one and the same concept. That is, he extracted the conceptual nature of each and saw they were the same. Each represented a dual-valued logic: the switch was either open or closed, meaning the impedance of the circuit was either infinite or zero, while logic operated on truth and falsity. Thus, in Boolean terms, any procedure in either logic or switching could be represented in terms of 0 and 1 and, therefore, could be manipulated by ordinary algebraic methods: "Any circuit," he said, without further ado, "is represented by a set of equations, the terms of the equations representing the various relays and switches of the circuit." Immediately, the converse jumps forth: any equation can be represented by the relays and switches of a suitable circuit. If the equation is a logical equation, then logic can be represented by the relays and switches of a suitable circuit. A laconic masterpiece, the rest of the paper explores these ideas, setting out the actual mechanical basis of machine-based logic. Conceptually, this work was of a different order from Turing's paper from the year before, which was purely theoretical, but it extended the ideas in directions Turing had anticipated. Shannon was translating the theory into action by showing how to screw switches and relays together so that they would represent a "perfect analogy" with the formal steps of logic. It was one of the defining achievements of the twentieth century.

We can start with the simplest circuit of all, a wire joining a transmitting switch P and some sort of detector, Q. A signal sent from P as a single, brief impulse will be detected more or less unchanged at Q. If the distance PQ is relatively long, then the signal will be attenuated by its passage, so the standard engineering response would be to boost the power of the signal. However, that also boosts the noise factor so that, over a very long circuit, the signal would eventually be lost in the noise. This problem is resolved by inserting a booster, known as a relay R, between P and Q. There is no limit to the number of relays, as they do not alter the signal at all, but selectively boost it over the noise in the circuit. Boosting requires energy.

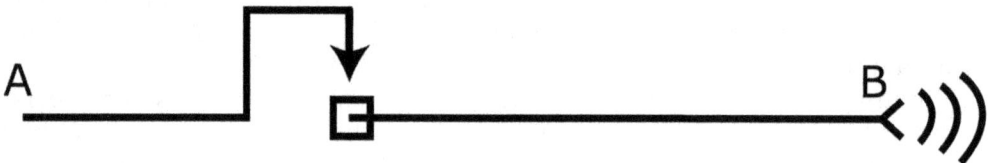

Fig. 2.1: A Simple Circuit

It is, however, possible to use switches and relays to change the signal so that where there was a signal, now there is silence, and where there was silence, an impulse is heard, i.e. the signal is inverted. An inverting relay converts a closed circuit (with zero impedance) into an open circuit, with infinite impedance, and vice versa (because he was using alternating current, he used impedance rather than resistance but the effect is the same). If, however, those values are represented in terms of *0* and *1*, then the inverter mimics the effects of the logical operation of negation of a value in a dual-valued algebra (the *1* used in a dual-valued algebraic notation actually means all or infinity, not the first unit in a decimal system, so its negation is *0*, not *-1*). Thus, an inverting circuit assumes the function of the formal logical operator of negation, or we could say that the logical operation hitches a ride on the physical machine, letting the machine do its work for it *without breaching the laws of thermodynamics.*

a) Signal Attenuated

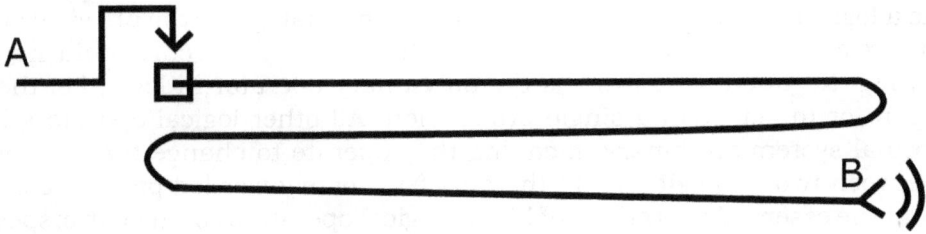

b) Signal boosted by relays at A_1, A_2

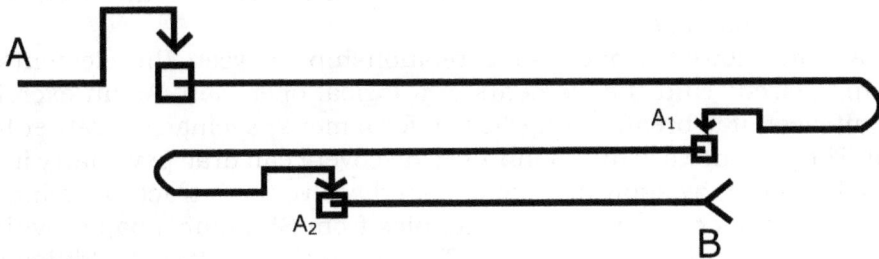

Fig. 2.2: A long circuit

This latter point is absolutely critical to any solution of the mind-body problem. In acquitting a logical function, the physical switching device does nothing that it could not otherwise do, even if it would never happen by chance. The physical switch is governed by the laws of the physical universe, especially the second law of thermodynamics. As a logic machine, however, its output is independent of this law: it makes no difference how we score its actions, each one uses the same energy (Shannon's 1948 theory of communication qualifies this point, as we will see later).

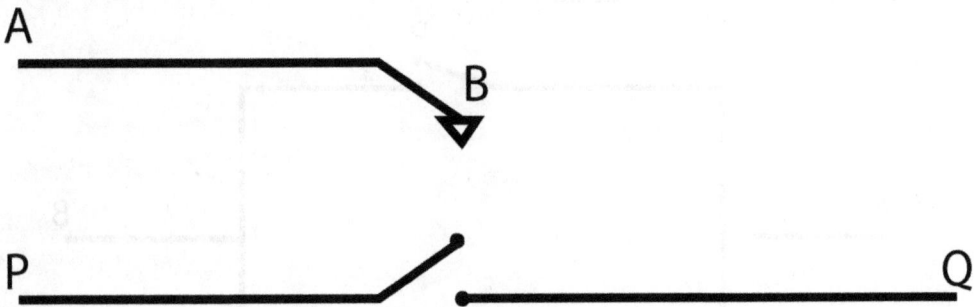

Fig. 2.3 Inverter: continuous signal in PQ is interrupted by activity in AB

Shannon described it thus: "The negative of a hinderance (impedance) X will be written X' and is defined as a variable which is equal to 1 when X equals 0 and is equal to 0 when X equals 1" (it is a dependent variable as the context makes clear). Crucially, he now draws the precise relationship between logic and electronics: "If X is the hinderance of the make contacts of a relay, then X' is the hinderance of the break contacts of the same relay." That is, he defined just those conditions under which a relay system could function as a logical operator, the essential point being that, given the physical state of the relay, its outcome could not be otherwise. This circuit could never be wrong. Negation, of course, is the only unary operator in logic, i.e. the only operator to act upon a single proposition. All other logical operators in the formal system are binary, meaning they operate to change the relationship between two propositions. In the next few, tersely-worded pages, he showed that the essential operations of binary logical operators could be transposed to mechanical form using switches and relays which cost only a few dollars at the local hardware shop. By the end of his seventh page, he concluded: "...it is evident that a perfect analogy exists between the calculus of switching circuits and this branch of symbolic logic." A perfect analogy: thus, the world shifted on its intellectual axis.

Shannon showed a one-to-one relationship between the elements of a switching circuit and the elements of a logical operation. As an exercise in pure intellect, it is breathtaking—even, for a mere psychiatrist, rather frightening. The good news is that Shannon's discovery can drag psychiatry into the new millennium, by showing how we can dissolve the intractable mind-body problem. Consider some further examples from Shannon's paper, which he put in diagrammatic form for clarity. The first is the concept of addition in the context of a dual-valued logic. Boole saw that the logical notion of conjunction, (A & B), was highly restrictive. The statement "A and B are true" could only be true in the single case where both A and B were true. If one or other (or both) were false, then the statement itself was false. In the algebraic form he devised, this was the same as multiplying the two values, where T=0 and F=1. The statement "A & B" has the same logical impact as "A.B" Shannon's contribution was to show that this was nothing other than the operation performed by two switches in parallel. If both were open, then the impedance of the circuit was infinite, i.e. no impulses could flow through the circuit. If either or both of the switches was closed, then the current would flow as the total impedance in the circuit was zero.

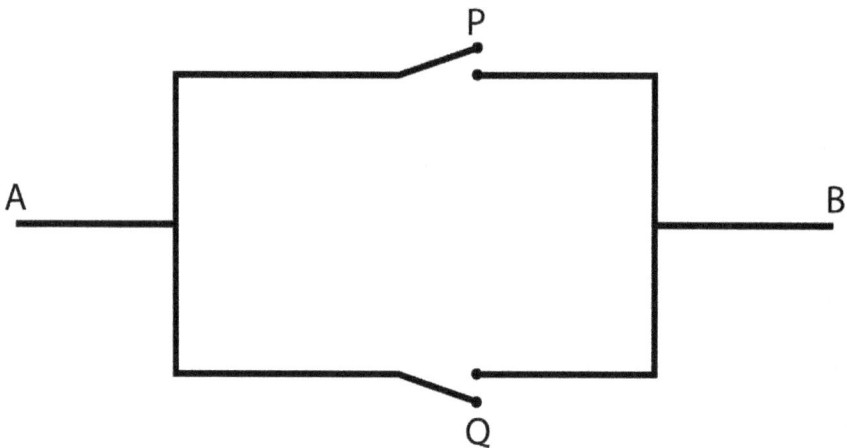

If either P or Q is closed, current will flow.

Fig. 2.4. The first logic gate: A ∧ B = A AND B

In short order, he showed that two switches in series subsumed the logical process of disjunction ("the proposition which is true if either X is true or Y is true") and demonstrated a number of logical theorems for which "perfect analogies" existed in the disposition of his switches. He ended the paper by showing how various arrangements of these switching devices could solve very complex formulae and problems, including one for solving prime numbers. That is, without picking up a screwdriver, he showed how mathematical problems could be solved by devices functioning wholly within the material realm. The final paragraph in his thesis stated sparely: "As to the practicability of such a device, it might be said that J.P. Kulik spent 20 years in constructing a table of primes up to 100,000,000 and when finished it was found to contain so many errors it was not worth publishing. The machine described here could probably be made to handle 5 numbers per second so that the table would require only about two months to construct." How could he be so sure? Because the fundamental validity of his case was beyond reproach; his derivations and conclusions were manifestly correct and required no further elaboration (his almost pontifical style was similar to Turing's).

His paper is remarkable. At barely twenty-one years of age, he helped lay the basis of the information revolution that has transformed human life in a few decades. However, he didn't devise anything new. All he did was recognize that a system he had used in engineering seemed to have an uncanny parallel in mathematics (or vice versa, we don't actually know). Thus, it was possible to map the abstract relationships of truth and falsity to the physical machinery of a suitable electronic circuit to build something that hitherto had been thought to be exclusively the province of humans and angels: a logic machine. A dumb machine working non-stop without time for sleep or meals or academic disputes, could do as well as or better than any professor of logic but in a fraction of the time and all for the price of running a couple of lamp globes.

It must be understood that his discovery did not depend on any random factors, either conceptually or in the actual construction of the circuits. The process of mapping or modeling consists of defining a point-to-point relationship between two entities of different scale or structure. We are all familiar with paper maps of the world, where the features of the sphere are projected on a flat surface, inevitably producing some degree of distortion but not enough to destroy the point of the exercise. There are many other types of maps or diagrams (such as an atlas of anatomy), but they all serve the same purpose: displaying in simplified symbolic form the relationships of the major elements of a structure. In the main, we still tend to reserve the word model for a three dimensional simplification of a larger entity, i.e. a smaller and less complex version. The purpose of a model is to allow the researcher to concentrate on studying the behavior of a limited number of the larger structure's subparts under different conditions. In order to qualify as a model, the new structure must exemplify the same essential functional relationships as exist in the larger entity, but with confounding elements removed. Thus, an ultralight airplane is not a model aircraft. Computer models, of course, do not exist in physical space but the principle is the same: a precisely-defined and ordered relationship between the major features of the object under study and the simplified version, which carefully minimizes distortion of the concepts involved.

In fact, Shannon went very much further, in that he mapped the entirely abstract realm of logic directly to the physical substrate of a system of circuits. There was no physical structure to be modeled. He wasn't building a model of a ship to float in a bath, his intuition leapt straight from the mental concept of a dual-valued algebra to the physical instantiation of that concept in switches and relays. The hard work lay in sorting out the finer points of the algebra but this apparently took him only a few weeks.

That, surely, was one of the transformative moments in human history. Fortunately for him and his bold idea, Shannon didn't suffer the same fate as a Galileo or a Darwin. His government was about to be sucked into the vortex of the Second World War, and it needed clever mathematicians and engineers to build controllers for anti-aircraft guns to beat the fast and maneuverable fighters that were taking to the air. Thus, he was given more or less what he needed to complete his tasks and never had to worry that his work would offend the Inquisition or the frosty bishops of the Established Church and their self-important friends at the Court of St James.

While engaged in this vital work during the war, Shannon met Alan Turing when he visited the US. Turing was working on the ultimate Allied secret, decoding the German Enigma code. No doubt, being young and enthusiastic about their respective fields, they managed to evade some of the secrecy restrictions but that is conjecture; what counts is that, when combined with the work of the Hungarian-born mathematician, John von Neumann, their work laid the basis of the information revolution. This is the third of the great waves of conceptual realignments that have allowed us to throw off the dead weight of ancient orthodoxy and cleared the way for the science we now regard as our birthright. It is true that these were revolutions in scientific thinking—recasting motion, energy and information as mathematics—but not in the sense Thomas Kuhn talks about revolutions in science. The Copernican revolution (which started well before Newton's birth), the chemical revolution, Darwinian evolutionary theory, Pasteur's and Virchow's novel concepts of disease, the atomic revolution and then molecular biology, these were technological applications of the three great conceptual realignments. It is quite feasible that many of these may not have taken place without the heroic reorientations in thinking described above.

2.3 Emergent Information

The significance for a theory of mind lies in the fact that particular dispositions of "mere devices" can solve problems that do not exist in any tangible form in the real world. Physical machines can be built to solve questions that are wholly mental constructs since they exist as information only, where "*...information is an assessment of some aspect of the universe by an entity with an emergent capacity to represent the physical universe in a symbolic calculus.*" The problem here is making some sort of practical sense of the term "emergent." This is potentially a dangerous expression; it has the capacity to appear to be giving an explanation when in fact it is doing no more than describing what we implicitly know, when the implicit fact (or factoid) is what we need to explain. In the rest of this chapter, I want to show that the proper use of the term "emergent" depends on a full understanding of what Shannon's switches were actually doing, because he wasn't thinking of human minds when he wrote his thesis.

Look at Fig. 2.1 again. It shows a wire joining two elements to make a circuit. The role of the switch is clearly understood, as is the detector; the role of the wire is often overlooked. Here, it functions as a conduit, a passive channel by which the impulses emitted by the signaling device are conveyed to the detector. It is a medium of transfer, but it does nothing else. In fact, it is a commodity; it could be replaced by any number of conduits and the effect would be the same. It could be replaced by glass fibers, or tubes of cream, or dogs tied in a line; the medium is irrelevant, as long as it does its job of faithfully transferring the signal. However, when we look at Fig 2.4, we see that something has changed. Between P and Q lies an array of switches and relays, which are anything but passive conduits. They take the incoming signals and manipulate them according to a predetermined calculus or set of rules, so that the final signal reaching Q is derivative: it bears a constant relationship to the originating signal but it is no longer the same signal. That is, between P and Q, the device assumes a totally different significance from "mere conduction" or, we would say, "a new function has emerged." Just by rearranging the circuits and interposing various switches, the function of the circuit from P to Q changes, from a conduit to a computing device or semantic manipulator. However, there is no discontinuity in the physical structure of the whole system. It is still composed of wires and switches and so on. An electrical impulse originating at P will make its way through the new circuit, bound throughout by the laws of the physical universe. What reaches Q, however, is a derivative signal. The circuit's capacity to manipulate a dual-valued calculus has "emerged" from the particular physical structure given it by its architect. As a matter of engineering, a small number of logic gates can be arranged in such a way as to reproduce all the logical operations of a Boolean algebra.

This emergent quality or property is totally dependent on the precise physical structure. If one switch malfunctions, or the polarity of one element of the circuit is accidentally reversed, then the device will not do its "job" of mimicking or underwriting the processes of logical operations. In the process Boole described, the logical operation is decomposed. In Shannon's development, each step in a logical operation is undertaken by the different elements in the circuit acting in a precise sequence, the net effect being that the "mindless machine" actually performs a whole logical procedure, except it doesn't. The machine does a physical job, it knows nothing about logic. Crucially, the nature of the physical elements does not change at any point between P and Q. The impulses are of exactly the same electrical nature throughout; they travel at the same speed from one step in the process to the next; they are transmitted or blocked according to the ordinary laws of the physical universe; and yet, at the same time, they are achieving something above and beyond "mere physics." By careful design, the signals in the circuit are generating a new realm, an informational realm which is insubstantial, unlocalized and immaterial. In these respects, we could even say it is a "virtual" realm that does everything that Dennett's "virtual machine" was intended to do, without the subterfuge. Nonetheless, even though it is wholly informational in nature (consisting of symbolic representations of the real world) and lacks the reality of a physical object, it can act upon the real world via the actual signals of which it is composed. The signal is still an electrical impulse even though its significance has changed. It is therefore real in the sense that it has real properties,

Thus, the carefully-defined circuit bridges the gap between the physical or material realm of matter and energy on the one hand, and the insubstantial realm of logic and meaning on the other. There is nothing accidental about its structure. If it didn't have just that structure, or a functional equivalent, it would not be able to generate the informational "space." Of course, only a being with its own emergent properties could build a logic machine, and recognize that that was what it was actually doing. Shannon's dog could never have achieved what her master did.

2.4 Machines that Think and Machines that Don't

The essential principle behind the first logic machines, i.e. machines that output logical relationships, was not their particular physical realization but the fact that they duplicated in glass and wire the precise relationships that underpin the dual-valued calculus. In this respect, what we call a logic machine differs from, say, a sausage machine because the fundamental principle of a sausage machine lies in just the physical relationships of the mechanism which takes in meat, herbs, bread and skin etc. to give the specific output called sausages. A physical machine, as described in the previous chapter, achieves its particular function because of the physical transfer of matter and energy through its mechanism. Because of the precise physicochemical structure of its mechanism, a sausage machine achieves a particular output *and no other*. The machine is built or exists only so that matter can travel through the mechanism, using different types of energy to transform the material input from one form to another. All the relationships in a physical machine are themselves physical: matters of temperature and pressure, chemicals and kinetics, pistons going in and out or pulleys up and down, of enzymes, fuels, materials, activities such as grinding, mixing, shaping, drying and finally packing, labeling and shipping. All of these processes are explained in their entirety by the fundamental laws of the time-space continuum, meaning the laws of physics, chemistry, biology and so on. Nothing that happens inside one of these machines, the way it is built or about its energy or inputs, requires a further explanation beyond those laws, just because there is no conceivable question about the structure or function of the machine that those laws can't and don't answer.

In the logic machine conceived by Shannon, or in any of what Turing called universal computing machines, what counts is not the physical state of the mechanism but the fact that its functional architecture precisely parallels the relationships of an abstract, content-free calculus (i.e. its operations stand in a one-to-one relationship with the operations of a logical calculus). In respect of its output, therefore, the function of the machine has nothing to do with the laws of physics; they are its substrate but not its goal. Given its input, meaning a physical representation or token of a value system, and its precise internal relationships, the machine is able to manipulate those values according to predetermined non-physical rules to derive novel conclusions which have no equivalent in the real or material world. While there cannot be a computation without a physical substrate, be it brain or PC, the exact physical substrate is irrelevant to the computation. It could be electronic or it could be built of feathers and dough, but all that counts is that the relationships of the dual-valued calculus can be given a physical representation in a suitable medium (i.e. one capable of storing the tokens long enough to use them). The tokens are then manipulated according to the rules of the calculus by a machine whose purpose is no longer an output determined by the laws of physics.

The value of the physical logic machine lies solely in its ability to duplicate in the material world the precise relationships of a dual-valued calculus. That is, the output of a computing system consists of values within a system of rules governing relationships, usually known as the logical operators. Crucially, those rules and values are completely independent of the physical world in which they are embodied: when compared to "the objective, materialistic, third-person world of the physical sciences" such as "...the physical principles, laws and raw materials that suffice to explain radioactivity, continental drift, photosynthesis...," they represent a duality of two "incommensurable orders of being." There are no logical relationships in a leaf. A leaf is not that kind of "machine" because its processes do not map to a dual-valued algebra. Yes, they can be *represented* in a decimal algebra but that relationship goes the wrong way.

Insofar as the brain is a physical thing with properties such as weight, color, shape and chemical consistency, and is composed of immensely complicated neurons which themselves have a ferociously complex internal architecture, all of which follows exactly "...the physical principles, laws..." of "the objective, materialistic, third-person world of the physical sciences," taking as its input oxygen and glucose and many other essential chemicals, to produce an output, then the brain is a machine. Insofar as the brain also has the capacity to manipulate the tokens of a dual-valued logical system according to a calculus which has no physical content, then it has an extra function above, beyond and not reducible to the physical structure in which that calculus is embodied. That is to say, the human brain is a true dualist system, where the physical structure and function of the brain, operating in the ordinary time-space continuum, can produce a novel, emergent and higher-order output which is at once utterly dependent on the brain's physical integrity but is also conceptually distinct and separate from that physical structure. The higher order output is an informational space which, by tradition, we call the mind.

If we wish to build a sausage machine, the *sine qua non* consists of certain critical physical properties that have to exist somewhere in its workings; without just those properties, sausages will not emerge. This is not true of a logic machine. There is no physical relationship which is a *sine qua non* of a logic or computational machine. A logic machine is what they call "multiply-realizable," an ugly expression meaning the same output can be achieved from many different physical structures.

Thus, when Dennett claims: "Somehow, the brain must be the mind," he is absolutely and irredeemably wrong, just because he has conflated the brain's dual functions. When he says that "accepting dualism is giving up" because it is "fundamentally anti-scientific," that it "is to be avoided at all costs" since it "wallows in mystery," he has missed the essential point that the brain is more than just a physical machine. It is *not* like a kidney or a heart, a leaf, a nuclear power station or a sausage machine, just because it is a dualist system *per se*. It works in two realms, the ordinary material realm governed by the laws of thermodynamics, and another realm governed by the rules of a two-valued logic (we assume; this point has not yet been proven but it is immaterial to my case). The fact that the propositional calculus is embodied in a physical form does not mean it is physical by nature: whether you are reading this essay on paper (or Braille), on a computer, an eBook or hearing it spoken, in English or in Urdu, by a human voice or a computerized voice system, is of no account, as the informational content is not constrained by the physical form. What matters is not the physical substrate of a logical system, but the nature of the relationships and values of any logical system that the physical machine can duplicate.

My conclusion is that it is not anti-scientific to claim that a mind is an informational space, generated by a brain, whose essential—indeed, only— function is manipulating logical relationships based on sensory input in order to facilitate the survival of the animal (human or otherwise). This, of course, is a case for dualism, but it most definitely does not mean, imply, connote, intend or convey any sense of the mind as a *substance*, real or otherwise, magical or not. Mind is a *function*, an activity or doing in a semantic (non-physical) realm. Because logical relationships can only be implemented in a switching device, the function of mind necessarily works back upon its substrate to control it. Without control, there is no relationship, only random sparking. That is, mind and its neural substrate interact, with a ceaseless flow of information from one to the other. This solves the mind-body problem because, in Shannon's formulation, information is a real thing, betokened by physical impulses (or marks, or colors, or anything, as long as they are dual in nature), and controlled not by the laws of the time-space continuum but by the rules of its own logical calculus.

The final point is that perhaps we should stop speaking of data processors, including the brain, as machines. It may be more appropriate to reserve this word for complex physical entities operating wholly within the laws of physics and chemistry with the goal of transforming matter and energy inputs into a novel physical output. Data processors do not have the requisite physical structure to qualify as machines (unless their input is electricity and their output heat and noise). Machines do not have the requisite logical structure to qualify as data processors.

2.5 Getting Rid of the Ectoplasm

Armed with this model, we can now examine Dennett's program to see how it measures against the standard of natural dualist interaction (the following points expand on the points listed in Chap. 1).

(i). "...YES," he says, "my theory is a theory of consciousness." As long as consciousness is a subfunction of the mind, there is no objection as he also talks a lot about minds (e.g. his *Kinds of Minds, 1996).*

(ii). "The prevailing wisdom... is materialism: there is only one sort of stuff, namely matter—the physical stuff of physics, chemistry, and physiology..." Agreed, but who claimed otherwise? Certainly not I nor any other modern dualist (I don't count Eccles [4] as a modern dualist). It should, of course, be understood that "mere physical stuff" does not exhaust the possibilities inherent in the term 'materialism.' By acting as though it does, Dennett is showing he is just a child of the fifties.

"...—and the mind is somehow nothing but a physical phenomenon..." Unless he has a new definition of 'physical,' this is not correct. If he wishes to make this claim, he must give some indication as to how mental phenomena will be realized in a physical system. I find his "multiple drafts" model [5] utterly unconvincing but so does he: at the very last paragraph of *Consciousness Explained*, he says: "My explanation of consciousness is far from complete....All I have done, really, is replace one family of metaphors and images with another..." My view is that the mind is not a physical phenomenon, it is an informational phenomenon, and this does give a means of realizing mental properties (such as sensation and emotion) in a dual-aspect physical system.

"We can (in principle!)," Dennett claims, "account for every mental phenomenon using the same physical principles, laws and raw materials that suffice to explain radioactivity, continental drift, photosynthesis..." At this stage, some suggestion as to how he proposes to do this would be very helpful; in the absence of any clues, he is guilty of making an unsupported ideological claim.

"Somehow, the brain must be the mind." Unless and until he can give some substance to the "somehow," this is just promissory materialism at best, and ideology at worst. In any event, I don't believe him when he says this. There is no conceptual path by which all mental attributes can be held to account in the physical realm, not the least because they aren't physical. He needs to show how the laws of the time-space continuum can give rise to the laws of a semantic system. I don't believe, for example, that the off-side rule in soccer derives in any sense from, say, the laws governing electron spin. To claim otherwise is purely fanciful.

"I declare my starting point to be the objective, materialistic, third-person world of the physical sciences." I don't see this as entirely honest, as it defines the really interesting bit (meaning the really difficult part) of mind out of consideration. Just as Skinner did, Dennett has given himself the task of accounting for the easy bit and pouring scorn on anybody who attempts the difficult task.

(iii). Consciousness is all sorts of things, but mostly it is about computation and information. That is his view. As a psychiatrist, I believe it is also about sensation, emotion, irrationality, human nature (e.g. violence, social bonding etc.) and other transcendentally difficult concepts.

(iv). "...we will try to remove the motivation for believing in these (special, subjective) properties (of our internal discriminative states)... by finding alternative explanations for the phenomena that seem to demand them." Again, this is just his intellectually lazy attempt to explain away the difficult bits that his "third person objective" approach can't handle.

(v). To paraphrase, 'Dualism always means substance dualism, which violates the laws of physics; therefore dualism is bad.' This claim is based on an excessively restricted definition of the word 'dualism.' "There is the lurking suspicion that the most attractive feature of mind stuff is its promise of being so mysterious that it keeps science at bay forever." In fact, I find the most attractive feature of dualism is that it offers plausible explanations of the frighteningly complex features of our perception of ourselves, i.e. the most complex entities in the known universe. For the rest, I believe his complaint that dualism is anti-scientific, mysterious and an intellectual dead-end to be simply wrong, just a bit of juvenilia that he overlooked in his regular bouts of self-criticism.

(vi). It is not true that Cartesian dualism fails because it implies an ectoplasmic hidden observer. The fault with naïve Cartesian dualism is an infinite regress, but this can be stopped by the usual means (e.g. as Dennett himself has outlined in Chap. 4 of [4]).

(vii). To paraphrase, 'Selves are good because they are abstractions that can be explained in terms of the same processes which result in snails' shells, beavers' dams and bower birds' bowers.' Again, my view is that he has fundamentally misunderstood the core concepts of biology as a physical science. He conflates mind and body just because he cannot conceive of a functional duality. This is his personal failure of imagination, not a failure of other people's philosophy. We can give an account of the development of mental capacities in children without mentioning any of the processes involved in snail shells or spider webs.

(viii). "This idea of 'mechanical' interpretation in the brain is the central insight of any materialistic theory of the mind..." My case is that the "mechanical" (i.e. biological) properties of the brain are not of the same order of nature as the mental properties which those biological properties subserve. They are utterly different but we need to give an account of each of them using natural principles, not just define one class of events out of existence. If he can give a reasonable account of how "mechanical" principles could account for, say, his own philosophical papers, he might start to sound convincing but, until then, his call for the brain and mind "somehow" to be the same thing is the call of an ideologue.

(ix). The notion that a monist theory of mind can succeed where a dualist theory must fail is based on several errors. In the first place, when all other monist theories have failed [1], there is no explanation of what the term "monist theory of mind" could mean. Second, the only reason to dispense with dualism lies in believing that it necessarily implies magical substances. The modern approach to dualism has nothing to do with magic. Finally, recasting the mind as an informational space leads to an immediate resolution of the mind-body problem as the body traffics ceaselessly in information. If the "Self" Dennett proposed (conceptually indistinguishable from that proposed by Eccles [4]) is itself an informational state, it can plug directly into the body in the manner I will explain in the following chapters but it most emphatically is dualist in nature.

(x). "The phenomena of human consciousness have been explained... in terms of the operations of a 'virtual machine,' a sort of evolved (and evolving) computer program that shapes the activities of the brain." "...when language came into existence, it brought into existence the kind of mind that can transform itself on a moment's notice into a somewhat different virtual machine... We are transformers. That's what a mind is, as contrasted with a mere brain, the control system of a chameleonic transformer, a virtual machine for making more virtual machines." If Dennett had not previously shown such ferocious antidualism, then this prescription of the nature of mind and its relationship to the brain would convince most dualists that he was one of them. With pellucid clarity, he says that the mind is a causally-effective, virtual machine generated by the brain which, just because of its semantic organization, can jump from task to task in precisely the manner outlined by Turing for his "universal computing machine." The very word 'virtual' means 'not the same as; similar to but substantively different from; of a different nature' and so on. The way Dennett uses the expression in this quote is absolutely consistent with a highly complex data processor generating a causally-effective informational space but it is not consistent with any sort of physical or biological machine or process.

He has expanded on this in a later work: "...language, when it is installed in a human brain, brings with it the construction of a new cognitive architecture that *creates* a new kind of consciousness—and morality." It is clear that, by architecture, he does not mean cytoarchitecture: cognitive means an informational state, one which can be written in, and written out. Thus, he means consciousness can switch more or less instantaneously from one state to another. In the brain, this is indubitable because it is primarily a hugely complex switching device. Immediately, this puts his formulation squarely in the area delineated by Shannon, meaning there is no direct relationship between the brain and the "new kind of consciousness," and especially, morality. Morality resides in the realm of information, presumably as a set of rules that can be changed at will. That is, Dennett's own formulation is not compatible with machines as matter-energy processors, only with machines as information processors. The mind as he sees it is therefore not of the same nature as "radioactivity, continental drift and photosynthesis." Those processes are governed by the set of physical rules. Manifestly, the mind follows rules that do not belong to the time-space continuum.

To my mind (*sic*), his concept of "a new cognitive architecture that *creates* a new kind of consciousness—and morality" is a very clear statement of dualism. What he is attempting to do is attribute to a physical machine properties that can only be instantiated by a sophisticated data processor *and which do not belong in the realm of physics*. "We can (in principle!) account for every mental phenomenon using the same physical principles, laws and raw materials that suffice to explain radioactivity, continental drift, photosynthesis..." Perhaps, but only by surreptitiously eliding the difference between physical and semantic, and attributing the properties of an informational space to the realm of the time-space continuum.

If he wishes to attribute to a virtual machine the properties that other people attribute to the dualist mind, then he must nominate the set of rules under which his virtual machine will operate. If it operates under the normal rules of physics and the rest of the material world, as do my car and the tree outside my window, then his virtual machine isn't virtual at all, it is hard, solid, weighty and ponderous just because the laws of physics can gain no purchase on anything that isn't hard, solid, weighty and ponderous. Absent mass and energy, they don't apply because they are the laws of mass and energy. If, however, his "virtual machine" doesn't operate according to the laws of physics, then it must operate according to a completely different set of rules. I believe he would opt for the latter, for a different set of rules but, if he does, then he is confirming that the universe is dualist in nature.

There is a further point to consider, one prized by naïve reductionists who see it as the *coup de grâce* of any claims for dualism. This relies on the concept that DNA carries information; but DNA is patently a physical system; therefore, they claim, all information is physical in nature, so therefore the mind can be fully reduced to chemicals with nothing else to explain (or something like that, the details vary). This is a profound misuse of the word 'information.' There is information, such as my communicating to you via this essay abstract issues of some degree of complexity, and there is "information," as when a key "tells" the door to open. Lock and key "information" is not information at all, as it relies wholly upon its nature as a physical machine to perform its task. A key does not hold any information as "elements of a semantic space" because a key isn't part of a semantic or informational space. We are now completely accustomed to speaking of genetic information, so I suppose that linguistic battle was lost years ago. Nonetheless, nobody should forget that the function of DNA in a cell is no different from the function of enzymes in the gut "choosing" which chemicals to absorb, or inflammatory cells "recognizing" foreign protein. Enzymes don't have a choice, inflammatory proteins don't have a clue and DNA doesn't inform. Claiming otherwise is a classic category error.

(xi) In chemical processes, such as DNA duplicating itself in mitosis or meiosis, in gene expression or in the immune response, we are using terms such as recognizes, knows, tells, and information in an allegorical sense, not a literal sense. Cells don't know anything. They are dumb machines, just as door locks are dumb machines, so it is wrong to say that a cell knows its target, tells its neighbor to release its messengers or recognizes when to activate the information in its genetic code. All of this is a gross breach of the rules of grammar and is scientifically misleading. A cell can only "recognize," "know," "tell," or activate the "information" in its DNA. That is, cellular activity is a simulacrum of recognizing, knowing, telling or informing, but it is not the real thing, not even a model of the real thing. The real thing consists of the manipulation of information in symbolic form in a semantic space, and the interior of a cell is not a semantic space. It does not contain any semantic elements because the laws of logic are not inscribed in the chemical soup of a cell. It is a chemical space, if we have to say anything. DNA is not a model of information suitable to explain the mind. Although, at first blush, it sounds sophisticated to talk of DNA in informational terms, this attempt to reduce mind to biology cannot succeed.

2.6 Minds as Biological Machines

The late psychiatrist, Samuel Guze, had no doubt as to the nature of his subject: "...one's feelings and thoughts are as biological as one's blood pressure or gastric secretion: feelings and thoughts are manifestations of the brain's operations just as blood pressure reflects the operations of the CVS and gastric secretion the stomach's function" [7, p130]. Thoughts, he continued, just are brain secretions, using the word in its common sense. He was not alone in holding this opinion, but was able to find support among some highly influential philosophers. John Searle has bluntly stated: "I think (dualism) is false..." [8, p11]. A few pages later, he dismissed all dualism as beyond the pale: "The way to defeat dualism is simply to refuse to accept the system of categories that makes consciousness out as something non-biological, not a part of the natural world" (p52). He has reiterated this view a number of times over the years, e.g. "As long as we continue to talk and think as if the mental and the physical were separate metaphysical realms, the relation of the brain to consciousness will forever seem mysterious, and we will not have a satisfactory explanation of the relation of neuron firings to consciousness" [9, p8].

Searle's view is that, without further qualification, the mind is biological in nature: "Above all, consciousness is a biological phenomenon. We should think of consciousness as part of our ordinary biological history, along with digestion, growth, mitosis and meiosis" [9, p1]. Elsewhere, he adds photo-synthesis and the secretion of bile to this list, leaving no doubt where he stands: "We must stop worrying about how the brain *could* cause conscious-ness and begin with the plain fact that it *does*" [10, p8]. "We live in one world, and all the features of the world from quarks and electrons to nation states and balance of payments problems are, in their different ways, part of that one world" [10]. "The smell of the flower, the sound of the symphony, the thoughts of theorems in Euclidean geometry—all are caused by lower level biological processes in the brain; and as far as we know, the crucial functional elements are neurons and synapses" [11]. Indeed, his theory of mind is known as biological naturalism. Dennett, of course, is equally uncompromising.

Searle's certainty on this point is a little perplexing as, in 1948 (i.e. when Searle was still in high school), the philosophically-inclined mathematician, Norbert Wiener, stated flatly: "The mechanical brain does not secrete thought 'as the liver does bile,' as the earlier materialists claimed, nor does it put it out in the form of energy, as the muscle puts out its activity. Information is information, not matter or energy. No materialism which does not admit this can survive at the present day" [12]. It is surely Searle's prerogative to disagree with Wiener; it is also Searle's inviolable duty to explain just why he disagrees with Wiener, not to ignore his case.

We need to be quite clear about what these renowned philosophers are actually saying, because it sounds to me that they are confusing provenance with nature. If they are saying that, as a matter of strict literal fact, the nature of mind is wholly and exclusively biological in the same way as bodily secretions such as mucus or semen are wholly and exclusively biological, then they are factually wrong. The nature of a witty pun is not of the same class of events as sticky stuff smeared on a paper tissue, because jokes, and all other mental events, have properties above and beyond those of bodily secretions. The universal set of biological properties does not coincide with the universal set of mental properties (I don't see any overlap at all). If, however, they are saying that the mind originates in the biology of the brain, so that it should be classed with all other biological phenomena to be explained by reductionist biologism, then they are also wrong, because language and other symbolic discourse cannot be reduced to its substrate. If (the only remaining option) they are saying: 'Because mind arises from the brain, and the brain is biological, then the mind is also properly classed as biological, even if it is a very strange sort of biology,' then their claim is trite. That explains nothing, it merely shifts that which requires explanation (the odd nature of the mentality of mind) from the large class of totally mysterious phenomena to a smaller but equally mysterious class of odd biological phenomena. When this claim is seen as the final outcome of careers as professional philosophers spanning half a century, it is somewhat underwhelming.

However, and even with the most benign charity, I don't think that is at all what they are claiming. Both authors like to pepper their works with biological snippets, showing that they actually try to read some biology. Both of them come from prestigious institutions where they have immediate access to biologists of the highest caliber. Unlike some authors in remote parts of the globe, they can saunter down to the nearest staff lounge and quietly ask a distinguished colleague to cast a critical eye over their works. Whether they do that or not, I don't know but, if they don't, they can't later claim to be misunderstood if what they say about minds and biology lends itself to an interpretation they don't like. In my reading, there is no doubt that when these authors say 'biological,' that is exactly what they mean. There is no room or scope for ambiguity in their reductionist claims. They are both adamantly opposed (in Dennett's case, virulently) to any suggestion that mind and body constitute a dualism of form or structure. Dualism, to them, is a ridiculous hangover from prehistory, a ludicrously anti-scientific and anti-rational myth that consistently and inevitably leads us astray from the task of discovering the true theory of mind which, they repeatedly state, is biological in nature: "Somehow," Dennett says, "the brain must be the mind." This says that the mind has no properties above and beyond those of the physical brain. By excluding dualism, they commit themselves irrevocably to the concept that mind is wholly and exclusively biological in nature.

I believe these philosophers are completely and utterly wrong, that they are both prisoners of their prejudices and their claims should be dismissed as the unhoned products of keen but uneducated eighteen year old minds that had just received what they thought were penetrating insights into the nature of the most intractable problem in human history. I'm sure we all had similar epiphanies at eighteen; not all of us had the good fortune to make a career out of it, though. Let's look at their case a little more closely.

Searle used the case of digestion as an exemplar of what he means by 'biological.' I agree: it is a very good example of what we mean by biology. Dennett's own example of snails secreting their shells is also of the same order of nature as digestion, so we can group Professors Searle and Dennett together in their espousal of the claim: Biology will explain all we need to know about the mind. First question: What is the nature of biology as an explanatory class?

A biological system is a case of self-sustaining, self-perpetuating thermo-dynamic instability; comprising a particular class of chemicals based in carbon, hydrogen, oxygen and nitrogen, with other elements in much smaller proportion; whose precise structure is determined by its DNA and RNA molecules. Lacking any one of these features, we are not talking about a biological system (viruses we're still not sure about and prions are out of it). So: in the case of humans, the property of speech is necessarily coded in our DNA. However, there is more to speech than a brain because what we say in any language is not, and could not be, coded in DNA. Language is infinite, the genome is not. Thus, language has properties that biological systems do not; biological systems are inadequate to explain the totality of language. Competition may well be coded into the genome but the Olympic Games are not. Territoriality is almost certainly based in our biological heritage, but the laws of intellectual property are not. The higher primate drive to form dominance hierarchies is genetically-based, the executive structure of a university is not, and so on.

In the case of biological systems, we are concerned with the precise disposition of the atoms making the molecules, and every unit of energy that passes through the system. In photosynthesis, we know exactly the fate of every photon that strikes the chloroplast. In the secretion of bile, we can track every last bile pigment from its origin to its destination. Let's look at this in more detail via a quotidian example:

Professor X is getting on in years. In the twilight of a long and illustrious career as a philosopher, he is invited to give the opening or closing address at some prestigious function his university is planning. Specifically, he is asked to summarize recent developments in his field for the benefit of incoming or outgoing students, to stimulate their little minds and give them something other than iPhones or student debts to think about. Prof. X is delighted by the invitation and calls his wife from work to tell her. She is equally pleased for him, and promises to cook his favorite dinner to help him get in the mood for writing his oration. That evening, having partaken of an immodest serving of Mrs. X's excellent culinary skills, he retires to his study to begin the task of writing his paper. Some hours later, his paper unfinished because of an unexpected knotty problem, he retires to bed. While his brain and its attendant mind are asleep, his bowel is anything but inactive. It keeps churning away in its mindless biological way, busily turning the evening's banquet into tomorrow's bowel action. Next morning, he rises, breaks his fast and, still pondering the philosophical problem, adjourns to the lavatory where he delivers of himself a generous testimony to the biological efficacy of the omnivorous bowel. Suitably refreshed, he repairs to his study where, in a burst of inspiration, he solves the problem and writes the kind of heartwarming talk for which grumpy alumni can be cajoled into shelling out a few extra dollars.

Now it is the case that we know a great deal about the anatomy and physiology of the bowel. We know how food is digested and absorbed, down to the last proton in every mouthful of food. We can describe in quite frightening detail the processes by which bodily wastes are excreted into the bowel, the myriad helpful bacteria who choose to reside there and how it all works together in perfect thermodynamic harmony to produce our daily fecal offerings (if it didn't, we would run the risk of blowing up like the fat man in *The Meaning of Life*). We cannot, however, say a word about how the brain "secretes" thoughts; that remains a total mystery. However, and I am prepared to lay the most generous odds on this proposition: Whatever the processes of thought involved in writing a philosophical paper, they are not of the same order of nature as H_2S production in the interstices of the colon.

So confident am I of my position that I will further submit that not even a flatulent paper by Professors Dennett or Searle would qualify as proof of their joint and several claims that mind and biology are of one and the same order of nature. Philosophy papers, or science, or religion or art or Claude Shannon jokes or rules of sport or GNP or plans for a birthday party or interest rates on defaulted student debts are *not* of the same order of nature as shit, and that is all there is to that. Those things have properties not shared with feces. Anybody who claims otherwise is guilty of the grossest ignorance: he is, we may even say, talking shit, but only by way of metaphor. It is not a literal claim to say that Dennett's or Searle's claim to understand the nature of thought as a biological phenomenon is shit, even when they say that their own theories are caused by processes conceptually indistinguishable from those that fill our sewers each morning. Information, which perforce includes all philosophy (good and bad), does not belong to the material world of the matter-energy continuum. Yes, it is natural but no, it is not "the same as" photosynthesis, secretion of bile, secretion of snail shells or even beavers building dams.

To quote Searle again: "The smell of the flower, the sound of the symphony, the thoughts of theorems in Euclidean geometry—all are caused by lower level biological processes in the brain; and as far as we know, the crucial functional elements are neurons and synapses" [17]. Yes, ultimately, these mental events are the result of biological processes in neurons and their synapses, but they are not *themselves* "lower level biological processes." They are, as he later admits, higher order processes; to be precise, informational processes that cannot be reduced to or equated with the commonplace biological processes that underwrite them, i.e. they represent a duality of nature. We think of theorems by means of our capacity to manipulate symbols, and symbols are not of the same order of nature as the physical medium that carries them. Thus, Prof. Searle's theory could have been written by any non-biological entity with suitable informational processing capabilities, but that only proves that the relationship between thoughts of theorems and brain events is contingent, not necessary, and so his broader claim fails.

Searle may think I am being unfair, that I am deliberately parodying his stance by not giving credence to the nuances in his claims: "Above all," he says, "consciousness is a biological phenomenon. We should think of consciousness as part of our ordinary biological history, along with digestion, growth, mitosis and meiosis.... We must stop worrying about how the brain *could* cause consciousness and begin with the plain fact that it *does*" [9, p8, his emphasis]. What he is doing here is arguing against substance dualism, but who takes that seriously these days? If he wishes to say that mental capacities are only found in suitably equipped biological entities, then he is making a claim for which he has absolutely no warrant. Maybe the next alien to drop in will be an android, who knows? Searle doesn't. But if he wants to say that the mind arises in some mysterious way from the workings of the brain, he is not exactly breaking new ground. The question for most of us is not whether it does, but how it does. And a preliminary to answering the question is to decide (finally) whether there can be a monist theory of mind. Look again at his injunction:

> "As long as we continue to talk and think as if the mental and the physical were separate metaphysical realms, the relation of the brain to consciousness will forever seem mysterious, and we will not have a satisfactory explanation of the relation of neuron firings to consciousness" [16, p8; 7].

This is not true. The claim that dualism is false necessarily closes the door if it turns out that it is not false. This book is about giving an account of the mental and the physical as separate metaphysical realms in terms that are *not* mysterious but aim to give "...a satisfactory explanation of the relation of neuron firings to consciousness." His injunction represents a failure of his imagination, not a universal law.

In my view, the mental and the physical do indeed represent separate ontological realms such that there cannot be a monist account of human behavior. We can, however, relate these realms quite easily using the principles outlined in Chapter 1, potentially giving us "...a satisfactory explanation of the relation of neuron firings to consciousness." Dennett's claim that "Somehow, the brain must be the mind" becomes "somehow, the brain gives rise to the mind," which is a much more interesting claim. I think we are now in a position to say just how this happens.

So much for elderly philosophers who have spent half a century trying to justify naïve opinions they formed in adolescence rather than submitting their ideas to open criticism. The only safeguard against persisting juvenilia is a ferociously self-critical attitude but, regretfully, self-criticism and becoming an academic celebrity don't seem to mix these days. With that, I promise never to mention either of these elderly professors again. Also, alert readers will have noticed that I have not addressed any of the claims for biological reductionism made by the late Dr. S. Guze.

2.7 Conclusion: *¡Viva la Revolución!*

By degrees, humans progress from the darkness of superstition to a rational world, guided (and driven) by "...our assumption that there is a comprehensible universe..." Our understanding of the features collectively called "the mind" proceeds from frank religiosity to something approximating rationality, but it is not a smooth or even a continuous path. The religious view, of a supernatural soul sent from heaven at conception to live in the head until its allotted span is over, dominates the intellectual landscape. It is the default position, as it were, of the vast majority of people throughout the world, not because of brainwashing, but because that's how it seems to be. As the Nobel laureate, Sir John Eccles said, "I can't imagine that this conscious mind of mine will some day cease to be." That, I suggest, was his failure of imagination. All he had to do was give thought to what happens when we go to sleep, or have a general anesthetic. I had one last week. From the time I felt the injection go up my arm to the time a nurse said "Wriggle across to the trolley," there was nothing, not even a perception of nothing. However, it is difficult to imagine nothing, which tends to confirm what Descartes concluded, long before anesthetics were invented.

As the broad field of science erodes the presumed factual basis of religious beliefs, many thinkers have extrapolated the secular trend and tried to assemble a non-magical model of mind. With rising levels of education around the world, more and more people are taking the view that the mind is not a magical entity but is the non-miraculous outcome of the particular structure and function of the brain. Mind emerges from brain, if you prefer; all that remains is to fill in the blanks. Unfortunately, the blanks are proving very resistant to conventional scientific inquiries: excitable people have been loudly promising the reductionist millennium for a hundred and fifty years. This has been especially true in psychiatry where, in my first lecture in my new career as a budding psychiatrist nearly four decades ago, the professor announced in ringing tones that the secrets of mental disorder were just about to tumble under the hammer blows of science triumphant. We're still waiting. For all the promises of the drug company shills, the much-trumpeted reduction of all mental disorder to brain disorder remains an ideological goal, not a scientific program.

In philosophy and psychology, the post-war period has seen a flowering of models, most of which disappeared as quickly as they appeared. The same themes persist as the tides of war ebb and flow in the endless battle between mindlessness and brainlessness [13]. In a 'brainless' model of mind, the mind is seen as totally independent of the brain, so that neurophysiology and other basic sciences are not considered relevant. The classic Cartesian model is the best example of a non-scientific concept of the mind as the free-wheeling but temporary inhabitant of a brain while, across the divide, the Freudian approach exemplifies exactly the same concept dressed in a lab coat. The modern version, of a cognitive psychology that owes nothing to neuro-physiology, is seen in many settings, usually among people who know no neurophysiology and are able to convince themselves it isn't necessary. The bad news is that the naïve cognitive model merges seamlessly with the fantastic, as a glance at the psychology pages in the telephone directory will prove. Naive cognitivism is not the way to go.

The most widely-followed 'mindless' model of mind was behaviorism, the notion that science had no right to attempt to deal with anything so ephemeral as a mind. Therefore, to construct a science of behavior, all the researchers had to do was establish a law-like linkage between the environmental stimulus and the behavioral response. That way, in Skinner's chilling words, science would be able to predict and control human behavior at all times. Fortunately, this went nowhere and even psychologists have (reluctantly) abandoned the idea that our behavior is so simple that watching a few rats or pigeons will tell us all we need to know about humans. Philosophy had its mindless phase, too, mostly over by the 1970s, but it lives on in psychiatry (and nowhere else). The main approach was to adopt an uncompromising hostility to the idea of the mind as a functionally separate but causally effective entity governed by rules of its own. It was this point they couldn't stomach, the notion that there may be more to the universe than the laws of the time-space continuum. The properties of the mind, they claimed, could be fully reduced to a special case of the properties of the brain. Therefore, a full understanding of the brain would automatically give a full understanding of the whole of human mental life.

Despite the elemental appeal of this approach to people who prefer their solutions cut and dried, it hasn't worked, and never will. This is a metaphysical claim, meaning there is no empirical evidence that can be brought to bear on it. Having said that, I don't believe the program to reduce mind to body was entirely wasted. Given the astounding progress of materialist science in the twentieth century, it was inevitable that somebody would say: "Well, we eradicated the question of possession states in infectious diseases, and showed that gravity keeps the planets in orbit, not angels, so why don't we get rid of the mind at the same time?" This step was inevitable, but what wasn't inevitable was the prolonged, ideological commitment to eliminating the mind from all consideration. True, for a large part of the past century, orthodox science did not have the tools to tackle the concept of mind but they were being developed. However, psychologists and philosophers (and psychiatrists, insofar as they think of these matters) were blinded to the possibilities by their need to be "more scientific than thou" in eradicating all hints of the deadly sin of dualism. By assuming that Descartes' formulation of mind as an unnatural substance was the only conceptual possibility, philosophers slammed the door to the radical new ideas being developed. They rejected the novel approach offered by Turing, Shannon and so many other brilliantly original thinkers, that information is an entity in its own right, a causally-effective part of the real world yet not the sort of thing you can poke with a stick.

The essential feature that converts an informational state into a causally-effective "thing" is that it comes equipped with the right connections to the material universe. This was the problem for Popper and Eccles: apart from poking its ghostly fingers in the cerebral modules to read them, they had no idea how their "Self" would interact with the brain. Conceptually, the connections are not difficult: since an informational space exists only insofar as it is generated by a material machine, then the connections just are the elements that generate the space itself. Information necessarily flows two ways, otherwise we would not be able to tell that an informational space had been generated: an informational space is not a black hole.

This has huge consequences for modern psychiatry, which has committed itself to the idea that all mental disorder is caused by specific brain disorders, i.e. there is unidirectional causality. If the concept of the dual mind is accepted, then it is immediately apparent that mental disorders can arise from disturbances of the informational state of the mind, independently of whether the brain is physically disordered or not. Mental disorders are programming errors, as it were, or even just wrong information (is the government *really* out to get you?), all of which can certainly occur in a perfectly healthy brain. Even the most serious disorders such as schizophrenia could be generated by this means. The only reason this idea is not accepted by orthodox psychiatry is because it flies in the face of their ideology—but science is not supposed to be about ideology.

By rights, a convincing account of mental disorder should proceed from a rational theory of mental order, usually known as a theory of mind. Conversely, a valid theory of mind should be able to predict the points at which a healthy mind will begin to malfunction. In any event, in the absence of a workable theory of mind, there will never be a plausible theory of mental disorder. I have suggested elsewhere that any theory of mind that doesn't generate a theory of mental disorder is incomplete, and proposed that this should be a standard test of all developments in philosophy of mind. However, before we can start the work of articulating a viable model of mind, we need to strip from our folk ideas of mind the accretions of centuries of religiosity, the dead weight of bad psychology, partisan philosophy, scientism, misplaced confidence in reductionist science, as well as the modernist fallacy, political prejudice and the like. That is, with respect to a formal theory of mind, we are in much the same intellectual backwater as the world was before Newton cut motion to its essentials, before vitalism was stripped from energy, or before Shannon and Turing turned information into a dual-valued calculus.

Perhaps this will be the final revolution: to formalize the processes of mind, stripping away the accretions of religiosity and using only formal equations to give a predictive science of mind. While I don't expect that we will be able to render mind in mathematical terms for many years to come, if ever, I believe that we are in the position where we can start the process of seeing mind as a natural dualism, part of the natural universe yet not part of the physical universe.

Mind as Algorithm

"Most of the things worth doing in the world had been declared impossible before they were done."

—Louis D. Brandeis

3.1 Introduction: Revolutionary Ideas

In Chapter 1, I briefly mentioned three of the most important conceptual revolutions in history, even though we don't normally think of them as classic scientific revolutions. Essentially, they reduced to mathematical form matters that had been considered central to our perception of the universe, but seemed unfathomably complex. In each case, the problem was not the concept itself, which was blindingly simple once pointed out, but the crushing burden of mysticism that had accumulated over millennia until the pure idea was no longer visible. The first of the modern conceptual revolutions is attributed to Newton, who was not altogether modern himself. In his education, he would have been taught the classic concept of motion as a movement to a preordained end. Thus, smoke rose, rain fell, moss grew sideways and the dead putrefied as part of their movement to their divinely-appointed ends. Motion was not as we see it, but it involved the concept of *teleos,* or the natural goal of being.

Of course, there were lots of problems with this: stars fell, disturbing the tranquil perfection of the heavens; water evaporated; iron rusted while gold didn't, and so on. Each of these phenomena was given an additional explanation, which led to further complications, until the whole tangled mess of ideas became little more than an arena for academic squabbling. It needs to be recalled that Isaac Newton was a very difficult and abrasive personality whose main interests were alchemy, nonconformist religion and academic squabbling. In a strong sense, he was a classic example of Kuhn's notion of the outsider who revolutionizes a field just because he has no strong emotional attachment to the status quo. His contribution was outlined in his magnum opus, the *Prinicipia Mathematica*, published in 1687. Stripping the accumulated junk of thousands of years of human fear and ignorance, he reduced motion to its essence, as summarized in the devastatingly simple formula of his Second Law:

$$F = ma$$

The acceleration of a body is a constant relationship between its mass and the force applied to it. This applied to all bodies without exception. It was therefore possible to calculate where a body would be after it had accelerated for a set period and, conversely, it was possible to predict where a moving body would be if no other force acted upon it. Of course, this latter conclusion was theoretical, as he had no way of testing a moving body free of gravity, but the principle was clear. A moving body would continue to move in a straight line unless and until some other force acted on it. Motion had nothing to do with *teleos*. It was the blind, pointless, undirected outcome of unvarying universal principles, applying in distant space equally as on earth. In short order, his new view of the world explained the orbits of planets, falling bodies and ballistics, and set the scene for the industrial revolution.

Within a hundred years, the world changed further as the power of steam was harnessed in James Watt's first steam engines and, within the next century, the power of electricity was tamed and understood in mathematical form. This time, however, there were many contributors as the notion of energy as a blind, law-abiding part of the natural world took over. Faraday, Gauss, Ampere, Carnot and many others added to the rapidly growing notion that energy had nothing to do with spiritualism. Until then, the concept of energy had been buried in the supernatural as people tried to explain the ability of living creatures to move and keep warm. Vitalism in its many forms, including Henri Bergson's *élan vital,* dominated the intellectual scene until Maxwell summarized the bare concept of electromagnetic energy in a series of equations. As the capacity for work in many forms, energy was now seen as a unitary concept rather than a collection of mysterious and unrelated notions.

This did not happen overnight: even at the end of his career, the great Pasteur was sure that biological energy was profoundly different from the physical forms. Eventually, the biochemistry he had pioneered was shown to be just a special form of chemistry and the mathematics of enzyme induction has since been clarified. There is absolutely nothing "vital" about biochemistry. At about this time, the Michelson-Morley experiment dealt a fatal blow to the notion of the ether as the medium of propagation of electromagnetic waves. Not long after, Marie and Pierre Curie isolated radium as a natural source of the mysterious X-rays Roentgen had discovered, just at the time Einstein's revolutionary concept of relativity transfixed the world of physics. Now, energy was seen as a purely physical concept, expressed in the most compelling and unassailable of all physical formulae...

$$E=mc^2$$

3.2 An Information Revolution

In the first decades of the twentieth century, during the heroic age of the physical sciences, another discipline was taking its first tentative steps. Many fields were converging on a single point: telegraphy and telephony, the mathematics of recursive systems, cryptography and cryptanalysis, high-order algebras and so on. From these arose the almost bizarre notion that information itself could be stripped of its historical accretions, with the residue subject to a rigorous mathematical formulation. At first, this was deeply shocking because there was felt to be a profound and inviolate relationship between the humanity of *Homo sapiens* and our capacity to conceive and communicate matters at the highest levels of abstraction and creativity. As described in Chapter 1, Claude Shannon showed that logic, the very essence of human rationality, could be duplicated on simple machines consisting of a handful of electrical relays borrowed from the local telephone exchange. A few years later, Alan Turing argued that, by the end of the century, we humans would be in the habit of talking of machines as though they had the same powers of thought and reason as we had always thought were ours alone.

In yet another astounding paper, published in the *Bell System Technical Journal* in 1948, Shannon outlined his views on the mathematics of communication. This paper was so revolutionary that few understood its implications. After a brief introduction, he stated his position:

"The fundamental problem of communication is that of reproducing at one point either exactly or approximately a message selected at another point. Frequently the messages have meaning; that is they refer to or are correlated according to some system with certain physical or conceptual entities. These semantic aspects of communication are irrelevant to the engineering problem. The significant aspect is that the actual message is one selected from a set of possible messages. The system must be designed to operate for each possible selection, not just the one which will actually be chosen since this is unknown at the time of design" [1].

This was little short of shattering: in a few, terse sentences, he snatched the entire concept of human communication away from priests, poets and polemicists, and flipped it across to engineers. Notice how deftly he deflated human egotism: "Frequently the messages have meaning..." What is clear is that he meant *sometimes*, but that's engineers all over. In case anybody missed the point, he followed with a lethal hook: "These semantic aspects of communication are irrelevant to the engineering problem." Communication, or information as it was later known, stood low in the order of things: it was strictly an engineering problem, in the sense, one could say, that delivering the food for a banquet to a great hotel, and removing the next morning's sewage, are engineering problems of a similar order.

In his formulation, there were five parts to any general system of communication, namely, a source, a transmitter, a channel, a receiver and a destination. The source and destination were usually people but could be any machine: communication was no longer the exclusive province of humans. The transmitter took the message and converted it mechanically into a form that could be sent through the channel (we would now say the medium of transmission) to the receiver, which decoded it by reversing the transmitter's function, before dispatching it to its destination. The choke point was the channel, and he showed how information could be measured in terms of the probability that a particular message would be chosen from the range available. His formula was:

$$H = -\Sigma p_i \log_2 p_i$$

The critical feature was that information restricted or negated uncertainty, which suggested a powerful parallel in physics:

> "My greatest concern," he wrote, nearly a quarter of a century later, "was what to call it. I thought of calling it 'information,' but the word was overly used, so I decided to call it 'uncertainty.' When I discussed it with John von Neumann, he had a better idea. Von Neumann told me, 'You should call it entropy, for two reasons. In the first place your uncertainty function has been used in statistical mechanics under that name, so it already has a name. In the second place, and more important, no one really knows what entropy really is, so in a debate you will always have the advantage'" [2].

Information, therefore, was negative entropy, which accorded it a natural place in the laws of the time-space continuum (roughly speaking, entropy is energy that is not available for work). That is, it had nothing to do with higher powers, prescience, the ineffable or any such folderol: for the first time in history, the concept of communication became amenable to an ordinary mathematical analysis. History itself was suddenly propelled in a new direction.

Having carefully excluded the semantic content of any message from his formulation, his concern was how a message gets from A to B, not what the message said. That was purely a question of predetermined codes, agreed between A and B for the specific purpose of making B aware of something about A's inner state. Shannon left this wide open: "...they refer to or are correlated according to some system with certain physical or conceptual entities." In broadest terms, the function of communication is to allow B to create a facsimile of some part of A's state, dependent upon a one-to-one relationship between those features of A's state and the copy recreated in B. Another way of phrasing this is that A's inner state is mapped upon B's inner state such that a facsimile of A's state is generated in B. Therefore, B *knows* (can act upon) what A intended in the message. That is crucial: there can be no communication of meaning without prior agreement on the tokens of communication, and nothing is communicated if B cannot apprehend the message as A transmitted it. Thus, if the message is smothered in random fluctuations in the channel (noise) or B has lost his copy of the code, then the facsimile is not created, and communication fails. As an engineer, of course, Shannon was very familiar with the problem of noise in the communication channels; as a mathematician, he left the question of the semantic content of a message to others.

From this work arose a very large part of the major revolution of the latter half of the twentieth century, the information revolution. But what about meaning? While Shannon brushed it aside, Turing mocked our sensitivities by betting that, since we can only ever guess what the speaker has in mind, we wouldn't be able to tell the difference between a human and a machine (with mathematics, we probably do know what the speaker has in mind but that can certainly be duplicated by a machine) [3]. This brings us to the question of mind and, of all topics encrusted with hoary and vexatious historical accretions, the most overloaded must surely be the human mind. Can we now perform upon the concept of mind the same operation as the revolutions described above? That is, can we strip from the concept of mind so many thousands of years of accumulated prejudice, misconception, fallacy, religiosity, political correctness and just plain junk, in order to reduce it to its barest elements? Can we, in fact, reduce mind to its essence, summarized in a linear equation (or even a hugely complex non-linear equation, let's not prejudge it)?

3.3 Stripping the Junk

Just before the Great War engulfed the civilized world, a young and abrasive American psychologist announced that his field also had to leap into the modern era, by ridding itself of all pretense of talking of mind. "I can state my position here no better," said John B. Watson, "than by saying that I should like to bring my students up in the same ignorance of (the mind-body problem) as one finds among the students of other branches of science." After half a century of confusion from the introspectionists, he argued that all talk of mind and mental contents, of consciousness and introspection, "bound (psychology) hand and foot" and blocked any chance of progress. Observable behavior was all that counted; all talk of unobservable intervening variables, such as minds, was a waste of time and energy. He aimed at a rigidly reductionist science of psychology: "The findings of psychology become the functional correlates of structure and lend themselves to explanation in physico-chemical terms." The only legitimate goal of a rational psychology was "...to learn general and particular methods by which I may control behavior."

Writing in 1916, after he became president of the American Psychological Association, he was sure it would be possible to devise such a psychology within a few years. As history reveals, Watson's optimism was a little premature. All he had at his disposal was a technique borrowed from the Russian physiologist, Ivan Pavlov. In fact, Pavlov conceived the conditioned reflex as purely a physiological tool of investigation which, he firmly believed, could never form the basis of a general psychology. Worse still, Watson hardly knew anything about it as he had only a few third hand translations from the original Russian to English via German to guide him. Nonetheless, in his eager hands, conditioning became the building block of a new view of psychology as a mindless, experimental science. Freed of its spiritualist bonds, psychology was to be fixed firmly in the same traditions of science as, say, Einstein's bold new nuclear physics.

At the same time, however, Freud's model of psychoanalysis had captured the attention of the elitist fringe of the academic world of psychiatry, not to overlook the chattering classes. Freud was also determined to rid psychology of any notions of spirituality by developing a huge and vastly complicated model of the mind as a quasi-hydrodynamic mechanism that could answer any and all conceivable questions about human behavior. Crucially, he insisted that his model was scientific, although his own, equally premature attempt at a "project for a scientific psychology" failed abjectly (Freud later tried to conceal it). What was his goal? He wanted to remove all poetry from the concept of mind, replacing mystical constructs with purely biological drives that could eventually be related to the brain. It was laudable, but totally misconceived. At about the same time, there were other projects to produce a rational, non-mystical psychology, notably the theory of radical behaviorism or operant conditioning proposed and developed by Burrhus F. Skinner. Once again, the author took an uncompromising stance against unverifiable historical accretions such as creativity, altruism, honor, freedom and dignity, replacing them with what he hoped were objective constructs based in valid laboratory research.

With the benefit of hindsight, when these models of a mindless mind fell by the wayside, they thoroughly deserved their respective fates. Since then, there have been others but we still haven't advanced very far in the goal to produce a non-question-begging, rational model of mind. My view is that this is because the goal of writing a non-mentalist or monist theory of mind has itself become just another historical accretion. That is, the twentieth century obsession with writing dualism out of the project for a theory of mind is as misdirected as writing it in by means of souls, nymphs or cosmic energies.

At different points in my various books and publications, I have argued that there cannot be a non-mentalist theory of mind, meaning any and all monist theories of mind are doomed. By monist theories of mind, I include all modern theories of psychology and of philosophy that are explicitly or implicitly antidualist. Similarly, we can dismiss all current dualist theories of mind that are self-consciously "scientific" without defining science, such as psychoanalysis and simple cognitivism, including all the fads known as CBT, DBT, RFT and all the rest.

If the mind is an informational state, we ought to be able to conceptualize it using the approach developed by Shannon, Turing, Wiener and such luminaries. My case, outlined in Chap. 1, is that the mind is an informational state and is therefore irreducibly non-material or mentalist in nature. This claim was presaged in 1948 by the mathematician and philosopher, Norbert Wiener: "Information is information, not matter or energy. No materialism which does not admit this can survive at the present day" (his use of the word 'material' is more or less what we would now call natural). However, we cannot even begin to approach this novel approach to mind from the correct stance if the path is cluttered by intellectual junk. It has to be remembered (with humility) that fashions change, and this applies to intellectual fashions just as it applies to women's hemlines or men's hats. In theories of mind, the driving impetus has always been the prevailing fashion, that is, people started with what they believed to be the correct conceptualization and then tried to hammer the observations to fit that model. All too often, the prevailing model has simply been political correctness. So, for millennia, all thought was directed to fitting the observations with the approved model of the immortal, faultless spirit pulling the strings, better known as the Cartesian model.

These days, it is fashionable to pour scorn on Descartes' meticulous reasoning in that he institutionalized magic. This is not quite the basis of Watson's antagonism to the study of the mind, which was that science had no means of obtaining reliable data on the mind on which to build a solid theory. Watson was, however, merely the child of his times. Marxism and other variants of what was called "scientific socialism" were fanatically hostile to any and all religious formulations of the mind. Indeed, in many parts of the world in those days, embracing anything like a religious view was enough to buy a bullet in the neck. Scientists were not immune to the waves of hysteria sweeping the world but were in fact part of it. Skinner's radical behaviorism took it even further, by providing what was thought to be a scientific rationale for revolutionary fervor.

Philosophy was no different. Armstrong, Smart and many others argued in favor of a radical physicalism for which, they believed, ordinary laboratory science would eventually provide the details. When this didn't seem to go anywhere, philosophers tried to shoe-horn an ersatz dualism into a monist case, otherwise known as functionalism. Manifestly, this has now failed, and the reason is simply that virulent hostility to dualism has now become *de rigueur* for anybody who wants to talk in public about the concept of mind. That is, an unthinking, knee-jerk type worship of the idea that "science is antidualist" is the latest political correctness driving philosophy, psychology and psychiatry. Meanwhile, in the next room, fully operational and hugely profitable dualist machines are beavering away, transforming our lives and turning their developers into the wealthiest humans in history.

At this stage of our intellectual and technical history, I don't believe it is either fair or historically accurate to blame people like Watson or Pavlov for the sins of blind, reductive physicalism throughout the twentieth century. Marx, for example, knew nothing about the concept of an infinite regress; as far as he could tell, the only intellectual accusation he could level against the church was that it employed preposterous magic to dupe and enslave the masses in order to enrich and strengthen an evil social structure. Therefore, if he wished to liberate the masses (and everything says that was his goal, not a new and worse form of slavery), then he had to attack the churches at their weakest point. This he did by adopting a stringently-defined scientism. Thus, until even the 1950s, the choices were seen as either a repressive, delusional religiosity known as dualism, or a progressive, rational, scientific, monist materialism. Apart from a handful of laboratories and university departments of mathematics, there were no alternatives. Granted, Wiener's peculiarly disorganized book proclaiming the new science of cybernetics became an unexpected bestseller, but that was only among the same intellectual gadflies who were also convinced that, when it came to ministering to their sensitive egos, psychoanalysis was the way to go.

By the late 1970s, however, things were changing. As radical antidualism was losing ground, philosophers tried to cross the attributes of dualism with a materialist concept of mind, from which unseemly mating came the hybrid known as functionalism. This was simply dualism by another name, a last-ditch attempt to save the face of the historical trend of anticlerical, humanist materialism. The very word 'scientific' had come to mean rational and progressive, as opposed to 'religious,' which meant irrational and reactionary. Thus, anybody who wished to be seen as forward-looking had to don the whole wardrobe of the left wing intellectual. As shown by the scornful response to spiritualism's last gasp, Popper and Eccles' mystical Self (1978), there were no half-measures. To be rational and progressive meant to adopt an unyielding antidualism; conversely, even to ask whether some form of dualism might be possible was to invite derision. Practically nobody asked whether it might be possible to find a path between the rock of magic and the hard place of sterile monism. Fortunately, the philosopher David Chalmers asked exactly that question, with predictable results [4]. However, he did that work nearly twenty years ago; has the world moved ahead since then? Without slipping into magic, is it possible to hold that there is more to materialism than matter and energy? I think it is possible and, to his great profit, so does Mr. Bill Gates. As do Mr. Larry Ellison, and the owners of Google, of Facebook, eBay and all the other purely informational systems that now dominate and facilitate the world's economies.

Let's go back to the eccentric prodigy, Norbert Wiener: "Information is information, not matter or energy. No materialism which does not admit this can survive at the present day." He said that in 1948, when all the modern philosophers who have eagerly jumped on the hybrid known as functionalism, were either at school or still to come. Not one of them can plead he didn't know there may be a "third path," as they now say. In particular, nobody who was studying philosophy of mind in the 1970s to 1980s was unaware of the explosive growth of the new information technology. Simply going into a library in those days was effectively a tutorial in how IT was transforming our perception of the world and of ourselves. Yet such was the power of the social drive to be seen as radical and progressive and rational and so on, that practically no philosophers or psychologists could bring themselves to admit that they had backed the wrong horse. In the fullness of time, antidualism has become a seriously misleading historical accretion in its own right. Anybody who disagrees with this claim must first show (without using a computer) that the algorithms of, say, Google, are not insubstantial information but are wholly and solely examples of matter and energy in action. As I have argued in the previous chapter, this would be folly in the extreme. To claim that information is just unqualified matter and energy is to betray a profound misapprehension of the nature of the universe, i.e. a profound ontological error. It is not possible to give an account of matters of information within the laws of the time-space continuum. Shannon didn't: he described the mechanics of moving information from A to B, and very specifically excluded meaning.

3.4 A Framework for the Mind as Information

For the purpose of discussion, let's assume that there is a place for a modern dualism, a 'third path' (not a 'third rail') between spiritualist magic and monist sterility. What would be the intellectual framework of such a theory? Stripped of its accretions, what would be its ontological status? My approach is that we can assemble a theory of mind as an informational space generated by the physical brain, one which stays entirely within the realm of the natural universe and therefore represents a real, natural entity not captured by the laws of matter and energy.

The case is simply that the formula for information ($H = -\Sigma p_i \log_2 p_i$) addresses an aspect of the natural universe which the other formulae ($F=ma$, $E=mc^2$) do not address. For example, it would be ridiculous to say that pure information could be accelerated by the application of a physical force. While the vehicles or substrates of information can be accelerated (stage coach vs. carrier pigeon vs. email), to claim that information is subject to the same laws as falling musket balls is to fall into a category error. This is because the category (or set) of natural events and entities is larger than the category (or set) of physical (matter-energy) events and entities. The physical universe (the time-space continuum) is a subset of the natural universe because the natural universe is composed of the set of the whole physical universe plus the set of the informational states deriving from ordered elements of the physical universe. In order to limit the universal set, I propose that there cannot be an informational state with no physical basis, i.e. spiritualism is not just impossible in practice, it is logically impossible (if spiritualism were possible, it would render the concept of the universal set absurd).

Because information exists only insofar as it has a physical basis, then it can travel back and forth between its own natural realm and the physical realm, controlling the physical realm as it goes one way, or modifying its own state as it returns. By formulating the mind as an informational space generated by the physical state of the brain, we arrive at a dualist system of mind and body, but one in which there is no mind-body problem because, by definition, information travels freely back and forth between mind and body *without transformation.* This way, we can satisfy the objections of, say, Ivan Pavlov, who wanted a science of mind free of religious distortions, without getting bogged in the posturings of latter-day ideologues who have not done the hard work of making room for information in their narrow ontologies. This is the first plank in the intellectual framework of a modern dualism.

The second plank is to try to define information without slipping into question-begging or circularity. There are dozens of definitions, probably none of them ideal, but I prefer this:

> Information is any coded or symbolic representation or assessment of some aspect of the natural universe, made by an entity with an emergent capacity to represent the physical universe in a symbolic calculus, that can be transmitted from a source to a receiver independently of the nature of the transmitting medium.

Note that this is closely aligned with Shannon's definition, given above. It immediately excludes from consideration every physicalist's favorite counter-example, DNA. An important and oft-overlooked point is that the word 'information' is simply a reification of the process of informing. Strictly speaking, there is no such *thing* as 'information,' any more than there are such *things* as, say, 'locomotion' or 'goodness.' To inform is to form a new mental state in another person, to form in him a new idea, or to reshape her mind. 'Information' is the set of instructions that passes from sender to receiver, from speaker to listener, writer to reader and so on, meaning it is the set of coded instructions which function to give the receiver a new (informational) state, thereby changing her mind. In this sense, cells and parts of cells do not inform, and therefore do not pass information. Moreover, the DNA of a cell will not function independently of the cell's subsystems: in the absence of perfectly-formed mRNA, there is no proteogenesis. I think this definition of information opens the door to most of what we want the concept to do without also letting too many hobgoblins through as well.

Now that we have a field of play for information, and can define what will or will not be allowed into that field, what next? Will it be like defining a new sport? "We hereby define a field 100m long and 50m wide for our Sport. Only humans will be allowed on that field, and any able-bodied person who does so and submits to these rules will be deemed a player." Thus, we exclude from the game excited dogs, angry bulls or humans hurling abuse from the side-lines. However, we now have to define an order or structure for our players, and give them something to do, as distinct from letting them mill around aimlessly and form gangs (that we call politics). This analogy indicates the point at which our new theory of mind takes its leave from the physical realm. The whole intent of Newton's equation is that it applies to one entity subjected to one force, whether that entity be a dust mote or a planet. Similarly, the Einstein equation reduces all the matter in a single thing of whatever size to its equivalent in energy. The point of a theory of mind, though, is that it is a metaphorical arena for the interaction of different informational entities. In a mind, an item of information representing a sound must interact with an item of information representing a memory to produce an item of information representing an instruction to the leg muscles. Unlike the physical realm, a mind cannot be reduced to a single entity. The notion of a mind holding just one item of information is absurd.

A theory of mind is not like a theory of alchemy, where the student poured different chemicals into a bottle, shook them and hoped gold would emerge. We cannot have a theory of mind where we insert items of information, shake them around and hope a rational answer emerges. The essence of any code or system of symbols is order: Shannon's radical concept of negative entropy again. Information is order, randomness is noise. A head full of disordered information is a head full of noise, i.e. it is mindless. So, to go back to the new Sport, the players have to go on to the field in a certain order, take up certain positions and obey certain rules as to what they may do to the ball or to each other. Just as the concept of sport implies a rigid structure and procedure, so the concept of mind implies a rigid mental structure. So far, so unexciting. The question now becomes: what is the nature of the structure that constitutes the mechanism of mind, as distinct from the contents of mind? It must not be forgotten that the structure of mind will itself be an informational state. It is like Turing's universal computing machine, where informational inputs (instruction set, program) told the machine what to do with its information. Just as we need a physical machine to manipulate matter and energy, so we need an informational "machine" to manipulate information. It is essential to keep the clearest distinction between the brain, meaning the physical substrate of mind, and the informational state known as mind. Given the above definition of information, they are utterly distinct. The mind itself will further subdivide into the mental mechanisms and the mental contents.

So we move to considering the structure of mind: we can start with our daily experience of being a mind. Our informational states readily distill into visual information, somatic information, memory, and so on. The easiest way of doing this is to stay with Chalmers' split between the conscious or experiential mind and the informational or psychological mind. Since I am using information as the basis of the whole mind, and the word psychology has too many implications, I prefer to split mental functions into experiential and cognitive. Experiential means any mental event that can only be understood through experiencing it, essentially the sensations and emotions. At this stage, they cannot be explained but can only be defined ostensively. Cognitive means any informational state that can be communicated, or any of the processes that underlie those states. It means the state of knowledge, or what we know or could know if we tried to remember or work it out, as well as the mechanisms by which we manipulate that state of knowledge. So, outside my window I can see a red car. I cannot communicate to you any sense of red without you having prior experience of it, for example: "You know what red is, it's the color of tomatoes and chilies." I can tell you why it's a car and not a tomato, and that it is 15m away. These are cognitive elements. The processes or mechanisms by which I recognize red, or round, or a tape measure, I do not know. Those processes are also cognitive matters, but they take place outside the realm of communicable mental events, so I will deem them part of the structure of mind, not the content of my mind. In order to see this difference more clearly, we can return to the idea of a physical machine outlined in the previous chapter.

In Chapter 2, I said that the essence of a physical machine is that it takes a material input and manipulates it according to the laws of the time-space continuum, including the laws of thermodynamics, to produce a particular outcome or product. At every point between input and output, the matter-energy relationships of the machine to the raw material are defined with utmost precision: "These relationships are not just approximately true or roughly correct, they are true to the nth degree. There is no room for error... If there is any imbalance of any sort in the equations, it will accumulate until, slowly or suddenly, the imbalances will overcome the structural integrity of the machine and it will either grind wearily to a halt or explode in a ball of flame. That is the nature of physical machines. Given their matter-energy relationships, it could not be otherwise." The essence of a physical machine is that it transforms the material input according to the laws of physics (including chemistry and biology) to produce something new.

By a tight analogy, the essence of a virtual informational machine is that it transforms the informational input according to the laws of logic, meaning it performs logical operations upon them. The parallel between physical and virtual machines is not just coincidence: by using the systems of relays defined by Shannon, now known as logic gates, there is a complete point-to-point mapping of the logical structure upon the physical structure. The structure of a physical machine is a series of ordered processes, all obeying the laws of the physical realm, to convert a series of physical inputs into a specific physical product. As a precise parallel, the structure of a virtual or mental machine is a series of ordered processes, all obeying the laws of the informational realm, to convert a series of informational inputs into a specific informational product. Just as the lid of a can of beans cannot go on before the beans are inside, so the sequence of steps by which a visual perception generates a knowledge state must follow a strict order.

The term used to describe a strictly ordered sequence of logical operations is 'algorithm.' Because the mind is a set of precisely-defined logical operations able to manipulate an input and integrate it with a range of other items of information, it should be seen as an algorithm. Empirically, the mind is almost certainly a collection of more or less loosely-related subroutines, each of which constitutes an algorithm in its own right and could be duplicated in a suitably large set of relays, or logic gates. The algorithm is silent until it has something to operate upon, just as a physical machine is silent until it is switched on and given some raw material to hammer or mix. The mechanisms of mind, or the cognitive processes by which we transform our informational input to produce experience and behavior, are forever outside awareness because they are not an input. I can recognize your face instantly, but I can never know how I do so. All I know is the outcome of that process of recognition.

Immediately, we see a basis for such concepts as human nature, personality and personality disorder, and Chomsky's universal grammar. Innate propensities or dispositions to act in certain ways constitute the elements of the algorithm. It goes without saying that some of these propensities or subroutines could be genetically-determined (cf. speech, or Seligman's notion of 'preparedness') while others are acquired (post-traumatic states). If I consistently react to, say, a particular sight or a class of comments in a standard way, then that habitual reaction just is my algorithm in action. The elements of an algorithm are defined in terms of their specific operations, although there are many levels of description. It must be understood that these proclivities are wholly informational, that is, they are not physical or biological in any sense of the terms. They have a basis in the brain's microstructure, but they operate exclusively at the level of coded information, working upon an informational input and utilizing only the laws of logic to achieve their output.

3.5 The Mind as a Series of Algorithms

We can define an algorithm as follows:
- A set of rules in symbolic form that operate upon an informational state in an ordered sequence to transform it.

David Berlinski was more specific:
- "An algorithm is... a finite procedure,
- written in a fixed symbolic vocabulary,
- governed by precise instructions,
- moving in discrete steps, 1, 2, 3...
- whose execution requires no insight, cleverness, intuition, intelligence or perspicuity,
- and that sooner or later comes to an end" [5].

The input is information and the rules (Berlinski's 'precise instructions') are themselves informational: we are talking about a wholly insubstantial realm that can act upon the physical world but which cannot be detected by any means other than its effects. Essentially, it does not exist in a material form, because it can be instantiated using many different substrates (electricity, marbles, neurons, feathers and dough...). That is, unlike a physical machine, an algorithm's ability to achieve its output is totally independent of its physical realization. The algorithm exists as rules only, and thus can be instantiated on many platforms. The rules must exist before the input arrives; they can be changed, but only as determined by other, predefined rules because, at this level, there is no random element and, as Berlinski emphasized, no wit. An algorithm is not even dimwitted: it is a witless application of rules. In the final analysis, each element of every subroutine in mental life must be related to a system of rules, and these must be instantiated in the brain's functional cytoarchitecture.

In one of his earliest papers [3], Turing considered the question of an algorithm that never stopped: how would we know if it contained an error? That may be of interest to mathematicians, but not to biologists: the role of algorithms in the human economy is to ensure survival, so an algorithm that does not produce a very rapid answer will not survive (obsessional doubt is a mental disorder in its own right). In mathematics and engineering, Berlinski required an algorithm to be finite and come to an end so that we may know by its outcome whether the procedure is correct or not. Biology is not so forgiving: the blood on the ground tells us when an algorithm was unsuccessful. Human (or any primate) algorithms err on the side of caution: better to be wrong and alive than right and dead.

Algorithms can be described at a number of levels:

1. *High level description* consists of an ordinary language or prose account of the goals, functions and outputs of the system as a whole.

2. *Description at the level of implementation* is a truncated prose description of the actual sequence of operations linking input to output. The purpose of this level is to clarify the actual steps involved in acquitting the function by showing that, because we already have a detailed description of the subroutines in each step, there are no omissions in the explanatory chain from input to output.

3. *Description at the level of formal operations* is a detailed account in code of the machine operations for each step of the process from input to output.

4. *Machine code:* This is the actual code used by the machine as it acquits the input instructions.

There has to be a precise, one-to-one mapping of each step of one level to the level below, so that we can trace without omission every operation involved in implementing the high level description. As we proceed from the high levels down the sequence, there is an exponential increase in the data involved in acquitting each step.

Examples:

1. *High level description.* e.g. "You can ask the computer to let you know when that book is available." "He was thirsty, so he went to the tap to get a drink."

2. *Description at level of implementation.* e.g. "Type in the accession number of the book you want, then press return. The computer will check to see if that book is on the list of current loans. If it is, it will then check to see when it is due back and it will ask you if you want to reserve it. If you do, it will ask you to key in Y to issue a notification to the returns site. When the book is returned, the scanner will check to see if there is a request notification and it will automatically email you." "High physical activity in hot, dry weather produced a quick rise in plasma osmolality due to hemoconcentration because of heavy sweating. Osmoreceptors in the suprachiasmatic region detected the change and interacted with a particular input from the buccal cavity caused by activation of surface receptors by high sodium levels in saliva. The organism has learned that only fluid can relieve this sensation, where learning is modification of behavior due to prior experience."

3. *Description at level of formal operations* translates, as it were, the operator's implementation instructions to a level where they can access the switching mechanism which constitutes the physical parallel of the logical operations that constitute the algorithm. We do not have any knowledge of this level in the brain.

4. *Machine code:* This is the actual code used by the machine as it acquits the input instructions. All modern computers use a binary code but we have no idea how the brain's functions are acquitted. We know that input sensory information is in the form of neuronal impulses, so it probably has a binary basis. Higher order functions also use the same physical system but are otherwise a complete mystery. Because we understand the biology of nerve impulses, we usually talk of their function in physical terms which tends to suggest that higher mental functions are biological in nature but this is incorrect. Physical neuronal activity serves the purpose of transmitting and manipulating coded information, such that inspecting the nerve impulses will not reveal anything about the information they carry.

The model of human mental function developed by the Soviet neuro-psychologist, Aleksandr Luria [6] some seventy years ago is exactly in accord with this approach. Using carefully detailed studies of brain-damaged soldiers from World War II, Luria showed that each human mental faculty could be decomposed into its constituent parts, and that these functions were highly localized within the brain substance. Actions do not arise complete, as it were, but are assembled sequentially in a step-wise manner, starting with an intention and ending with the coherent, integrated behavior. Physical damage at any point in the sequence has a predictable effect on the particular behavior, just as damage at a particular point on a car assembly line will produce identical defects in each vehicle that emerges from the factory. Because techniques of non-invasive investigation of the brain were still rudimentary, Luria's main concern was motor and sensory function, but the same concepts apply to emotional behavior and cognition. An incoming sensory message is broken down and analyzed, then instructions are sent to different brain centers. Subsequently, an intention to act is formulated, and suitable behavioral programs are activated to achieve the specific goal.

The idea of a production line is not inappropriate, except this one is insubstantial, not physical. It consists of a set of tightly-defined rules in an informational space generated by the brain's switching capacities. The rules are thus information themselves, and they act upon an informational input to transform it, just as a physical machine acts upon a physical input to transform it (each machine stays within its own realm to do its job). What shifts this from the realm of wishful or magical thinking to reality is this: the rules are physically-embodied. Each rule consists of a preset array of switches in a very large and complex switching device (better known as the brain). The input data, coded in the form of neuronal impulses, enters the switching device and proceeds through it to emerge in a new form, having been manipulated by the switches according to their predetermined pattern. By changing the sequence of the data flow, the switching device changes the form of the outflow, giving it a new significance, or meaning, as we prefer to say. However, the switching device can itself be reset or modified by other information, and each new state produces a different but entirely predictable change in the data flow passing through it.

The fact of the physical setting of the switches being significant in determining the outcome leads people to presume that the nature of the process itself is physical but this is not so. The switches are switching *something*, and that something is ephemeral information. The physical switches are only the means for achieving a task, not the task itself. I carry a ladder to the side of my house and climb it to the roof. The ladder is the means to achieving the task, it is not the task itself. A pigeon carries a message tied to its leg. The pigeon is physical, the piece of paper is physical but the message is not. I could send the message via telegraphy, we cannot transmit a pigeon by telegraphy. Never confuse the medium with the message. The medium is most emphatically *not* the message.

Thus, if we were to talk about 'rules' without having some notion of how these are embodied in a physical system, we would be guilty of magical thinking. Conversely, if we talk of the rules as being of a physical nature themselves just because they are implemented in a switching device, then we would be guilty of physicalism, the opposite sin of spiritualism. We have to find a "third path" between magic on the one hand, and matter-energy on the other, as Wiener insisted: "Information is information, not matter or energy." It means expanding the definition of materialism to include matter and energy, *and* the informational states that control them. Recall that the impulses in any switching device (neuronal or otherwise) have two distinct functions: as non-physical symbols and as physical causes. Within the switching device, impulses represent or symbolize, for example, truth and falsity although, at the neuronal level, these concepts are meaningless. However, when they leave that particular structure and pass from neurons-as-switches to neurons-as-conduits, the impulses lose their symbolic function and assume a trigger function, i.e. they can activate distant organs. Berlinski summarized this in more lyrical terms: "What gives to the program its air of cool command is the fact that its symbols function in a double sense. They are *symbols* by virtue of their meaning, and so reflect the intentions of the human mind that has created them; but they are *causes* by virtue of their structure, and so enter into the rhythms of the real world" [7].

The significance of the neuronal impulse having dual roles is that it confers on the brain the ability to acquit two functions, one symbolic and the other an ordinary physiological role activating the effector organs. This inevitable and immutable duality of function lies at the very core of the brain's computational capacity, thereby affording and committing us to a dualist explanation of complex human behavior (which is equally true, I firmly believe, of many other animals). So long as the neuron carries this duality of function, it constitutes the point of interaction, the point of contact between the one realm and the other. The form of the neuron is such that it permits the informational realm to influence the physiological body, and vice versa. The twin roles of the neuronal impulse, as symbol *and* cause, provide continuity between the informational and the physiological aspects of the healthy human, solving the mind-body problem in its classical formulation and thereby negating the drive to devise a monist account of mind. Without this capacity to formulate symbolic representations of the external world, manipulate those symbols and then to communicate the decisions back to the physical realm, we would function at the level of sea slugs, with no computational capacity, thence no complex behavior, and no mental life.

Some people may complain that this sounds very robotic and, in one sense, it is. The purpose is to show that, regardless of its nature, each human action can be broken down into a lengthy series of intervening steps, each of which can then be explained in naturalistic terms. This way, we do not beg the questions we are trying to answer. For everyday human actions, meaning actions of the same order as those shown by other animals, this mechanistic process is almost certainly true, but a theory of human mind has a more important question to answer: will it also account for executive functions and creativity? At this stage, the answer is that it can do so in principle but the details will be devilishly complex, not the least because it is perfectly feasible that we may never know the ultimate codes the brain utilizes.

We can look again at Berlinski's definition of an algorithm, which is essentially the basis of a Turing machine: "An algorithm is... a finite procedure, written in a fixed symbolic vocabulary, governed by precise instructions, moving in discrete steps, 1, 2, 3... whose execution requires no insight, cleverness, intuition intelligence or perspicuity, and that sooner or later comes to an end."

His term "finite procedure" means only that the set of rules has a beginning, a middle and an end. In biological terms, an infinite procedure is incomprehensible. The "fixed symbolic vocabulary" is a problem because it doesn't exist in nature. In biology, the instruction set is recursive, meaning a vocabulary emerges from a switching device but is then used to program it. I think this is a very complex issue as we are born without anything approximating a vocabulary, but we can make meaningful decisions very early in life, such as crying for food. In the new-born, that is almost certainly just biological but, somehow, by a 'bootstrap' process, the crude, all-or-none behavior of neonates is transformed into the creativity of a Mahler or the homicidal paranoia of a Saddam Hussein. Part of that process is the further development of the networks of neuronal switches which continue growing until adolescence (when many are culled) and part of it is due to acquiring language. People whose brains are damaged by childhood deficiency diseases or who are denied the opportunity to learn a language do not develop to their full (genetic) intellectual capacity.

We also run into another difficulty here because of what I have previously termed the "innate cognitive system." This is the cognitive capacity we share with other primates, e.g. the capacity to recognize a particular behavioral display as a threat, fear of heights or the instinctive negative reactions of little girls to frogs. We would say that this is genetically-determined but the "vocabulary" is, as it were, hard-wired into the brain because of its high survival value, i.e. something we might call human nature. These behaviors are fixed at birth and, while they can slowly change as a result of experience, they cannot be reprogrammed just by learning a few new words. Because of the genetic influence, we would expect to find considerable variation in the strength of these reactions.

Berlinski's next three points are closely interrelated. The procedure is not *governed* by precise instructions, it *is* precise instructions. Any algorithm that does not consist of a set of precise instructions coded into the switching device is either a sloppy algorithm (i.e. it will give an inconsistent output) or not an algorithm at all, in that it is little better than random or stereotypy. Similarly, just as an assembly line in a car factory has to proceed through discrete steps in a very precise order (don't put fuel in before the fuel tank is fitted), so a logical switching device has to proceed in a fixed order of discrete steps just because the algorithm has no brains of its own and cannot recognize when something is wrong. If some data cannot be manipulated, it doesn't ask its neighbor for advice or give up and go out for a smoke, it just keeps on going, which was the basis of Turing's concern known as the Halting Problem (some people will object to this, as large-scale commercial programs can scan themselves for errors and correct them. However, that exception proves the rule as the scanner represents an auxiliary algorithm, external to the one that has failed).

Next, Berlinski specified that execution of the algorithm "...requires no insight, cleverness, intuition, intelligence, or perspicuity..." because the algorithm just is the instantiation of the processes that constitute these faculties. At base, cleverness is a particular algorithm in action. It is not wrong to speak of a person (or a machine) as "clever," in the sense that Skinner despised, because having that particular algorithm gives him a propensity to act in a clever manner when the occasion arises (i.e. when there is a suitable informational input). In a similar vein, it is not wrong to speak of, say, a bulldozer as a very powerful machine, even when it is switched off, because, when the time is right, it has a suitable mechanism that allows it to act in whatever manner it is that we deem "powerful." Finally, the algorithm must come to an end, which is what finite means.

At this point, we have to guard against the tendency to assign to some unproven state of affairs the "really difficult" part of a theory of mind. It is not good enough to say of something like current sensation or emotions, "Oh, don't worry, that will all be explained by a dedicated algorithm." There is, however, another body of evidence we can bring to bear on this question, namely, mental disorder. In Chapter 1, I suggested: "...a convincing account of mental disorder should proceed from a rational theory of mental order, more commonly known as a theory of mind. Conversely, a valid theory of mind should be able to predict the points at which it will begin to malfunction." Being able to predict malfunction is extremely important: if we have some complex mechanism but we have no idea how and why it breaks down, then we don't understand it at all. Unfortunately, the complexity of the human brain is such that we do not know why its function breaks down. However, if the phenomena of mental disorder are consistent with the notion of the mind as an algorithm, then we may just be making some progress (even though consistency is weak support).

3.6 "I'm Going Out of My Algorithm."

"...a valid theory of mind should be able to predict the points at which it will begin to malfunction." What do we know about malfunctioning algorithms? The first thing we know is that, even in the absence of any physical disturbance of the data-processing system that supports it, it is perfectly valid to say that an algorithm can malfunction and deliver a disordered output. The simplest case is when the informational input is wrong. The second case is when the parameters of the algorithm itself are disordered, meaning an incorrect answer emerges. The third is when some part of the output serves to disturb the normal function of the algorithm. We can easily find examples of these types of disorders in mental disorders, but this is the essence of the biocognitive model of mental disorder, so we will consider it in detail later in this book.

3.7 Conclusion

Anybody offering dualism as a valid theory of mind has the difficult task of showing precisely how a thought or perception can lead to bodily changes. As a generalization, the explanatory principle is this: as irreducible mental elements, thoughts and perceptions are the contents of an informational space generated by the brain. At the same time, the brain and body are conduits of information where all bodily actions are caused by information. Therefore, information can readily travel from body to mind and back again with no breach of the laws of thermodynamics. To reprise Berlinski's view: "...symbols function in a double sense. They are *symbols* by virtue of their meaning, and so reflect the intentions of the human mind that has created them; but they are *causes* by virtue of their structure, and so enter into the rhythms of the real world." The same *signal* (meaning fusillade of nerve impulses) can be a *symbol* in one part of the brain and a *cause* in another. I will give a more detailed account of this in the chapter on the Challenge Hypothesis.

Strictly speaking, Shannon's epic work was a theory of signaling, which is not surprising in an electrical engineer who had telephony as his exemplar. In mind-body terms, the signal changes its significance as it moves through the brain substance and out into the periphery to the effector organs. The physiological basis of nerve impulses does not change at any point; only its functional role changes and, theoretically speaking, that is a simple matter of switching. Critically, we cannot explain symbols or causes in terms of each other. Like Orwell's sausage and a rose, they occupy different realms of discourse such that their explanations do *not* intersect. To speak of one in terms of the other is a major category error. Or, in Wiener's words: "Information is information, not matter or energy. No materialism which does not admit this can survive at the present day."

4

Brains
That Think

"The future has a way of arriving unannounced."
—George F. Will

4.1. Introduction

Now that we have established some basic principles to cover the case of "machines that think," we can move to the cluster of questions surrounding the idea of whether humans think. Do humans think? The cautious answer is that some do, some of the time, so what is the nature of thought and other mental events? Given the context of the human brain, how do these things come to pass? And if people are acting without thinking, how can they manage this quite remarkable achievement? What are automatism, dissociation and personality disorder? These are not trivial questions, to be "explained away" or dismissed as primitive ramblings in the face of a universe we don't understand. If we wish to explain mental disorder, we need to answer them.

4.2. Accounting for Thought in a Dualist System: Preliminaries.

The first two chapters were a long but essential diversion on the path to resolving the problem of the dualist mind. We now need to revisit some of the material in my earlier publications, especially as it relates to the notion of a natural dualist model of mind, as proposed by David Chalmers. Chalmers sees no place for a monist model of mind and has therefore mounted a case for dualism, but he deliberately excludes the magical or substance dualism of Renee Descartes. For Chalmers, the dualist mind arises from or supervenes upon the brain by psychophysical laws which, in the fullness of time, we can expect to know in detail. In his view, there is nothing magical or supernatural about the process of supervenience, and it is not incoherent to speak of a mental realm which is of but not part of the physical universe. This, he claims, "gives us a coherent, naturalistic, unmysterious view of consciousness and its place in the natural order" [1, p165].

Consciousness divides readily in two aspects, the realm of phenomenal experience and the psychological or cognitive realm. The experiential mind is the inner, subjective world, the compelling but ineffable sense of 'what it feels like to be something.' He restricts the term 'psychological consciousness' to the knowing, informational and reportable sense of selfhood which I can convey to you, but he prefers not to label it 'computational consciousness' as this presumes we know its nature. In effect, this is a bicameral model, where *camera* means 'box.' Both 'boxes' arise from the brain's switching capacities but they are functionally separate. The experiential mind is knowable but not causally effective whereas the cognitive or knowing mind is causally effective but not knowable (i.e. its workings are not open to introspection). However, by talking of 'boxes,' I do not want anybody to assume that the mind occupies physical space. That is completely wrong. The totality of mental life is insubstantial, unlocalized, formless, weightless and cannot be detected by waves or other emanations for the very simple reason that there aren't any. The mind is not a physical entity in any sense of the word as it does not occupy the material universe of matter and energy. It is an informational space, and the only way we can detect it is via its connections to the effector organs of the body. It is not contradictory to say that an "insubstantial, unlocalized, formless" entity can act upon the real world: the question is not whether it can do so, but how it manages this remarkable feat.

In the following sections, I want to use the concepts developed in the opening chapters to show that the mind is an informational space generated by the brain by processes that we accept as reality in other settings (i.e. I am not proposing anything new or magic), and how it connects with the body on the afferent and efferent sides. There are thus two parts to my case.

4.3 How to Generate a Biological Informational Space,
Part I: The Wetware

The brain constitutes the nexus of perceptual and effector neuronal tracts. It consists of a large number of hugely complex, intensely interconnected nuclei and a bewildering variety of afferent and efferent tracts. It has been said that the human brain is the most complex thing in the known universe, and it is in fact so complex that we will never understand it. I'm sure the first of these superlatives is correct, just because there is a lot of universe we have still to explore but I disagree with the second. There is no reason to believe that the whole of the biological CNS (or the rest of the body) operates by anything other than the various laws of the material universe as we are coming to understand them. The brain itself is "just another organ to be dismantled" and, as our technology improves, so does our understanding of the 1300gm organ called the brain. However, it also operates in the informational realm, whose laws will certainly be difficult and perhaps we may only understand them in principle.

Because of the success of the reductionist program in the biosciences, we know what neurons are, how they function, how they are connected, even down to the level of being able to detect specific chemicals being manufactured in the soma and transported to the peripheries. We know with great precision the concentrations of the ions in the brain, how they are shunted in and out of the cell by their various membrane pumps to maintain the concentration gradients on which neuronal function depends, on and on. With something like seventy-five known transmitters, we know a great deal about chemical neurotransmission at all levels of the CNS, although it is clear there are more transmitter substances still to be discovered. We know that all neurons, afferent and efferent, spinal and cerebral, function according to the same principles first worked out for squid giant axons and later for mammals. While the brain is ineffably complex, there are no mysteries in the organ itself. Nobody can point to a part of the brain and say: "Aha, that part is so very different from the rest of biology that the mind must reside there."

Let's look at just one of the many processing systems in the CNS, vision (this is possibly not the best example but it is well-known). The peripheral receptor, the retina, has a dense layer of sensitive nerve endings responding selectively to energy in the form of light at a particular wave-length. When light falls on the retina, it stimulates action potentials in the optic nerves, which carry the data from the retina back to the brain stem. Processing of the input actually begins at the level of the retina, so that the information transmitted back to the brain is highly derivative. In the CNS, the information enters a cascading system of nuclei, undergoing further refinement at each point along its way. Finally, it enters the cortex proper but we cannot track its progress after that. In due course, a set of instructions is dispatched from brain to effectors (larynx, hands, feet etc) which allows the observable behavioral response to be initiated.

In its macro- and microarchitecture, the CNS is very similar in form to that outlined for calculating machines in Chapter 1. In both cases, brain and calculator, an afferent conduit brings data in the form of impulses to a processing area where it is manipulated before being dispatched via exit pathways to the peripherals. The physical form of both afferent and efferent conduits is essentially identical; they could be swapped one for the other, or replaced by some other type of conduit, and it would not alter the ability of the calculating part to do its job. They are mindless and totally passive tubes, blindly receiving impulses at one end, then squirting them along the tube and out the other end. Lying between the conduits are switching mechanisms, metallic or silicon-based in the case of man-made calculators or neurons in the case of living creatures. These are no different in form or function than the conduits themselves, and operate strictly according to the same principles. An impulse in the incoming conduit directly triggers an impulse in the first stage of the computational circuits just because they are of the same form, if not identical. There is no gap, conceptual or physical, between the two systems. However, the switching mechanisms are arranged in ways that distinguish them from their conductive brethren; the function of the intervening switches and relays, or neurons, is to manipulate the incoming data according to predetermined procedures, or algorithms.

It is absolutely critical to this model of the brain that at no point along the way does the nature of the informational flow change. At entry and at exit and at all points between, it is in the form of highly complex volleys of neuronal impulses spreading throughout specific parts of the brain. These impulses do not change in form at any point in their progress. They are generated strictly according to the same principles as all other nerve impulses anywhere in the body, and anywhere in nature. Impulses do not leave the body and there is no gap in their transmission where we could be excused for believing that the information has left the CNS, perhaps to travel to some spiritual "Self." Nonetheless, something is done to those impulses as they travel along their respective paths. There is no doubt that, say, the eye and foot are joined in some way, but their conjunction is not of the same nature as simple reflex arcs such as the knee jerk or the corneal reflex. We could not, for example, join the optic nerve to the sciatic nerve in the expectation that a driver will be able to drive faster if he bypasses all those tangled neurons in his brain. That would delete something vital that happens between the eye perceiving a red light and the foot hitting the brake.

So, even though there is no change in the physical nature of the nerve impulses between eye and foot, there is a change in their significance or import. That is, afferent impulses are manipulated in precise ways within the brain substance before being sped on their way via the efferent tracts, but there is nothing random about the manner or process by which they are changed. A highly coherent process of manipulation hones the efferent discharge so that the body behaves in a precisely directed way to achieve its targets. The processing of this information takes place in dedicated brain centers, whose microanatomy is rapidly becoming clearer as enormously complicated switching systems. While progress is rapid these days, the task will keep neuroanatomists in jobs for decades to come.

The mode of processing of the information traveling through a human brain is conceptually not different from that in a frog's brain. In turn, frogs' brains are operating by much the same principles as Shannon's switching and relay circuits. In both brains, neurons are switched on or off, just as the circuits in Shannon's system were switched on or off, in order to vary the outcome. The whole point of seeing the brain as a switching device is that it takes a relatively simple input and selectively produces a graded or nuanced output so that the organism's behavior matches the environmental demands as closely as possible. Regardless of its form, an entity that cannot adapt its behavior to meet fluctuating environmental contingencies will not survive. That is what switching devices do, be they mechanical, electronic or biological.

In principle, there isn't much more to be said about brains as switching devices. We can talk about the finer points of competitive reuptake of neurotransmitters, of how neurons are blocked or facilitated by different chemicals acting on the genome, how synaptic outgrowth is stimulated or retarded and so on, but it would be quicker (and more enlightening) to read a proper text on neurophysiology. Several points should be emphasized as the term "switching device" can be misleading. Firstly, people tend to think of the individual neuron (of which we have something of the order of 100,000,000,000) as a single switch, but this is not the case. Each neuron receives about 2,000 inputs from other cells, each of which acts on the receiving neuron to produce either excitation or inhibition. These appear to summate according to a Boolean process. That gives us something like two hundred trillion connections per human brain. The individual neurons are not to be confused with the individual switches in Shannon's model. Each neuron is a microprocessor in its own right: we have something like a hundred billion microprocessors in our heads, each of which could have up to hundreds of functional logic gates. Since each neuron can fire up to a thousand times per second, we are dealing with an organ with very prodigious computing power.

Second, the brain shows a distributed modular structure, so that each behavioral outcome is assembled according to a specific functional architecture superimposed upon the cytoarchitecture. While functions are localized to recognizable nuclei (e.g. input from the ears does not impact on the visual circuits), there is no single point at which a neurological or psychological function "resides." We cannot point to The Speech Center, or The Sadness Center, any more than we could point to The Sports Center, The Center for Personality or The Center for Patriotism. Human behavior is ineffably complex and infinitely variable, with each identifiable unit of behavior being the outcome of myriad factors computed in real time. There is thus no such thing as a category of human behavior, as all conceivable behavior is distributed dimensionally. While everything we know about neurons says they function as digital processors rather than analogue (which hormones do), the final outcome is so nuanced as to constitute a dimension rather than a category. I can move my finger to any of an infinite number of points within its range. My voice can vary infinitely while a complex function such as attending to a task can only be conceptualized as a dimension of behavior. Modern psychiatry, which insists that there are categories of behavior (all the while fudging the issue in practice) is thus taking a direction diametrically opposed to the reality of human behavior (and to this theory, for what it is worth).

Finally, there is so much going on in our heads at any one instant that we could not possibly attend to it all. Survival depends on as much of our inner processes being automated as can possibly be managed. This leaves the rest of the brain to deal with the really important stuff. This applies to relatively simple behaviors, such as walking and running (which certainly aren't simple in practice, just ask the people trying to design robots that move over rocky ground), as well as the more typically "higher cerebral functions" such as speech. While I am talking, I do not have to plan what I say, I have an idea of what I want to convey but the actual words come out before I have time to think of them. Even more amazingly, they are almost always in the form of grammatically correct sentences. The tone of my voice varies appropriately and even my breathing is timed so that I run out of breath at the end of a sentence, not in the middle (people with certain forms of brain damage can lose this ability, with quite devastating effects on their capacity to communicate, even though they can read and write).

All of this is done for me; I don't have to worry about how to stand upright, my motor system does all that for me; I can catch a ball on the run; I can sing without knowing how I hit a particular note; I can write poetry without knowing how I get the rhythm and rhymes; I can recognize your face in a crowd and discern what you are saying in the midst of a hubbub; I can tell if I have seen a face before; I can tell when something sounds fishy, without knowing why, then find the error even though it might amaze me; I don't choose to be amused or angry or sad, these moods sweep over me and I am the passive victim of my own mental states. Sometimes I like them and don't even consider why they have arisen, sometimes I don't, and wish they would go away but they won't. A very large part of human behavior is essentially automatic; we can override it but it's better not to. Most of the time, we are only going along for the ride. This is essential to understanding how mental disorder arises but, first, we need to look at what the brain is doing when it processes data.

4.4 How to Generate a Biological Informational Space, Part II: The Thoughtware

The essential feature of any switching device is that it switches on and off. It isn't the case that every switch in its circuits is closed all the time, or open all the time, because then it isn't a switching device, just a conduit or a blockade. So what determines the state of the switches in such a device? In Shannon's original paper, the circuits were built in a particular form just because they mimicked the algebra of the equations he wanted to duplicate. He could have had others, but those were the ones he needed, so he arranged his switches and relays to produce just that result and no other. They were the first mechanical logic gates; the only way to reprogram them, i.e. to function in a different way, was to take them apart with a screwdriver. They were expensive to build and run and were prone to breakdown. It was soon recognized that electrical logic gates would be a vast improvement, not least because they could be changed from one state to another simply by turning their elements on or off.

Here, Turing's work was critical: he had showed that if the instructions were coded into the input tape, then a single computing machine could mimic any single discrete state machine via its universal capacity. There were thus two completely different aspects to the informational state of a circuit. In the first place, there was the incoming data, which represented something of the world. Second, there was the information state written into the circuits themselves, telling them what they should do to the incoming data. He called this the instruction set but we now know it as the program. The program consists of the set of instructions for the machine to follow when it has incoming data to work on. Each step has to be specified in minute detail as the machine has no knowledge itself (or of itself).

Does the brain have a similar informational state? We know as an empirical fact that there is a constant, massive and highly-detailed data input to the brain from a range of sensory organs. There are also "law-like organizing principles" or rules at work in manipulating that data and determining the behavioral output. While we cannot specify these rules, or where they are located in the brain, we know they exist just because human behavior is not random; whatever acts to organist it constitutes an instruction set of some sort, i.e. a behavioral program. For the present, we can't go any further than that as we don't know the codes involved but we also don't need to go any further. We can be fairly sure that long-term learning results in differences in the ease with which neurons transmit impulses, either facilitating or blocking them. With these principles, we can start to make some progress in assembling a non-question-begging, naturalistic theory of mind.

Returning to Chalmers' bicameral or dual aspect theory of mind, he assigned the sensory and emotional functions to the experiential mind, and the knowledge-based functions to the cognitive or psychological mind. As described, the greater part of the cognitive functions is beyond introspection. The processes by which we decide the activities that keep us alive are forever outside our ken. Incoming data are computed for us, very rapidly, on demand and in real time, to give a precisely targeted response to the world. The suggestion, widely bruited by post-modernists, that we do not have an accurate knowledge of the real world, cannot be taken seriously. Even a post-modernist can tell when his glass is empty or his oysters have gone off. Our survival is utterly dependent on a supremely accurate, up-to-the-moment assessment of what is happening "out there." Without it, we would die.

In the biocognitive model, the knowledge-based part of the mind, the part that recognizes and names sensory data then decides what to do and calculates an appropriate behavioral response, is nothing more than an informational realm generated by the brain's neuronal switching circuits. There is no difference in principle between the brain and the calculating devices described by Shannon, as above. Afferent neurons carry impulses reflecting the external environment; these passive conduits enter parts of the brain which function as high-speed switching devices of unimaginable complexity; while in these parts of the brain, the afferent digital impulse is no longer "just an impulse;" it becomes a token of, or is translated into, the bearer of a truth value in a dual-valued logic. Once it leaves the switching or computational section of the circuit, it loses its truth value because, as Shannon showed, truth value becomes void in the absence of a switching capacity. If there is no choice, then truth has no meaning, as every dictator knows.

While we know a great deal about the mechanisms of memory in primitive animals, and increasingly in the white rat, our knowledge of how rules of behavior, including speech, are stored and activated in the human brain, is little more than guesswork. Perhaps a rule is just a matter of preselected and preset switches, or it could be a set of impulses dispatched to the computational regions on demand, the exact nature is not critical. The essential principle is that the coded rules and the incoming sensory data interact as cascades of impulses in a complex, interconnected neural network. In this form, rules and data from different sources can interact without hindrance: information from a particular rule can control how a unit of peripheral information is manipulated. There is no change in the status of the sensory data, it does not leave the brain nor is it transferred to a special part of the brain other than the dedicated sensory cortex. As coded neuronal impulses, it can interact with pre-existing information such as memories, rules of behavior and, most importantly, rules of conduct that do not exist at a verbal level. For example, everybody has an accent; it never fails (but it sometimes lets us down). The process of generating vowel sounds is completely non-conscious, we have no idea how we do it (one year old children can copy a particular vowel sound immediately, implying some very powerful analysis and computation), but it is powerfully controlled by rule-like regularities.

It has to be understood that rules are activated and do their work entirely outside the range of introspection. We are appraised only of the outcome of a rule being activated, in that we "know" what to do or say, but we do not know how that decision was made. I do not know why I laugh over something, the humor simply bubbles up whether I want it or not. There is, therefore, a great deal of what Freud would have called "unconscious motivation" in that a very large range of rules is constantly being brought into play and then switched off, every second of our waking lives. How much of what really counts in human behavior is outside our comprehension? My guess is that as much as 99.9% of our behavior takes place without us giving it a moment's attention. Why, then, would we bother saying that we decide what to do when it is decided for us? The answer is that we own our rules, we recognize them as part of what constitutes the sense of self, an assemblage of rules, experiences, likes and dislikes with which we are familiar and comfortable. I do not see any metaphysical element in this type of construct. Also, bear in mind how often, after having done something he regrets, a person will claim "It wasn't really me." It was him, the only difference is that now he feels guilty.

While coursing through the brain's processing centers, the significance of each impulse lies not just in its ability to spark the next neuron into activity (as in a peripheral nerve), but in its ability to carry a truth value that can be manipulated and transformed: "Thus, a (neuronal) circuit assumes the function of a formal logical operator, or we could say that the logical operation hitches a ride on the physical (neuron), letting the (neuron) do its work for it *without breaching the laws of thermodynamics*" (from Chap. 1). Clearly, any diffuse physical disturbance of the neuronal switches will result in degradation or even the loss of the informational output of the particular circuit. Typical disturbances include infective products, drugs and alcohol, concussion and brain swelling, metabolic disturbances such as hypoxia or hypercapnia, hypoglycemia or liver failure, hyper- or hypothermia and sleep deprivation (whatever its mechanism).

In addition, there is a further cause of perturbations of the brain's capacity to function as a smoothly integrated switching device, and this is the brain function itself. Unlike Shannon's (and Intel's) switching devices, the brain functions only within remarkably narrow physiological limits. One of the limits is known as the level of arousal, a physiological function mediated by the reticular activating system of the brainstem. As every student knows, a drowsy brain does not perform very well but an over-aroused brain is also a handicap. If too many signals are entering the brain, it begins to malfunction in predictable ways. Unfortunately for humans, by acting recursively, the malfunctions themselves can become cause for further malfunction, leading to what in other contexts is called "chaos" in the informational system. This phenomenon has been charted as the Yerkes-Dodson curve, described in Chap. 13 of [2]. In a cognitive psychology, the Y-D curve is an essential part of any explanation of mental disorder but it must be understood that the agitated brain is functioning perfectly normally in every respect other than its over-arousal.

It is most likely that the phenomenon of self-reinforcing over-arousal arises because the brain is not a single organ but is a large number of separate, neuronal organs that just happen to be located in the head together. Some operate quickly, others are slower. At normal levels of arousal, they all work in concert because that is what evolution has "designed" them to do. At higher levels of arousal, their integration starts to break down as, say, throughput from one module or subroutine starts to overwhelm the next. Under conditions of excessive stimulation, their smooth symphony becomes discordant and the output we regard as "normal mental function" begins to disintegrate. This is all that the term "mental breakdown" implies.

In the model proposed by Aleksandr Luria [3], the knowing or computational mind is composed of a huge number of subunits, some of which operate fairly independently while others are closely-integrated minor players in a larger scheme. These are empirical questions that do not affect the general account of the nature of mind being developed here. For a relatively simple matter, such as reaching for a door knob, we don't have to explain anything, as practically all animals exhibit similar behavior. For a complex example such as language, there may be as many as hundreds of subroutines contributing to the final outcome. If these are not working in harmony, speech becomes garbled and disorganized

The other half of the bicameral mind, the experiential mind, remains a mystery. The question "Why can we experience anything at all?" actually consists of two questions. The first is: "What is the mechanism by which we experience anything at all?" while the second is: "What is the reason we experience anything?" (essentially, Socratic efficient and final causation). To answer the second question first, the glib response is: "We experience things because the primates from which we descended had the same faculty." It did not arise *de novo* just because *H. sapiens* burst on the scene. Our forebears had the faculty because it conferred survival value. If they didn't have the faculty of, say, smelling, they would have had another which served the same function of providing specific and valuable information about the external environment. Every sensory ability gives us a remarkably accurate representation of the outside world, so accurate that you might think our lives depend upon them. Which, of course, they do.

As for the second question, the mechanisms that generate sensory experience remain totally beyond us. We do not know how to decompose sensation as the first step to a reductive explanation (as we do with cognition). I am in two minds (as they say) over this issue. Part of me says: "The fact that reductionist explanations work for cognition does not mean they will work for sensation, so try something new," while another voice says: "Don't give up just when we hit the really difficult questions." At this stage, all I can suggest is that sensation arises as the result of some extremely sophisticated, recursive informational processing by dedicated centers in the brain such that it generates an illusion of "something happening" (Nagel's 'something it is like to be experiencing'). This does not set up an infinite regress as I am myself the illusion (but I am not the victim of an illusion).

While the brain definitely has prodigious computing power, I seriously doubt that the sensory experiences I am now having arise just because of massive, real-time number-crunching. Rather, it seems to me that we would have this capacity just because of some very parsimonious real-time computation; birds give every behavioral indication that they have similar sensory experiences, but they don't actually have many neurons in their little heads to compute with. Operating within exceedingly narrow ranges of matter-energy in time spans of milliseconds, the brain can compute a remarkably accurate facsimile of what is going on "out there." It has to, otherwise the organism wouldn't have time to respond to threats using the brain's remaining computational capacity. That, however, doesn't explain why we have any sensation rather than none. As I have shown previously, it isn't causally effective, so why does the phenomenon of sensation persist? I have suggested it has something to do with memory, that this form of sensation constitutes the entry point to memory but, from the psychiatric point of view, it doesn't change anything. It is the states of overwhelming distress that count, not so much their internal causation. In a natural dualist model, they arise by computational activity in the brain that generates a specific, recursive informational space.

The causally effective mind is a silent, high-speed computation incorporating incoming sensory data, general rules and behavioral programs already in memory, as well as other contingencies. In fractions of a second, I can recognize an event, determine a response and initiate the appropriate behavior, all without the benefit of internal speech. Throughout my life, I have acquired a myriad rules governing most aspects of my existence, from speech to sport, from cooking to economics by way of philosophy and telling jokes. These rules govern my behavior most of the time even though I often don't know when I learned most of them or even that they are actually present—I don't think of them from one year to the next. I can't recite a list of all the rules I use to govern my life and, in ordinary daily life, I am not aware of how they are selected for action, even to the extent of sometimes surprising myself with my behavior, but I have to accept that they are mine. I can tell the difference between doing something of my own volition and doing it under duress.

The question then arises: what reprograms a computational module so that it can give a different response to incoming data? Why, for example, do I get excited about a news item today when the same material yesterday didn't interest me? The answer is: another computational module, in an endless circular cycle, back to the moment I was born and even before. There is a ceaseless interchange of information between the modules such that they constantly modify each other in response to the demands placed upon them by the exigencies of getting through each day alive. And the day I die, it will stop, for all time.

This process is not the same as Spinoza described: "There is no such thing as Freewill. The mind is induced to wish this or that by some cause, and that cause is determined by another cause, and so on back to infinity." Firstly, I am saying we do have freedom of choice, determinism is false. I prioritize my decisions, changing them moment to moment according to my perception of my surroundings and my endlessly varying needs. Second, on his account, all current behavior of all living humans arose from a single cause way back then. The brain is capable of an infinite output; we do not go back to an infinity of time but back to an infinity of potential causes. The infinity is now.

It is not clear if we will ever be able to know the exact codes by which information is carried in the brain. Perhaps we won't, but I doubt that it matters, anyway. If we want to know why a person did something, all we have to do is ask him. He may tell you the truth, or he may lie to you. Only a being with mental capacities can deliberately tell falsehoods and only another being with mental capacities can discern a lie.

From this cognitive model of a bicameral mind, we can derive a formal account of mental disorder as a primary, psychological dysfunction in a perfectly healthy brain. There is no contradiction in the idea of *mens insana in corpore sano*. Given the infinite complexity and subtlety of the modular computational brain, the crude reductionist notion of a "chemical imbalance," beloved of biological psychiatrists, is facile in the extreme.

None of this is conceptually difficult or novel. This model does not invoke the supernatural to get over some difficult points of the theory, nor does it smuggle forbidden elements in to complete the chain of explanation. Every principle involved is either open to direct experience, including by introspection, or has been developed and used in other contexts with no significant objections from the usual critics. The only potential objection so far is whether some of the principles from physical data processing can be applied to human cognitive function, but that's the purpose of developing novel theories, taking them as far as possible, then subjecting them to stringent criticism. For a newcomer to these ideas, the notion of the dualist mind is often shocking, but remember that it has only been for a minute part of human history that it was considered disreputable, and, even then, only by a tiny proportion of the academic population. The hugely overwhelming majority of humans who have ever lived (including most academics, such as physicists) do not have the slightest difficulty with the concept of a dualist mind. That doesn't justify it, of course, but it does suggest that those who accept monism as the natural stance need to have some very convincing arguments. So far, I have seen very little in the way of arguments. Ideology, yes, but of reasoned arguments, precious few.

Even for those for whom dualism is the natural or default stance, the idea of a natural dualism often seems counter-intuitive. In their joint book, the neurophysiologist and Nobel winner, Sir John Eccles, said: "I can't believe that this mind will just cease to be." To which his colleague, the philosopher, Sir Karl Popper retorted: "I find the idea of immortality quite terrifying" [4]. This theory states that the experience of being something, what we know as mind, is a virtual construct, an informational space generated by a healthy brain by means of its staggeringly large computational networks. The mind is not *in* an informational space, it *is* an informational space, and informational spaces are both wholly virtual and causally effective. The mind therefore exists only so long as the brain keeps computing data: no switching, no mind, just as happens in general anesthesia. In the absence of computation, the informational space ceases to be, the image of being alive collapses and where there was something, there is oblivion.

The only difficulty lies in accepting that the mind is wholly a self-sustaining illusion of activity. It is indeed virtual, which also means "something giving the appearance or effect of a real entity while lacking the essential properties or form of any real entity; an image or mirage." The informational space we call the mind just is an illusion or virtual space. It is private since we cannot enter another virtual realm, we can only infer its presence by its effects. This virtual machine known as the mind requires a healthy, fully functional brain before it can spring into existence but, once awake (as we also say), the virtual machine runs the brain to suit itself. Of course, my mind doesn't cease to exist just because I am asleep. Parts of my system of rules are still operating at a primitive, effective level, entirely independently of my state of consciousness (arousal): I don't wet myself just because I am asleep, and some sounds will wake me immediately while I can sleep through jets taking off nearby. Approaching the question from this direction, the notion of self-aware computers is entirely feasible.

4.5 The Nature of Thought

It is probably easier if we start with an account of what thought is not, and see what is left:

4.5a. Thought is not an emotion. An emotion is one of a range of experiences occurring in inner subjective space with an ineffable visceral quality that is entirely real to the subject but that cannot be communicated or shared in any way. Essentially, they are internally generated sensations. Emotions are not essential to life but serve powerfully to reinforce patterns of behavior with strong survival value. Emotions can reinforce positively (i.e. increase the probability of a behavior recurring in the future) or negatively (reduce its chances), or they can increase the chances that a behavioral gambit will be successful (anger), but they are rarely of neutral value. As a wholly subjective experience, emotions have no informational content that can be communicated to another person; we can only define or communicate them ostensively. The whole concept of emotion is critically important in psychiatry, so we will come back to emotions in due course.

4.5b. Thoughts are not memories. We may use the term idiomatically, such as "I thought I left it here," but that has no technical value. We need to distinguish very precisely between memory and all other mental events just because memory is so important in its own right (I place great stead on *not* devaluing the currency of language; we should come back to this point as well).

4.5c. Thoughts are not beliefs. Anything that I believe forms part of my total informational state, specifically decisions I reached in the past (a millisecond ago is in the past). A belief is a proposition or item of knowledge that forms the basis for an action. The only difference between a belief and other ephemeral bits of information is that it isn't ephemeral. Since we are capable of changing them, you could say that beliefs are ephemera that last. Beliefs are of central importance in a cognitive psychology so we will need to reconsider them at length.

4.5d. Thoughts are not inner voices or verbalizings. I can "say" to myself: "Oh, I must post this letter," but that only signals I have already made the decision to post it. A person who "says" to himself "I shouldn't have done that" knew at the time he should not have been doing it but chose to ignore his self-awareness; now, the guilt has got him. All decisions are very fast and silent in that we cannot introspect them in the process. Decisions arrive, as it were, ready-made. They are not dressed in language but are simply an unspoken knowledge of what to do, and even this can be but the merest shadow flickering on the edges of awareness. When I reached for my computer mouse a moment ago, I did so without anything approximating inner speech; I don't even recall thinking about it, my hand just went out and moved it. And guess what? I just did it again. Damn. I wish I could catch myself in the act of making a decision, then I would have a better idea of why I do things. But then again, as the Duc de la Rochefoucauld said, nearly 350 years ago, why should I bother? *"Tout le monde se plaint de sa mémoire, et personne ne se plaint de son jugement."* Everybody complains about his memory but nobody ever questions his judgment. The notion that our decisions are made outside immediate awareness is absolutely central to this whole theory of mind, and thence to mental disorder, so we will come back to this point at length. Meanwhile, we can consign inner voices or verbalizings to the bin. They are just clutter among the mental furniture, idle amusements and fancies of no causal significance. Anybody who is really busy doesn't waste time talking to himself in his head.

4.5e. Thoughts are not mental imagery. "I was thinking of Babylon" means I was manufacturing and then dwelling upon imaginary scenes or fantasies of that almost mythical place. When, by night during the Second World War, Tolkien wrote his compelling stories, his head was full of an imagined world. He rehearsed it and polished it until, with what was happening at the time, it may even have seemed a little more real that the world in which he was living. If somebody said to him, "What are you doing?" he could have said: "I'm thinking of the wizard, Gandalf." By that, he would have meant "I have an image in my head, not of reality, but consisting of a series of mental pictures which together tell a story." A yearning youth may say "I can't stop thinking about X," meaning he is constantly rehearsing in his head a series of mental images, some memories, others (probably most of them) just amusing and gratifying fantasies that trigger emotions he enjoys. It can go the other way, of course, a person may say "I can't stop thinking about X," where X was a terrible event. The images come back with a horrifying reality and generate intensely unpleasant emotions which he cannot control. We have to distinguish between mental imagery and thought because of its unwilled nature, so we need to return to this point, too.

4.5f. Thoughts are not sensations. Sensory experiences are imposed upon us by external reality. They are not under our control, as imagery is, and we would never say we "think" our experiences: "Are you in pain?" "Well, I'm certainly thinking that I'm in pain." "I'd like to examine your shoulder, can you think up a pain for me?" While our senses can be misled, we have no capacity to change them at will. We can and frequently do change memories of sensations but that's different. Perception, of course, is central to any cognitive theory so we better add this to the list of topics to be revisited.

4.5g. Thoughts are not hallucinations. A hallucination is an experience, perceived as though through the sentences, which has the full quality and conviction of a veridical percept but with no independent basis in reality. A pseudo-hallucination is an experience perceived as through the senses with most or all of the quality of a veridical percept but which the subject understands is either lacking some essential quality or the conviction of a genuine impression of reality. These experiences are not under the subject's control, especially when they are terrifying, as is so often the case. We will have a lot to say about hallucinations when discussing the psychotic disorders.

Is there anything left, or is that all of the mental furniture? I can think of only one thing, which is inherent in just that statement: "I can think of only one thing." It may be clearer if I had said, "No, I can't think of anything." Thinking is the term we apply to decisions we have reached (or failed to reach).

- "I can't think of anything to do." This means only that I can't make a decision.
- "You children turn that TV down, how am I supposed to think?" How can I make decisions with all that racket distracting me?
- "I think I'll go to the Kasbah." I have decided to take my next holiday in an exotic location.
- "I think you need to stop spending so much." Well, that's my conclusion, now let's hear your lame self-justification.
- "I think Smith is an idiot." I believe he is, I decided that some weeks ago.
- "I thought you were in Samarkand." I believed that yesterday, but it seems I must revise my decision.
- "I can't think what I'd like to buy." The middle-class agony: forced to decide between affordable but unfashionable and fashionable but unaffordable.
- "I've been thinking..." I have been pondering the pros and cons of various options and have come to a decision you probably won't like.
- "I'll think about it." I will review the material and make a decision in my own time so don't bother me.

The problem here is that decisions are very fast and always beyond introspection. We do not "think our way through a decision," unless we mean dismantle it into minor decisions, but each of those is then acquitted silently and rapidly, as we cannot introspect them. Effectively, decisions are an instantaneous informational state. Their information content may then form the basis of further behavior but we won't be able to introspect that, either.

When we strip away the different types of mental events that we use each day, there really isn't much work left for the verb "to think." It is a lazy verb, one we use loosely because it saves us having to think too hard about our use of language (as in that sentence). There is no place for this verb in a technical theory of mind. I believe we can say everything we need to say about mental operations, using more precise terms, and never once mentioning the words think or thought. As with consciousness, the word 'thought' is an empty screen on which we individually project our prejudices, never checking on what our neighbor believes but immediately assuming he is in full agreement with oneself.

That means there isn't anything left to be given the name "thought."

What, then, is the nature of thought? It's nothing.

At least, that's what I think.

5 | The Nexus Between Brain and Mind

"Where in my thesis is there a weakness that someone else might find—because I sure better find it before they do, because if they find it and I'm not prepared, I'm in deep trouble."

Carl Sagan, talking of PhD candidates.

5.1. Introduction.

It is reputed that, sometime in the late nineteenth century, a man named Buckley announced that he would walk to China. "So?" you may ask, "happens all the time," except that Mr. Buckley was then a native of the fair city of Sydney, and there is a lot of water between Sydney and China. Undeterred by the scoffing and derision, he set off but was never seen again. He thus achieved a kind of fame in the Antipodes, where a person who has no chance of success in some scheme is told he has "Buckley's chance." William James was of the view that anybody attempting to resolve the mind-body problem had Buckley's chance: "Nature in her unfathomable designs has mixed us of clay and flame, of brain and mind, that the two things hang indubitably together and determine each other's being, but how or why, no mortal may ever know" (*Principles of Psychology*, Ch. VI).

In my previous publications, I outlined essential principles by which James' flame may arise from the clay and then act back to control it. The first four chapters of this book set the scene, so now I have to justify my claim of a theoretical resolution of the mind-body problem. We will be relying on several areas of knowledge, none of them developed by me. All the principles are in use in other fields of knowledge: there is nothing new in this thesis, just a different way of looking at old problems that leads to the resolution we need. This is a bold claim so those of you who are reading a borrowed or purloined copy can scoff now, while anybody who paid full price can only hope you get value for money.

The first area of knowledge is the vast and ever-growing field of the neurosciences, but I can't claim to be keeping up with developments as it moves too fast. The second is the principles of information theory developed by Turing, Shannon, von Neumann and so many others. Again, I am not an information theorist and sometimes make a mess of the updates on my Linux system. Third, there is the field of philosophy, especially of mind, science and language. Once more, I'm not a professional philosopher. My undergraduate units were decades ago and hard core philosophy papers certainly tax my ageing brain. The penultimate is the sprawling field of "human studies," including psychology in its many forms, sociology, epidemiology, general medicine, history and politics, not to overlook "near-human" studies such as ethology, primatology and so on. We mustn't forget basic chemistry, physics and biology, but mathematics now gives me a headache. Finally, there is my own discipline (and I use the term advisedly) of psychiatry, in which I can claim some expertise (although I am certainly not an academic). The real test of any resolution of the mind-body problem, meaning the ultimate test of any theory of mind, is that it must generate a plausible and testable theory of mental disorder.

That is, I will be relying on very broad swath of human knowledge, without being an expert in any of the preliminaries to my theory of mental disorder. Does that give me Buckley's chance? Then read on.

5.2. Preliminaries

In data-processing machines, there is no conceptual discontinuity at any stage between the point of entry of the data input and the point of exit of the final instructions at the interface with the peripherals. Data enters the processing system at dedicated points via sensors able to register just that particular form of energy. The sensors are in fact transducers, converting the data into the common codes of the system to send it through the system. At no point is there a change: it remains in the form of the codes until the peripheral is reached. While in the "common currency," any and all forms of input data can interact with information already in the system (instructions, memory etc) in an emergent informational space. Critically, instructions are encoded in the same form as the data they are to process, otherwise there could be no interaction. There is nothing supernatural or anti-materialist about any of this: once data from a range of different sources has been transduced into the system's codes, the data-processor is able to manipulate it to achieve an unexpected but rational outcome.

The data processing machine uses the laws of the physical world to create and acquit a higher-order function or virtual machine which is itself related to but separate from the physical realm. The realm of information constitutes an emergent state which exists only while a suitably-constructed switching machine is actually engaged in switching data. The emergent virtual machine can only interact with the physical world if the switching devices in its computational substrate are connected to suitable conduits, usually the same type as the switches themselves. This also applies to two separate informational spaces: they remain completely private until they are connected by suitable conduits.

Data flow can be detected at any point in the system by probes but, unless the codes used by the system are known, any signals detected remain meaningless noise. Once within the computational section of the machine, data are manipulated according to the semantic rules of the system and are therefore able to drive the system to work against the laws of thermodynamics at the expense of increasing entropy. The entire system exploits the natural laws of the material universe to achieve ends which are thermodynamically vanishingly unlikely, but never impossible.

It is common for people to claim that, since a physical machine can acquit conceptual tasks of the highest order, therefore, conceptual matters are themselves physical. This is a variant of the monist argument but it misunderstands the actual case. The switches of a data processing machine *function* in the physical realm, according to the laws of physics, in order to *implement* logical operations in an informational realm, according to the rules of its semantic system. In classic terms, the function of the physical machine constitutes the efficient cause of the computation, while the semantic instructions constitute the final cause. The two realms are incompatibly different and can only interact at the point where the computational neurons contact the conduit neurons.

All data processors operate at exceedingly fine tolerances, so that any disturbance of the physical system will quickly be evident in the system's output. The more complex systems almost always have a high level of inbuilt redundancy such that minor physical faults can be bypassed, either by physical or by informational means. Because of the nature of the informational "space," a complex system may well have the capacity for self-assessment and self-rectification but this is optional and certainly not necessary. A system may have no capacity to inspect its own data stores but would still function perfectly well. All of this is a natural and predictable consequence of the concept of information-processing as an ontologically separate realm from the physical world that implements it.

The human brain meets all these criteria. It is a hugely complex data processor with an afferent input, intervening computational systems, and clearly-defined efferent tracts that activate peripheral effector organs. The "common currency" of the human nervous system, neuronal impulses, is initiated at the level of the distal sensory receptors, when specific energy inputs are transduced into data flowing to the central centers for processing. In their passage from input side to output, the impulses may undergo many changes of neurotransmitters at different points in their tracts, but the significance of the impulses as carriers of information does not change at any point: in health, neurons are capable of being influenced by impulses from their neighbors, and impulses can influence neighboring neurons. The actual form of transmission between neurons is of great interest but it is not significant in terms of the brain's capacity as a data processor. Neurons themselves could be replaced by silicon microprocessors and the new owner would not be able to tell. It is feasible that we will eventually devise self-aware computers with the capacity to experience perceptions.

5.3. Transducers in Brief

All peripheral sensory receptors (meaning peripheral to the CNS) exploit specific energy fluctuations to extract information from the surrounding environment. The eyes detect electromagnetic radiation in the range 380-700nm; the ear detects pressure waves in the range 20Hz to 20kHz; there are vibration sensors, gravity sensors, chemical sensors (olfaction, gustation), pressure sensors and so on. Energy impinges on dedicated sensors which convert the energy flows to neuronal impulses. Each form of energy has a specific detector; each detector is activated by a specific form of energy. Energy fluctuations are converted to neuronal impulses by different mechanisms but the common feature is the ability of the incoming energy to trigger an impulse by acting on ion pumps in the neuronal wall. By a cascade of effects at the molecular level, an excitatory potential is initiated which can then generate a spike potential. The spike potential is now in the form of the "common currency" of the CNS. It is transmitted via conductive neurons (conduits) to the computational zone of the CNS where it is manipulated by instructions coded into the processing neurons interposed between the afferent and the efferent conduit neurons.

5.4. Data Processing in the CNS In Brief

Neurons influence each other according to defined anatomical pathways. Individual neurons can affect their neighbors via specific excitatory or inhibitory transmitters at synaptic junctions. Excitation is almost always very brief but states of physiological inhibition can last much longer. Ultimately, all neurons must return to *status quo ante*: in formal terms, energy is expended by the CNS in processing data but no physical work is done. Extracting information from the noise of the environment results in increased entropy. Data processing consists of ordered (non-random) processes of excitation and inhibition of interconnected neurons located in the cortical modules and subcortical nuclei and their connections. Data processing in the cortex results in an emergent informational space which is functionally totally dependent on, but ontologically separate from, the physiological integrity of the brain. During waking life, there is a constant, two-way flow of information from brain to mind and back again. In normal health, the informational space (mind) acts recursively to control the switching activity of its physical substrate (brain).

5.5. Human Mental Function in Brief.

The emergent mind is a composite of contingently-related functions whose only commonality is that they are generated in the head by the same neuronal processes. Human mental life divides readily in two classes, the experiential and the knowledge-based, or cognitive. The perception of being alive and able to sense or experience the universe is phenomenologically distinct from the capacity to know the universe and act upon it. Perception is vivid, private and ineffable while cognition is silent, fast and communicable. Perceptions can be of the external environment or of the internal environment. Emotions are unusual perceptions in that they are both activated and perceived internally, and are therefore private.

The cognitive functions are the basis of all action or output states, including motor behavior, speech, emotion, and control of the internal environment via the autonomic nervous system. On the basis of external perceptions, decisions are rapidly made and enacted in order to ensure the organism's survival. These decisions are influenced by acquired rules of behavior (learned behavior), as well as a large and diffuse system of innate cognitive rules common to all higher primates. In humans, the adaptive cognitive system has the capacity to function rationally but the influence of the innate cognitive system means that much of human behavior is more or less irrational. Cognitive processes cannot be introspected; we are apprised only of their outcome, e.g. a sudden increase in the heart rate, reaching for a cup, recognizing blue or knowing that 12 x 12 = 144.

5.6. Personality in Brief

Personality is the sum total of interactions between the individual and his environment throughout his life. Because this definition is encyclopedic and interminable, it must be abbreviated to be of use. Our interest lies in using past behavior to predict future behavior, by discovering the characteristic or predictable patterns of the stable adult mode of behavior which serve to distinguish the individual from his peers, i.e. to discern his system of rules. The patterns of behavior that erase individuality, such as language, ethics and other social-conforming behaviors, are excluded from the definition. Personality defines individuals where culture defines groups, so personality becomes: *The sum total of rules that generate the characteristic or predictable patterns of the stable adult mode of behavior that serve to distinguish the individual from his peers.* Many of the rules that govern the unique patterns of behavior in an individual will have been acquired pre-verbally or by implicit learning and may not be accessible by introspection, but they are nonetheless real and influential in determining behavior (unconscious motivation or latent processing). Some rules in the innate cognitive system may have a genetic basis but can still contribute to personality as they help distinguish the individual.

When the total system of rules in an individual produces behavior that meshes smoothly with the society's expectations, and functions harmoniously to produce a predictable emotional state that facilitates his behavior within the society, we will deem that person a normal personality, even when his society's rules are inhibitory or destructive. If, however, his rules bring him into conflict with his social surroundings or produce excessive inner conflict and distress, sufficient to impair his personal or social performance in his cultural context, then that person is defined as having a personality disorder, even though the social practices he breaches may be destructive. Since much behavior is culturally determined, personality disorder is context-dependent.

Since behavior is determined by a myriad rules, all behavior will be infinitely variable. Just as there are no discrete categories of intellectual ability, height or skin color, there are no discrete categories of behavior. Thus, there can be no categories of personality disorder even though, as a matter of convenience, we speak of artificial clusters of similar behaviors. Personality disorder is not an illness in any sense of the term. The brain is functioning within its normal limits but, because of inconsistent or self-contradictory rules, the behavioral output is classed as disordered. Because the system of rules does not become stable before early adulthood, we refrain from diagnosing a personality disorder before age eighteen. Children can display disturbed behavior for the same reason of inconsistent rules, but they don't have a brain disorder.

5.7. On the Nature of Mental Disorder

The term "mental disorder" (prev. mental illness) is reserved for changes in the individual's total mental state resulting in substantial distress or impairment of function but with no physical brain impairment. In some forms of mental disorder (anxiety, depression), the individual experiences an exaggerated and inappropriate variation of normal mental life; in others (psychosis), mental function is so severely disturbed as to render meaningful contact with the social environment difficult or impossible.

By virtue of the mind being an emergent informational space, human mental life is not reducible to its physical substrate. Mental disorder of any type is therefore not reducible to a physical "cause." It is feasible for some types of mental disorder to be seen in progressive brain disorders but these will are reactions to the primary process and will appear and fade as the physical disease progresses.

In a complex system with self-referential abilities, primary disturbances of data processing are to be expected. These can take the form of disordered sensory input, disordered data processing because of inconsistent rules, or breakdown of integrated function at any point due to excessively high or low data flows. Because no individual knows the full extent or nature of the rules governing his behavior, there is, in reality, little chance that mentally-disordered people will be able to state with certainty all, some or even any of the causes of their problems. To many individuals, the experience of a mental disorder may well seem to be a visitation from the unknown.

The informational space works for self-maintaining normality (homeostasis) but is not immune to bouts of self-perpetuating abnormality via feedback systems. The vicious circle is the crucial concept for understanding how the mind can fail while the brain remains healthy. As Pythagoras said, "Give me a fulcrum and I will move the world," so, today, it is no longer outlandish to conceive of a tiny error being amplified and magnified until it brings the whole edifice crashing down.

5.8. Treatment of Mental Disorder

Mental disorder therefore becomes a primary psychological disturbance of integrated mental function. Because of conflict between the individual's rules of life and his social setting, distress builds to the point where it becomes self-sustaining. Treatment of mental disorder starts with assisting the sufferer to settle to the point where he is able to begin a rational process of self-exploration to understand and rectify the factors contributing to his distress. This process may involve providing a place of refuge, a supportive social milieu, and the use of medication to reduce arousal to the point where the therapy can begin. Apart from exceptional cases, the use of drugs merely to provide long-term suppression of symptoms has no theoretical justification. In theory, all mental disorder should be resolved by psychotherapeutic means; recurrent mental disorder or chronicity simply says that the cause hasn't been found and therapy should continue. In the event that a person declines therapy, or actively evades effective treatment by dissimulation, then treatment should be withdrawn and the individual becomes responsible for the future course of life.

The vexed question of incarceration and compulsory treatment of mental disorders cannot be decided by fiat or for political convenience. The larger society should not forget past enormities done in the misguided belief that it was for the mentally-disordered person's benefit. In considering this question, it is always necessary to distinguish clearly between what is good for the disturbed individual, and what is for the society's benefit, or the benefit of commercial or professional interests. There is no rational basis for denying all individuals the right to end their lives, just because the measures needed to prevent all suicides will become so burdensome that they destroy any reason to continue living.

5.9. The Social Reaction to Mental Disorder

Because the human cognitive capacity confers on us the ability to dissemble, and because the experience of mental disorder seems so alien, those in the immediate social environment of a mentally-disturbed person are at liberty to question whether he is being genuine in his complaints. As in the case of crime, the complainant must be given the benefit of the doubt so, until that question is settled, the society is still required to provide him the same care and assistance as any other person whose life has moved beyond his personal control. In the event it is determined that he is genuine, then that assistance should continue to the same extent as available to any person in that society with a physical illness. There can be no presumption that a person complaining of mental symptoms is acting with the intention of deceiving or defrauding his society. As a group, mentally-ill people have more in common with normal people than they have points of difference. They are no more capable of controlling every aspect of their lives than the rest of us.

The question of the guilt of mentally-disordered people who commit crimes also cannot be decided by fiat. It is not possible to say that all mentally-disordered offenders were acting deliberately with full conscious control, nor that they are all automatically excused their offenses. Each case has to be considered on its merits. No benefit will accrue to mentally-disturbed offenders, or to the larger society, if they believe that they can escape the consequences of their actions by virtue of a diagnosis but a society that punishes mentally-disordered people for reason of their condition has no virtue.

In the following chapters, we will consider each of these points in more detail.

<table>
<tr><td>

6

</td><td>

The Cerebral
Wetware

</td></tr>
</table>

"The total possible consciousness may be split into parts which coexist but mutually ignore each other."
—William James, *Principles of Psychology*

6.1. Introduction

Life begins at the edges. Life is lived on the edge. The term 'transducers'
applies to the peripheral (external to CNS) sensory receptors that detect
energy changes in the external environment and use those changes to generate neuronal impulses, the "common currency" of the CNS. I won't spend
much time on receptors, they're not of direct significance to a theory of mind
although they are important in that they all illustrate a number of essential
points. Firstly, there are many different types of sensory receptor, all of them
keeping a metaphorical eye on the narrow band of energies, including chemicals, that are keep us alive. Some of them are designed to let us smell or taste
the difference between food and not-food, some are short-range risk receptors
(touch, thermal energy) while others are long-range receptors that tell us
danger is approaching. Second, each type of input is specific to a particular
receptor; the receptor can respond to that form of energy alone, and does so
by unique changes in the chemical shape or constitution of the receptor proteins. Third, a change in the receptor protein will eventually activate an
excitatory post-synaptic potential which may lead to an actual neuronal
impulse.

Any standard textbook of physiology will give full details of the structure
and function of the receptors. I use Pocock and Richards [1] and Bear,
Connors and Paradiso [2] for the neurosciences. Wikipedia has a very nice
picture of the rhodopsin receptor molecule [3]. Bear has 30 pages on the eye,
so there's not much point in my trying to summarize that for physicians, who
may want to skip the next few pages. The point of this short chapter is to

outline a way of looking at human function, where a central processor takes all incoming and stored information, rapidly computes a variety of decisions in a range of systems and sends those decisions speeding to the effector organs, all in much less than the blink of an eye. Motor behavior, speech, emotions, physiological functions, these are all seen as output states, on the output side of the brain's decisions. That is, all output states are the result of decisions that we can understand as the comprehensible, predictable outcome of the various inputs and the existing rules.

This puts a totally different emphasis on, say, emotional life. In the bio-cognitive model, the idea that emotions simply well unbidden from the depths or out of the blue is impossible. This idea appeals to psychiatrists, of course, who want to have a model of mind as mysterious and unknowable, so that daily experience *seems* to support the notion of intense, unpleasant emotions caused by physiological disorders acting outside awareness. Thus, the expression "free-floating anxiety" is often tossed around, as though there were a quantum of some hot internal miasma, like an angry cloud of static electricity floating around inside that sticks to different mental events and makes them painful. This is puerile. In nature, anxiety is the most widespread of all the emotions; if we can't understand that one, psychiatry has no chance as an intellectual discipline. The expression "free-floating anxiety" means only that the psychiatrist hasn't taken a proper history (or, more likely, doesn't know how to take a history from a frightened patient).

6.2. Receptors

In brief, a receptor consists of a highly specific detector protein that is remarkably sensitive to energy inputs within its range. Photodetectors in the retina consist of a complex of unstable chemicals that react to photons by depolarizing the neuronal membrane and activating an impulse. This is wholly an electrochemical process and has nothing to do with what we call the mind. In essence, the photoreceptors "harvest" the energy in light but, instead of using it to build new chemicals, as chloroplasts do, the energy triggers the first step in a process of mapping the external environment in the CNS. Because light energy travels in straight lines with such a small wavelength, it gives a remarkably accurate "picture" of the external environment to any organism with sufficient information processing capacity to "read" it. By that I mean, the retinal architecture is such that, when the energy is converted or transduced, it yields a pattern of information which gives the organism a precise and detailed assessment of what is happening "out there." Rhodopsin responds to light in about 200 femtoseconds (1fsec = 10^{-15} seconds), so the organism is effectively seeing things as they happen.

There is, however, no picture in the head. If I see blue, there is nothing in my head that turns blue. The visual image the brain derives from the visual input does not exist in the real or material world, it exists only as an informational "space" (but not *in* an informational space, as that implies an infinite regress). It is a product of the brain's capacity to switch huge amounts of information very quickly to produce an artifact or facsimile of the real world as a private, immaterial space, thereby constructing the mind. The artifact *is* the informational space; the informational space *is* the mind; the mind *is* the artifact. The brain generates the artifact, so I am an artifact but, within certain limits, I can tell my brain what to do. If there is no light of about 450nm impacting on my retina then, much as I may want to, I can't see blue (we can explain after-images in physiological terms). There is no such thing as "blue" in the real world. Nature is colorless. Blue exists only in informational spaces generated by brains, and not just human brains. It is asking too much of evolution to believe that chimps don't see blue.

6.3. Data Processing

A great deal of processing takes place in the retina itself, with reciprocal repression and potentiation of adjoining photosensitive zones serving to exaggerate the differences. We respond selectively to sudden changes in brightness, such as at edges or with movement. Once an impulse is generated in a fiber in the optic nerve, nothing happens until it reaches the CNS as the afferent nerves function as conduits only. However, when an impulse reaches the actual processing zones of the CNS, its function changes: showers of impulses percolate as information through cascades of switching mechanisms to implement an instantaneous informational space which eventually con- stitutes the sense of "being something." The informational space is not projected *to* something, it *is* the something. I don't inspect my informational space, I *am* my informational space. Where my brain goes, there goes me, too, but it is important not to think of the informational space as some sort of gassy chamber floating above the brain (forget astral traveling). A switching machine and the informational space it generates do not coincide because they occupy ontologically different realms. If the brain stops switching data, then the informational space ceases to be.

People often say: "The mind depends on the physical state of the switches of the brain. Therefore, the mind is physical in nature." This is another example of naïve materialism, which conflates the provenance of the mind (i.e. what it comes from) with its nature. There is not a one to one relationship between the state of the switches and the outcome of the computation; there are, as Turing showed, many ways a universal computing machine can be programmed to achieve the same output. The output is dependent upon the fact of switching but it is independent of the physical state of the individual switches.

All of this talk of neuronal switching mechanisms presupposes a very detailed understanding of neurophysiology. An impulse travels down the axon to the synapse where it activates the transmitter vesicles to discharge into the synaptic cleft. In fractions of a millisecond, the transmitter diffuses across this tiny gap, 20-50nm wide. There are known to be dozens of neurotransmitters, each of which can either excite or inhibit the post-synaptic dendrite. Consider the simplest form of transmission, where there is a one-to-one relationship between pre- and post-synaptic impulse traffic (Fig. 6.2). The two neurons are acting as a single conduit with an interposed relay but, since there is no switching, no informational space is generated by this relay process. The relay may be more complex, e.g. a single impulse in pre-synaptic neuron A may fail to trigger a post-synaptic impulse in neuron B. However, two impulses in

Fig 6-1 a) Simple circuit: neurons as conduits

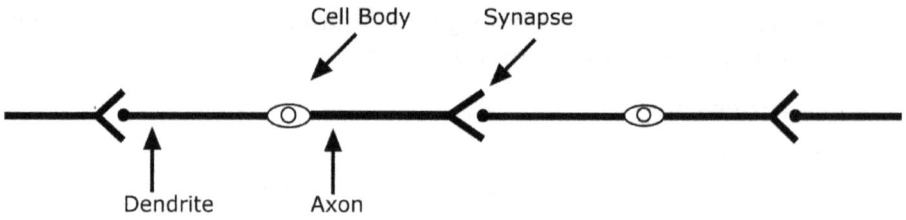

Fig 6-1 b) Complex circuit: neurons as switching circuits

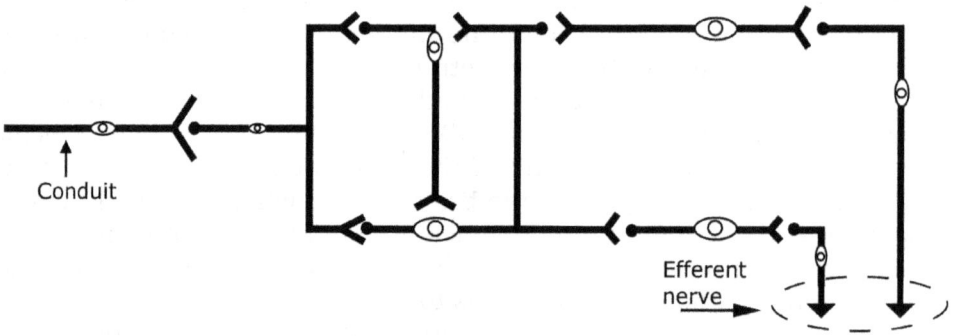

Fig. 6.1 The difference between neurons acting as conduits and neurons acting as switches.

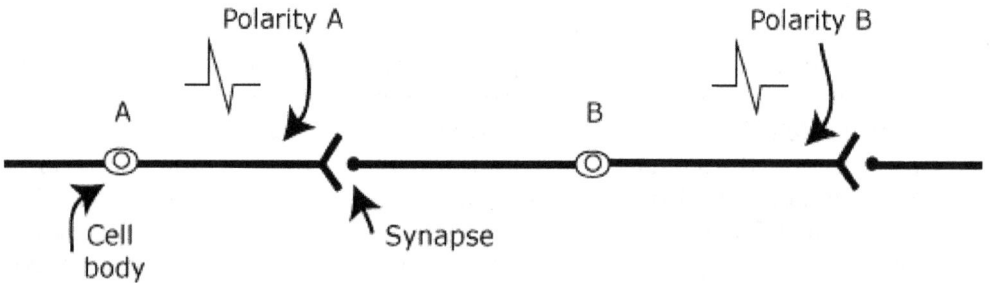

Fig. 6.2: One-to-one relationship between pre and post-synaptic neurons

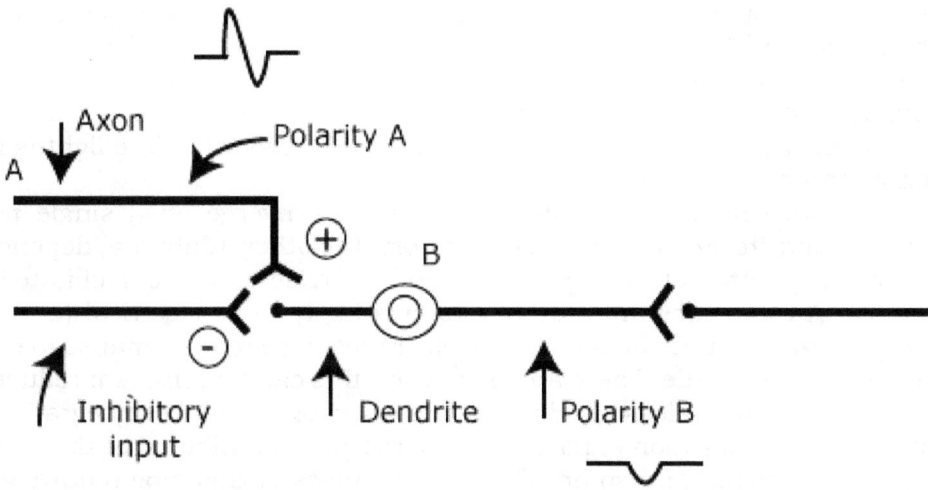

Fig. 6.3: Two neurons converge on a single post-synaptic dendrite

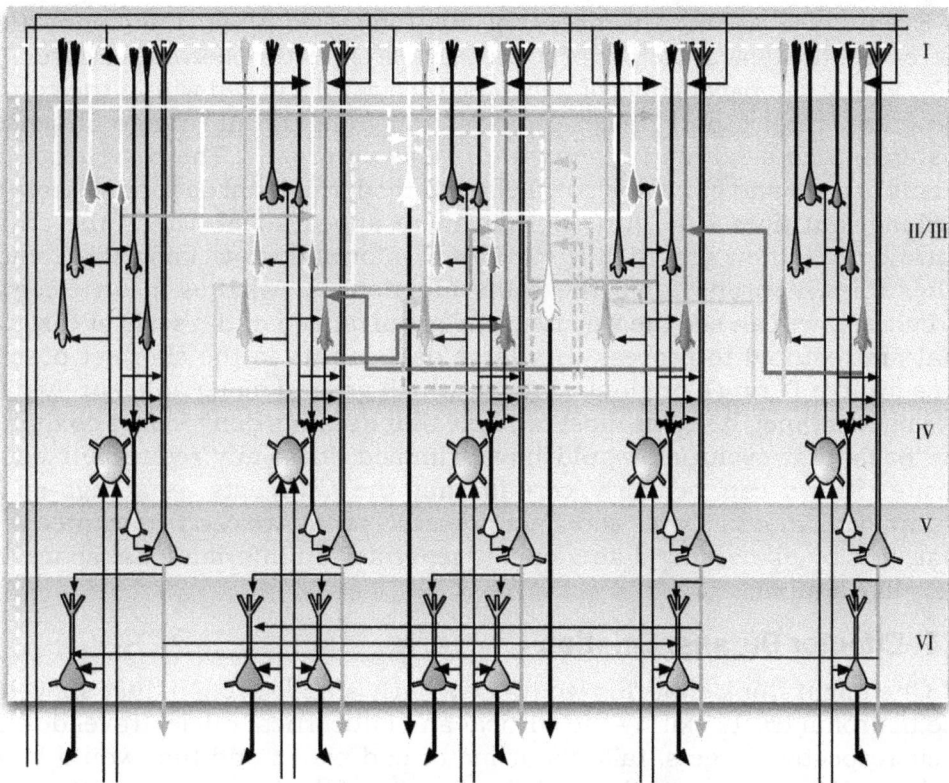

Fig. 6.4: Stylized model of human cortex [1]

---

[1] From: George D, Hawkins J (2009) Towards a Mathematical Theory of Cortical Microcircuits. *PLoS Comput Biol* 5(10) (with permission).

rapid succession in A may trigger an impulse in B while three in rapid succession may block B again. In a simple system, this allows discrimination. Say the sensor connected to A is a red light detector. A pink light triggers one impulse, bright red triggers two and dark red triggers one (or maybe three). We would then say of the system: "Yes, it certainly knows when the light is red, it's not stupid."

At a more complex junction, two neurons converge on a single post-synaptic dendrite (Fig. 6.3). One is excitatory, the other inhibitory; depending on how they interact, the post-synaptic impulse may be facilitated or inhibited. A transient inhibitory blockade is likely to be electrical (i.e. brief hyperpolarization) but chemical changes are required to the synapse to effect a longer-term blockade. There are many ways this can be achieved: reduction of neurotransmitter release by different means, rapid reuptake or degradation, reduction or stabilization of post-synaptic receptors, inhibition at the level of the neuronal soma, and so on. Chemical changes of this type require gene activation and expression. This potential multiplicity of causes for a single effect means the notion of a single biochemical "cause" (and, worse still, of a single pharmacological "cure") of mental disorder is highly unlikely as an empirical fact.

Eventually, as the numbers of neurons and their interconnections increases, the typical picture of cortical cytoarchitecture becomes clearer (Fig. 6.4). Vastly complex arrays of neurons, precisely localized within the cortical structure, receive and process information from the full range of sensory systems, then send instructions to the effector organs. The complexity just seems to grow and grow; the parallels with modern digital data processors are striking, but does it go further than mere appearance? That's the critical question. We know that the CNS traffics in information; we know that, among other roles, neurons fulfill the same function as switches in an electrical circuit and we can see the way neurons are arranged in the sorts of cascades that are required to process very large data inputs in the shortest possible time (unlike Turing's original concept, which ground along at leisurely pace, one bit at a time). It seems most unlikely that neurons don't in fact do that, on the basis that evolution would have trimmed down any redundant neural tissue. So we can be fairly certain that the CNS acts as a high-speed, multimodal, massively parallel data processor; what we can't guarantee yet is that, just by processing data alone, it generates an informational space that feels like a mind.

6.4. Effector Organs: Emotions

One might think that this would be a fairly simple section, just show how the neuronal tracts exiting the cortical and subcortical nuclei travel down to their respective targets, talk about motor end plates and that would be the end of it. However, skeletal muscle is only part of the output state of the brain. Yes, there is the endlessly complex system of respiratory and laryngeal control that governs speech, or ocular control with its seemingly simple saccades to keep track of a moving object (they are anything but simple), not to mention running down a set of stairs as an exercise in coordination or the fine motor control of the fingers in typing, etc., but there are other systems of equal importance. For example, emotions are an output state of the brain, and emotions lead to hormones.

"An emotion is one of a range of experiences occurring in inner subjective space; with an ineffable visceral quality that is entirely real to the subject but that cannot be communicated or shared in any way." An emotion is an inner perception. It is generated by a cognitive act, which is usually not in full awareness, and is then perceived recursively as an experience, i.e. the direction of causation is:

Cognitive realm → Activity in subcortical nuclei (outside awareness) → experiential realm via cortical regions.

This is not immediately intuitive: people will usually say "But I don't cause my emotional storms by an act of will. If I could do that, I would will them away, believe me." This is true: we do not choose to laugh at something, the humor just erupts and we are, in a sense, the victims of our own tasteless humor (I certainly am). Similarly, I do not choose to get angry over the rubbish that comes over the news each night, irritation flares up and the only way to settle it is to go and do something else. Affection is not willed; people do not choose to feel frightened ("I'm so bored. I know, I'll have a panic attack, that will help pass the day") nor have we any control over grief following a loss. So why say emotions are the result of a cognitive act?

The answer is that we do not consciously will 99.99% of our actions. We speak, without knowing just what the next word will be. I use a hammer to hit a nail. I am not aware of undertaking a formal judgment of exactly where to swing the hammer or how I actually strike the nail, it just comes. A fieldsman is running after a high ball, he jumps and, single-handed, catches it, rolls to the ground and leaps up, throwing the ball accurately back to the wicket keeper. He has no sense of thinking over what he is doing, it just happens, but he wills it and does not doubt that every movement is his and his alone. I lift up my right arm. I cannot catch myself in the act of deciding to lift it, but it happens anyway. My fingers are typing rapidly but I have no sense of willing them to do their job, they just do it. I recognize the sound of lorikeets flying overhead. I did not have to work out what birds they were, or even that they were birds and not dogs, this decision was made for me.

So it is with emotions. I perceive an event or thing and, before I can know it, I have a decision about that event and the appropriate emotions have been activated. I turn and see a small child just about to chase its ball into a busy street. Immediately, I feel a rush of sick apprehension and I start to run. This is done outside awareness, it is not "conscious" in the sense of some sort of inner speech. Words would only get in the way. All this takes place at a primitive level, with little subtlety or finesse involved. Human emotional reactions are coarse, not much different from chimp emotions, in fact. We would like to think we have finer control due to more factors involved in generating the response but the emotions themselves aren't much different.

Incoming information interacts with a set of beliefs and attitudes to generate the decisions that trigger an emotional reaction. The signal to the subcortical nuclei is of the same nature as the signal to, say, lift an arm, i.e. a barrage of impulses in a specific corticofugal tract (or tracts). The experience of emotions is closely associated with activity in midbrain and thalamic nuclei but the instructions are cognitive, issuing from the highest brain centers. After the event, we can usually put words to the factors involved in the decision but rules governing emotions are often learned implicitly so it may take some time or assistance before the individual can accurately identify the (many) rules and other factors involved. Except for the factors that we can't identify, such as when one person finds a comic hysterically funny while the next person sighs in boredom.

The general principle is that, as mental events, all emotions, even crippling emotions, have a mental cause although it may not be obvious. This is determinism in action (cf. Schopenhauer's Principle of Sufficient Reason: "Nothing is without a reason"). This concept stands diametrically opposed to the orthodox view in psychiatry, that intense emotions are totally mysterious, pathological upwellings from the cerebral depths which cannot have and do not need explanation but should be suppressed and not experienced. Unfortunately, it is very often the case that emotions need to be experienced before their causes can be understood, so suppressing them means that the psychological factors that generated them remain intact and, in all probability, will lead to a recurrence. It is often difficult to be sure of the exact nature of the information that leads to unpleasant emotions, a lot of it was learned pre-verbally or implicitly, and it is also active before the emotion is experienced. Thus, trying to work backwards in a state of agitation, to discover some vague, half-remembered notion that has risen briefly, done its damage then disappeared just as quickly, can be very difficult. Indeed, it can be so difficult that a lot of people think it is impossible, that emotions are forever beyond comprehension and probably embarrassing, so that talking is a waste of time. Regrettably, a lot of modern psychiatrists also believe it.

How many emotions are there? This is an important question; as a lumper, I am not inclined to believe there are as many as there are poets or hysterics in the world. I see evidence for a small number of basic emotions, which combine under the influence of the cognitive set to produce an infinitely wide range of experiences. My reason is that each emotion has a specific cerebral substrate; there is not enough room in the head for a thousand emotions, each with its own dedicated bit of brain. Thus, we recognize humor, anger, the very large group of fears, sadness, joy, wonder, and perhaps a few others. Suspicion is a good example of what an emotion is not. Even though psychiatrists talk of a suspicious affect (mood state), it is a composite of apprehension and repressed hostility rather than a pure emotion. Guilt is the same, a combination of self-loathing and fear of punishment. Interestingly, when women say they feel guilty, they usually mean fear of punishment (getting into trouble, such as disapproval, hostility directed at them etc) while men usually mean self-hatred and regret.

It is very important to untangle emotions very carefully, because the exact emotion is the clue to the cognitive causes. It is useless to say "I'm stressed," because that word has absolutely no meaning. People who talk about "anxiety and stress" are showing that they don't know what they're talking about. Similarly, it is wrong to conflate sadness and the condition known as depression. A person may be gripped by a terrible sense of sadness and loss that seems to have no end, but it is still not depression because there is no guilt or lack of self-worth. An emotional response is caused by an interaction between the individual's perception of his world (which may be very distorted, even by emotion) and his personality, i.e. that huge, half-hidden mass of rules and injunctions, often unnamed, often frightening in their own right, which generates responses to events as they occur. In order to sort out the rules, we have to work back from the emotions as the subject experiences them and the events, to construct the rules that must have in play to cause just that response and no other. Simple in theory, not always so easy in practice.

6.5. Effector Organs: Vegetative Systems

We are accustomed to thinking of motor activity and speech as behavioral output states; with a bit of reorientation, people get used to the idea that emotions are a just a private output state; but a lot of people have difficulty thinking of autonomic or vegetative activity as an ordered output state. This attitude is a little bizarre: if the CNS didn't have control over our bodily functions, what would? So, I have to give a highly contentious lecture to a group whom I know are, shall we say, not entirely receptive to the message I want to give. As the hour approaches, I get a message to back-pedal, that the group is actively hostile (they are psychiatrists, of course). Walking to the lecture room, I feel that familiar thud-thud I used to get before oral exams in high school: the old ticker is speeding up a bit. Why? I do not mean Why as in Aristotelian final cause, we all know from daily experience what the flight and fight reaction does, but Why as in efficient cause. What is the mechanism by which merely entertaining an idea of a future action can stimulate the body to the specific level of activity that is needed for the successful completion of that action? Answering this question demands a resolution of the mind-body problem.

The empirical fact of the fight or flight reaction is beyond dispute; all that is lacking is a mechanism that translates thoughts to pounding hearts. We will consider this critically important question in the next chapter but one. The next chapter will consider what we can loosely term the "thoughtware," the informational content that tells the output side of the "wetware" what to do.

6.6 Conclusion

One of the guiding principles behind the biocognitive model of mind is that it all makes sense. There should be no loose ends in the explanatory chain, no missing gaps in the sequence, no mysteries. From the time a person sees something to the time he has finally forgotten about it, everything has to make sense, even when it doesn't appear to make sense at first (especially then). The first step in understanding anything is to know what we are dealing with, and how it should properly be oriented. Psychiatry has to rid itself of any notions that its mental subject matter cannot be understood in terms of mental causes. The cause of a mental event is a prior mental event, perhaps even hundreds of them, and these have to be understood in terms of the complex interaction of other prior informational events. If we say "It's all mental, stupid," then we are overlooking an important point, that a lot of what takes place in the head to generate the overt mental event is actually "not quite mental." It is informational, but often cannot be introspected.

So there is a difference between overt, fully conscious mental events (and I have my doubts about even them) and the underlying informational flows that generate those overt events. That doesn't mean we can't, with time and effort, render the informational flows more obvious, it just means that the human mind evolved to make very rapid, safe decisions, so it doesn't need anybody interfering with its processes to do that. If chimps can decide to move to a quieter part of the cage without "mental talk," so can I. Except, with mobile phones and computers, I can't seem to find a quieter part of my cage.

7

The Mental
"Thoughtware"

"We all have a tendency to think that the world must conform to our prejudices. The opposite view involves some effort of thought, and most people would die sooner than think—in fact, they do so."
Bertrand Russell, *The ABC of Relativity* (1925)

7.1. Introduction

One of the many remarkable features of the seminal paper by Alan Turing, in 1937, was his proof of the possibility of building a machine that would duplicate human mental activity. In one remarkable move, he changed his "discrete state machine" to a "universal computing machine." The way he did this was to configure the informational state of his first machine so that it mimicked the range of all possible computing machines. It became universal, not because he built it so big that it could do anything, but because he changed the way it ran itself "inside." He rewrote its instruction set in such a way as to "fool" the machine into "thinking" it had a universal capacity (be wary of anthropomorphosis). He gave each possible configuration a number, actually a set of numbers, that would mimic the activity of each machine built to handle just one of the range of conceivable tasks.

In doing this, he was building on the work of one of recent history's more mythical figures, the Austrian-American mathematician and logician, Kurt Gödel (1906-1978). At the age of 25, shortly after he had completed his doctorate, Gödel published two theorems that eventually turned mathematics upside down, but not immediately because practically nobody understood them (for a marginally comprehensible account of Gödel's work, see Douglas Hofstadter's revised version of the little book by Ernst Nagel and James Newman [1], which almost succeeded at the impossible, popularizing Gödel's monumental intellectual achievement).

Most of this, of course, is utterly beyond a mere psychiatrist, not that it matters as the point is this: Turing was able to use Gödel's concept to implement his notion of an unlimited computing machine. Reconfiguring the internal informational state of a very limited machine would allow it to mimic the internal computational state of any possible machine and, thence, to generate any possible output. A corollary is that, in a sufficiently complex data processing machine, a particular informational state can always mimic any possible physical error (as an aside, I have always taken this to be a lethal objection to the reductionist idea that all mental disorder is necessarily due to a physical disorder of the brain). With no breaches of the physical laws of the universe, and certainly no little miracles, a finite machine could be built that would give, essentially, an infinite output. In few words, this is not a bad description of the human brain.

7.2. The Concept of Human Nature

Bearing in mind that the human brain is only about three times the size of the chimp brain, what is the nature of the informational content of the human brain that converts it from something that is comfortable in trees, to something that can conceive of infinity? The difference between human and chimp intellectual ability is not just due to raw computing power. The difference has to be, as Turing understood so clearly, a matter of how the information is organized and how it is processed. In certain vital respects, the human and chimp behavioral repertoires have far more in common than they do differences. In other, equally striking but completely different respects, we leave them, well, in the trees. But first, let's look at some of the similarities:

7.2a. They are social animals. Essentially, they cannot survive alone and always aggregate into long-term social groupings. These social groups are held together by bonds of an emotional nature which they reinforce by a variety of ritual behaviors. When a bond is broken, by death or other separation, they evince a characteristic reaction known as the loss or grief reaction. Within the group, they act cooperatively for the benefit of the group and often demonstrate altruism. However, their affection for their species is limited, in that they also show clearly-defined xenophobia, the fear of strangers or outsiders, and will usually attack an intruder on their territory. Away from their territory, they are much more circumspect and are inclined to react submissively to strangers or to flee from contact.

7.2b. Within their social groups, they form dominance hierarchies. These are most clearly defined among males, for whom a higher status confers rights to the available females, but females and juveniles also form their own hierarchies. Between social groups, where their territories abut, there is constant jostling and friction as the groups seek to establish and maintain dominance.

7.2c. They are highly territorial. They establish territories and then defend them aggressively against interlopers of their own species. Their territoriality extends to possessions and, for males, over their females and offspring. If one of them is removed from its territory and placed in a neighboring territory, it will show a mixed reaction of fear and aggression until accepted or driven away. As soon as the individual crosses the border to its own territory, the fear abates and aggression will dominate.

7.2d. They are generally aggressive in their relationship to the natural and social environment. Anything that causes heightened arousal is likely to trigger an aggressive response, mostly directed at the object that has provoked the fear but the aggression can also be displaced to other objects or to their own kind. They fear change and show a strong desire for stereotypy or repetitive, ritualized behaviors. It is not unfair to say they are creatures of habit with a restricted appetite for novelty.

7.2e. They show a well-developed sense of curiosity and will indulge in exploratory behavior when placed in non-threatening new surroundings or if some novel task is presented to them. Closely associated with this, they show a sense of fun and play.

7.2f. They have a wide range of innate fears, i.e. fears that are fully active at the time of first exposure to the stimulus. These include heights, dark spaces, certain types of noises or shapes, especially anything that resembles a primal threat such as the shape and movement of snakes and large predators. They are generally comforted by familiar noises and movements, and apprehensive of silence. They use physical contact to reduce anxiety, especially with their offspring. This appears to be based in innate abilities to recognize characteristic features of their own kind, such as facial recognition, the touch of fur or hair compared with scales or slime, the sound of species-specific vocalization, either of reassuring or frightening kind, and so on.

7.2g. They can communicate via learned or acquired behaviors, generally of a verbal nature but also by bodily means. They also exhibit a number of stereotyped behavioral patterns, which are not dependent on prior experience, mostly in the context of intense emotions, e.g. crying, grief, happiness, threat, submission, etc.

And now for chimps...

This list shows that, cognitively, there are many behavioral attributes, common to all higher primates (including *H. sapiens*) which could not have arisen by chance. Hair and fingernails did not arise by chance in each primate species but are genetically determined, so it seems reasonable to assume that some typical primate behavior contains an element of genetic control, much as the reproductive behavior of birds is imminent. We are talking about the activity and effects of an innate cognitive system. Immediately, we have a number of epistemological problems. For example, how can we transpose a cognitive assessment ("I am no longer in my territory") to the class of heritable dispositions? What is a heritable disposition? How can genes influence the sort of behavior that seems to require an intervening cognitive variable in order to complete the chain of causation between perception and behavioral response? These are not trivial questions but go to the heart of this project.

I am not making the sort of claim popular among reductionist philosophers and psychiatrists, that the behavior of avoiding a foreign territory is of the same order of nature as the excretion of urine by the kidneys; rather, I am saying that the objective behavioral phenomena displayed by higher primates are most explicitly *not* of that nature; they are ontologically different, and *ipso facto* problematic. We can, as many philosophers have tried, attempt to redefine the ontological gap out of existence but it never works. Mind and body are irreducibly different.

7.3. The Innate Cognitive System I: Decisions.

The goal is "to transpose a cognitive assessment ('I am no longer in my territory') to the class of heritable dispositions." In order to do this, we need to provide a causal explanation, by transposing a *high level* description to a description at the *level of implementation*, then to the *level of formal operations* and finally to *level of the machine code,* because the level of the machine code is heritable whereas the others aren't. In principle, this level is the same in humans as in squids.

A **high level description** would be of the order: "Oh dear, I've just wandered across the border, I'd better nick off before one of those ugly monkeys that lives here sees me."

At the **level of implementation**, it would be something like: "The organism detects it is in unfamiliar territory. Immediately, its level of arousal starts to rise, quickly becoming uncomfortable so it looks for a means of reducing it. Familiar territory reduces arousal. With its motor activity rapidly increasing due to the arousal (aka agitation), the organism scans the surroundings for signs of the last known point of familiar territory and quickly moves in that direction. As it reaches familiar zones, its arousal starts to decline so the behavior calms and becomes more normal, such as foraging or seeking reassurance from its fellows by means of some ritualistic behavior or other."

Description at the **level of formal operations** is not available to us at present. It would be something like the sets of coded instructions from the perceptual apparatus to the various effector systems in the body. Effectively, it would be a set of instructions from one brain subsystem to the next, which we can render in English (jargon) as follows: "Unfamiliar territory detected, scanning local environment but no sign of familiar faces or doors. Unfamiliar doors detected. Alarm systems activated; all aggression systems disabled; foraging and sexual exploration systems inactivated; low level emergency escape systems implemented; revert to medium level avoidance behavior" etc. The expression "alarm systems activated" means the reticular activating system switches to a higher level, resulting in cerebral alertness (as detected on EEG) with sympathetic autonomic arousal, also known as the fight or flight reaction. The heart rate and breathing rate increase, blood flow is diverted from vegetative functions to the brain, lungs and somatic musculature, and so on. The organism starts to scan the environment very closely, using all sensory modalities, and is relatively over-reactive to any signs of danger while becoming unresponsive to signs of food, sexual release, pain etc.

What this means is what computer engineers are doing when they say things like: "Oh yes, the detectors are talking to the peripheral activators now, checking to see if they've got any info on this problem. They'll flick us an answer shortly... Here we are, they say the problem's in the No. 2 unit. Strange, No. 2's telling us it was checked a week ago. OK, let's see what records are saying." Subunits do not think or talk or have opinions or have any such anthropomorphized faculties; we might say they "think" and "talk" and have "opinions," but that's all. A module in a larger system simply receives information, checks it against its instruction set, manipulates it and dispatches it, all of it done mindlessly and exactly in accord with the principles established by Turing three quarters of a century ago. There is no intelligence to be found by decomposing intelligent operations.

At this level of explanation, we have dropped below the level at which intelligence emerges; all we have is a bunch of cerebral subunits that take whatever message they are given, roll it over a set of instructions and shove the answer down the Out tube. Where it came from, what it means and where it will go, they have no idea and, more to the point, they don't care as they don't have the wherewithal to know what those concepts could possibly mean. Intelligent behavior is assembled from unintelligent sub-behaviors. Meaning emerges from subsystems that don't know what they are doing. Intelligence is not a thing that resides somewhere in the brain but it is a function that is assembled from lots of little subfunctions, each of which comes from sub-subfunctions, and so on. If I take a car apart to look for the Car inside, all I will have is a box of immobile spare parts. If I start to put them back together, there will come a point at which I can say: "Hey, look, turns out there was a car in this box."

Now we move to the level of the **machine code** which, in biological systems, means the level of interaction of the signal with the neuron's subcellular machinery: how does a signal influence that machinery? A signal is two things: it is a physical event (an incoming spike potential), and a significance. To be precise, it is a significant physical event. Its significance lies in the way it can transmit information in a form that can be manipulated while, as a physical event, it can act upon the cell. At this level, information consists of no more than instructions to a sub-unit to act or to remain inactive. We have reduced knowledge to mere instructions. The signal arrives at a receiving neuronal dendrite in the form of a pre-synaptic spike potential; as a spike potential, it is able to trigger the release of neurotransmitters or to activate gene expression. Thus, the instruction inherent in the impulse is implemented either as a new physical event (post-synaptic transmission) or as a new entity (gene expression leading to new proteins). At the level of the machine code, neuronal impulses do not carry meaning in the way we talk about it at the highest level. Meaning has been broken down or decomposed (*not* deconstructed) to the level at which it is no longer correct to talk of the impulses carrying meaning. All they carry is instructions but, if the instructions are entered according to a particular code then, when they are reassembled, something clever has been achieved.

This, then, is the **level of the molecular resolution of the mind-brain problem**, the level at which a signal from the external receptors activates a sub-sub-subfunction of the subcellular machinery. The subcellular organelles, being wholly physical, can only be activated by a physical event, meaning an impulse: I can shout at them as much as I like, but they won't answer until a spike potential gets them jumping. However, the physical event has a dual role, in that it also constitutes an item of information (a bit?) about the external environment. The impulse only arrives *because* of the information it carries. It is not a random firing driven by the neuron's physical needs but a controlled firing driven by the whole organism's informational needs. On the other side of the synapse, the processes are reversed and all the separate little impulses wandering around the computational parts of the system are reassembled and squirted down the conduit to the effector organ. At that point, it becomes appropriate to say "Well, I can see where those signals are starting to mean something" (as in: "Hey, look, I found a car in this box"). It's a bit like a giant oil tanker turning. The boatswain swings the wheel and, half an hour later, they are on a different course. There was no instant in that half an hour when anybody could say: "It turned just then." Turning is a process, assembled from an infinity of instantaneous vectors; individually, they are nothing but add them together and the giant ship heads in a new direction. So it goes for mentation: making a decision is a process, not a single event.

What does this have to do with baboons rolling back their upper lips in threat displays, or humans amassing bigger fortunes than they could spend in a hundred lifetimes (hierarchy, or perhaps territoriality)? It has a great deal. It tells us where the programs for these activities are encoded (not 'where' as in this particular part of the brain, but 'where' as in a particular point of the conceptual system). We can go back to our primate who has just wandered into neighboring territory. He looks around but each item that he sees fails to trigger a 'familiarity' response (whatever that is, the details don't matter). In the absence of regular familiarity responses, his arousal level starts to rise because familiarity responses exert a transient inhibitory effect on the ARAS. The process could, however, be the exact opposite, in that unfamiliar items could exert an excitatory effect on the ARAS, so that the net effect is the same. The details of the implementation of these concepts are not all-important at this stage, the object is to see whether complex, higher order functions can be explained in lower order terms.

So: a male baboon or a young adult male human (who, on the behavioral level, are much closer than baboons would care to admit) sees another of his kind approaching. Our organism knows he is still on his home turf (the environment is triggering familiarity signals in him) so his anxiety level is low. How does he know the stranger is another of his kind and not a dolphin? Primates are so proficient at detecting faces from among confusing signals (noise) that we know they are preprogrammed to do so. That is, the raw data flow from the eyes activates a preconfigured response which may start at the level of the brainstem, long before the data flow arrives at the association cortex. It is similar to the effect of a baby crying: the inherent pattern of the sound waves acts at a very basal level in the CNS to trigger a sense of apprehension; in women, this sense can readily be assuaged by nursing (or it may cause a rising sense of apprehension which can be resolved by the oxytocin released in nursing); in males, it has no such innate outlet so the apprehension continues to rise until it is resolved, either by escaping or by aggression.

However, our male is now standing face to face with another of his kind, and his level of agitation is rising. It is rising because he needs to dominate the other male as an evolutionary imperative (males low down the social scale don't get females) but the primitive part of his brain, where all this activity is taking place, doesn't know anything about social hierarchies or even about the future of the species. Bits of brains don't know anything. What happens is that a specific type of input signal activates a particular behavioral program just because there is no other possible response: the neuronal tracts activated by a species specific set of input signals (face + facial hair + scowl + hostile sounds from a male throat) travel directly to the brain centers which activate the hormonal systems needed to engage in aggressive behavior. Presumably, this activity takes place at a level similar to the way certain grating or scraping sounds can make us shiver uncomfortably. We will look at this again when talking about the Challenge Hypothesis in Chapter 8.

Everything has to be given an account in less complicated terms. In order to explain mentality, we must, as Philip Johnson-Laird noted, reduce it to the level of an automaton. This does not mean, as many people who should know better have taken it to mean, that in explaining mentality, we try to explain it away. By explaining the precise cellular mechanisms of your pain, I have not explained it away. It still hurts, where 'hurts' is an emergent function in a sentient system. Explanation means that we decompose mentality to its elements so that, when we reconstitute it, we know exactly the sequence of intervening steps that occur to produce the effects that were previously so mysterious.

So (once again), we have two males of the youthful persuasion, equal in height, weight and sexual needs, suspiciously eyeballing each other on a narrow path where only one can pass. Neither wishes to submit because submission inhibits sexual arousal; the act of submission in any male primate suppresses testosterone production, and high levels of testosterone feel good (are positively reinforcing, in Skinner-speak). The sight and sound *and* smell of the other male triggers a particular behavioral response at a level far below anything we could call rational, conscious deliberation. This is crude, primitive brain stuff straight from our primate heritage, where a specific sensory input bypasses the highest cortical centers, going directly to insensate brain centers whose function is to arouse the organism to fighting pitch with the least possible delay. The brainstem centers are preset, as it were, or pre-programmed to respond to, say, sounds of a particular frequency, or odors of a particular kind (whoever was aroused to fighting pitch by the smell of violets?) or certain colors, shapes, and so on. We are genetically programmed to strike first and agonize over the finer points later (which victors never do). Anything less than this endangers survival, and evolution is all about survival of the fittest.

"What does it mean to say preprogrammed?" you ask. "Isn't that just smuggling mentality into the brainstem?" No, it is not, because we can give a cellular (non-mentalist) account of the intent conveyed by the word preprogrammed. The idea of peripheral sensory receptors responding selectively to signals in the environment raises no concern: that idea is inherent in the term receptors. A receptor that responded to everything is not a receptor at all, just an open door. From all possible physical messages that impinge on it, a receptor is preprogrammed to respond to just one (it 'selects' the message from the noise); the selected message is sent forward, the rest bounce off. The receptor is "designed" (by the random processes of evolution) to respond only when a highly specific form of energy at a particular intensity strikes it. In the case of dermal mechanoreceptors, deformation of the physical shape of a particular molecule that constitute the receptor produces an electrotonic charge that activates the afferent neuron.

Every receptor follows this principle: the critical element of the receptor organ consists of a highly sensitive (read: highly unstable) molecule that is easily deformed by a specific energy input but by nothing else. The specific energy (pressure, light energy, chemicals, etc) allows a sudden change in intracellular ionic concentrations and is thus able to provoke a discharge, leading to an afferent impulse. The same type of effect occurs at the next step: brain stem neurons respond selectively to the afferent impulses reaching them. One pattern of impulses (let's say those triggered by the sound of a loud male voice) will activate the target neurons whereas another pattern (from a female or child's voice, or a submissive male voice) will not. Groups of neurons in the receptor area react more powerfully to particular frequencies; they "recognize" those frequencies, in anthropomorphic terms. If the receiving neuron is activated, it sends a signal to whatever centers subserve arousal and physical aggression; if it is not, then no aggression results. So a loud male voice "means" aggression to the hearer.

"Right," you reply, still not convinced, "if you have not smuggled mentality into the brainstem, surely you have cut the ground from under your own feet by giving a very clear-cut reductionist account of human mentality? Doesn't behavior become a matter of dumb molecules doing what they are programmed to do, just as the epithelium of the gall bladder is programmed to secrete bile? Aren't you admitting the truth of the very program you have been at pains to deny?"

No, the principle behind this is not problematic: complex behavioral patterns can be broken down into simpler behavioral units, and these can be given a rational account in terms of the physical machinery of the body. They do not, however, correlate in one-to-one relationship with their neuronal substrate. The relationship is contingent, not necessary. The physical machinery of the neuron is doing more than just acting as a conduit, it is carrying a significant impulse. Don't forget to keep the distinction between the informational input and the ensuing behavioral output. We are actually talking about the connection between the two. This is not reductionism in the sense of believing that the properties of the atoms that comprise the body determine the behavior of the body as a whole unit. We are decomposing complex behaviors into less complex subunits in order to understand how they summate within a powerful switching system to produce the final, observable outcome. We cannot, however, relate the property of "significance" to the physical machinery of the neuron. Significance is determined at a higher level than the physical. It is determined at a symbolic level, with the qualification of a two-level system of cognition, the innate and the adaptive.

For example, our male-type creature, growling and swaggering on the narrow path, would not have been aroused if he had come across a photograph of the other male nailed to a tree. He would still perceive a face, and it might make him jump a little at first, but a disembodied face would not provoke aggression (except a bit of posturing for the benefit of any females who might be watching: "My gosh, imagine him putting his election poster in my territory. If I ever see him in the flesh, he'll be sorry..."). If the photo had been upside down, he would have been less aroused, but more if it had been in color. A voice echoing through the trees or down the street would be more effective at arousing him but that's what hearing is: a long-distance alerting mechanism. The smell of another man is effective at levels we really don't understand (the smell of a milky baby or a fish doesn't do it) and so on. So all these stimuli come together and, as a whole, they precipitate an aggressive behavioral response that, separately, they can't achieve. It is the gestalt that counts, not the elements. The gestalt exists only as a pattern of codes in an informational space generated by the brain. Granted, the innate cognitive system constitutes a very limited informational space with little ability to project beyond the next few moments, but it is the minimum we needed for survival.

"OK," you counter, "but you still haven't answered the question. Why is this not just reductionism à la mode, reductionism by subterfuge? For all the cognitive lipstick, it still grunts like a reductionist pig." Once again, the answer is no, it is not reductionism by subterfuge. If it were just a case of "dumb molecules doing what they are programmed to do, just as the epithelium of the gall bladder is programmed to secrete bile," then wherein lies human creativity and other abstract functions? I can say to myself: "I've had enough of doctoring, I think I'll be a gardener." The gall bladder can't suddenly decide: "I've had my fill of bile, I think I'll make ice-cream." Firstly, the precise matter-energy relationships of the cellular machinery in the secretory pits of the gall bladder cannot make ice-cream. It's bile or nothing. Second, gall bladders can't decide anything because they don't have the switching power. That type of machinery doesn't exist in them.

Don't forget we are talking about the innate cognitive system, not the adaptive cognitive system. This is one very dumb system, it comes to us more or less unmodified from *H. erectus*. Human nature (because that is what the innate cognitive system is) is nothing more than higher primate nature. This is the system that drives humans to the depths of irrationality, like nuclear arms races, genocide, institutionalized greed leading to GFCs and so on. We are not yet talking about the truly abstract, adaptive cognitive system (Turing's universal computing machine) that allows us to devise natural logarithms (that are promptly used to build bigger nuclear missiles; what the adaptive cognitive system devises, the innate cognitive system debases). So yes, in one sense, this is a form of reductionism, but it is informational reduction, not "mere reductionism" because its mechanisms can be over-ruled by an informational input from higher centers. In human mental function, reductionism comes to a halt at the level of the elementary symbolic functions; it can't go any further, because the relationship between the symbols and their physical substrate is contingent, not necessary. To rephrase that, physical reduction will stop somewhere as there is a final point beyond which it cannot proceed. These "final particles" were once named atoms, from *a* (not) and *tomic* (can be broken or cut). A-tomic particles, particles that cannot be cut, hence atoms; but we goofed, we set the limit too high and a-toms turned out to be very tomic. But it would appear that the a-tomic level for an informational entity is the level of symbols; if we try to go below that, we destroy the informational level itself.

"It's just a matter of switches being open or closed," you object. "In your schema, symbolic computation becomes a matter of mechanics, a matter of which path the impulses can take through a maze. That, surely, is a matter of 'mere physics' in that, if a switch is closed, they get through but if it is open, they don't. Why is this necessarily non-physical or immaterial in nature?" Fair question. Sometimes the response is something like: Gold is a physical substance but something about it makes it different from, say, lead. It has two aspects, one a cluster of physical properties, and the other a cluster of mental attributes. Our neuronal switches are the same, in that they have physical properties and mental attributes.

You jump on this: "Pure word play," you scoff. "All you have done is shift that which requires explanation from the switches or the gold into the head. This is exactly what Skinner tried, with his 'creativity-inducing environment.' You'll have to do better than that." I agree, so here are two responses to the "Switches are physical, therefore what they switch has to be physical" objection. First, switches are indeed physical but what they switch is not. They are not switching impulses as just any old impulses skimming around the brain, they are switching impulses that carry a precise significance in terms of a set of predetermined rules. These impulses are set in action by semantic imperatives, by the meaning the organism needs in order to survive. That duality, of the physical impulse and the "something else" that the impulse carries, is at the core of the concept of information processing. If we could not have Shannon's "perfect analogy" between the switching functions and the laws of the particular semantic system, then we wouldn't have any sense of being alive, of being something that a dead thing is not.

Second, you could, if you wished, go through the calculator and change the settings on all the memory cells to your heart's desire, but it would never calculate again. It would only spew out garbage because, unless you know the correct codes, you could not reprogram it. And the codes are lodged in a human head, as a bunch of irreducibly mental properties, so we're back to where we started. You cannot get rid of the mentalism, which is precisely what Skinner tried, but failed to do. By trying to reprogram the calculator with a screwdriver, all you are doing is setting up an infinite regress, chasing the intelligence further and further down the road, but it's always there, lurking in the background, smirking at your efforts to stamp on smoke. It is not possible to get rid of mentalism by redefining it as physical. Chalmers said something like this: "You can redefine consciousness as a ham sandwich, but that doesn't get rid of the hard problem of consciousness."

"One more objection," you say. "You said DNA is just crude, lock-and-key 'information,' not information at all. Its function depends wholly on its physical structure which cannot be divorced from its medium. Remember sickle cell anemia, in which hydrophilic glutamic acid (MW 147) at the sixth position in the β-globin chain of hemoglobin is replaced with hydrophobic valine (MW 137). A tiny physical change in a giant molecule of MW 64000 causes it to fail. So why should just one change in a switch not cause the computation to fail? That, surely, proves it is all, at base, nothing more than physical?"

No, it doesn't. It proves that codes are utterly dependent on their physical substrate but it doesn't prove that codes are, in themselves, physical. Once a machine is set up according to a code, such that its functional output is determined by the code and not by the machine's operations as a physical machine driven by the laws of thermodynamics, then any alteration in the code itself will cause the machine's output to degrade. We could, of course, randomly reset as many switches as we like and, as long as we used the same code to counteract or contradict those changes by resetting other switches, then the output would not be affected. We can reset any computational machine to produce any output, or we can reset the machine to negate those changes, but we can't reset any physical machine to produce any output. Geese can't lay golden eggs but humans can *think* about geese laying golden eggs. There is the difference, geese exist in the material realm while thoughts of geese are immaterial.

A code does not exist until it is written on something. The idea of a code without a physical medium is the stuff of magic. That is why the mind, as formulated here, does not survive death. However, the mind is something the brain is not, because minds have properties that are not also properties of brains, and vice versa. Mental properties are not magic, they are natural, predictable, just as the properties of a computer are predictable while it is still on the drawing board (if anybody uses drawing boards these days). But their expression in a physical medium does *not* mean that the message is physical *in nature*. The repeated attempts by so many philosophers, psychologists, neurophysiologists and psychiatrists to elide that difference, to conflate mental and physical, have led only to fractious squabbling and wandering in circles. The mental and the physical are not the same, and no amount of hammering and hacking will make them fit in the same box.

We need to press on, to give an account of the higher order system that can (sometimes) over-ride the crude system that evolved in East Africa two million years ago. I am not suggesting the innate cognitive system isn't important, because it is: if anything can destroy the human race, it will be because we have relinquished control over this primitive system. But first, a digression to another ancient part of the mind: sensation.

7.4. The Innate Cognitive System II: The Experiential Mind.

Is sensation a digression on the path to abstraction? Following Chalmers' lead, I have characterized the mind as bicameral, a dual system within the mental-physical duality, where the silent, high speed decisions of the cognitive system are of a fundamentally different nature from whatever it is that happens to produce the experiential mind. The cognitive system is itself a duality, of the innate and the adaptive, but the experiential mind, the fun bit, seems different. We can divide it functionally if we wish, into the exteroceptive part and the emotional part, but that seems a little artificial as there is nothing to suggest that the mechanisms behind the faculty of, say, pain, are any different from the perception of a sense of anxiety. At this stage, it seems like perception is perception, whether by sight or as an emotion, while any differences are a matter of programming. The difficulty is that the experiential mind is also very old: I don't see the slightest reason to suppose that, when a chimp looks a fruiting banana palm, it sees any more or less than when I look at the same tree. Agreed, I have a great deal of information that the sight of a banana can bring forth, such as the fact that all five hundred million existing banana palms are clones of just one plant a long time ago, but that's not of the same class of events as the experience of seeing a tree. The experiential mind has been around a long time, long before we acquired the intellectual machinery to work out the principles of cloning.

What *is* the nature of experience? In a sense, this defines us: our daily lives are dominated by our sensations. The information we use in the battle to survive just chugs along underneath, quietly making its boring decisions and allowing us to devote our attention to having a good time (or struggling with a bad time, it depends on where you were born). In a few words, I can't explain the nature of experience. It is just that, an additional modality that allows us to think we are something, as distinct from computers which don't have any such inner life. As far as we know, they don't have a life at all, any more than a lump of steak has an inner life, any more than a bit of fingernail or a tree or a microbe or a rock. In fact, I'm not sure if you have an inner life, but I have to act as though you do, and if I act that way, I can predict what you will do with considerable accuracy. If I assume you are having much the same experiences as I am having, "putting myself in your shoes," as they say, then you are no more a mystery than I am to myself. Still quite a mystery, but a predictable mystery. So back to the nature of experience, the central point of this section.

In fact, there is no central point or, more accurately, there is but I don't know it. I can make only a number of peripheral points. The experience of a sensation of any kind remains a brute fact, a raw given not open to further analysis or explanation. I see a banana: end of discussion. How I *know* it's a banana and not a canary is a matter for the cognitive system, and a fairly elementary part of it, as chimps can certainly tell the difference between a banana and a canary (bananas don't squawk when you bite them). Go back a step: I see yellow, or I see a color that I can't name (I can always tell the difference between a color and a sound) but I have the experience and cannot decompose it in any way. There is always a brute fact blocking further explanation. Birds can respond selectively to yellow, and can discriminate finely between shades of yellow; can they also "see" yellow, as we can? We know they can discern shapes with remarkable accuracy, and can detect the slightest movement in their central visual field, equivalent to a single leaf in a forest moving half its diameter at a distance of two hundred meters, but is it of the same rich, fulsome nature as our experience of yellow? Imponderable at this stage of our knowledge. All we know is that, with their few visual associative neurons, they easily achieve the same levels of visual discrimination as we can.

It would seem, then, that the experience of seeing yellow is the product of an ancient part of the brain, a part capable of generating an immensely complex illusion in its own informational space on next to no computing power. Very interesting. It says that people who are trying to devise the concept of self-aware computers using massive computational power are probably heading in the wrong direction. It's like playing chess: it doesn't really matter how much computing power you have, if you try to solve the problems by brute force, any computer will wear out before it finishes a single game. It's not the computing power, it's how you organize it, which is exactly what Turing worked out long before you or I were born. The brain generates an informational space, and this informational space constitutes the experiential realm of mind. It's an extremely fast (split second changes in real time), incredibly accurate (Was that a leopard hiding on the next ridge or just a shadow in the grass?), multimodal (Yes, I can hear you and see you) system with an amazing range of sensitivity. Hearing is so sensitive, a power range of approximately one trillion times, that we use a log scale to measure it.

Conclusion #1: the sensory sphere is not a unity, it is comprised of a number of functionally and logically independent modalities. Whether and what I can hear is totally distinct from whether or what I can see. The experiential realm is actually a dozen or more contingently-related realms with a lot in common but not enough to say they are necessarily a unity. Each sensory experience is generated separately from all others but we tend to lump them together for convenience, just because they are so different from the bit that we see as uniquely our selves, the capacity for abstract thinking.

Conclusion #2: We presume that the cortical machinery used for generating one sensation is similar to that used for another, meaning we haven't been able to find a major difference between the various sensory areas in the brain. But we don't expect any: different experiences are generated by how the data are manipulated, not by being processed on neurons with different qualities. If I connect my second cranial nerve to my eighth, I will "hear" what you look like. Transplant a bunch of auditory association cortex to a hole in Area 18, connect all the loose neurons and you will still see perfectly well. You will not have a patch of sound in the middle of your visual field. Sensations are generated in a fairly primitive part of the brain: in hypoxia, the computational faculties are lost first. A confused person (medical confusion, that is) can still see long after he is unable to string two words together. Damage to Area 17 produces cortical blindness, but there may still be discrimination at more basal levels. Strictly speaking, the experience of seeing yellow is irrelevant to the task of discriminating yellow, as any industrial robot proves.

Conclusion #3: The experience of a sensation does not draw heavily on the brain's computing power. It must be a clever, recursive property of the relatively small numbers of neurons involved, a programming trick, we might say in another context. Of course, it would be: evolution would soon grant an advantage to the organism that could generate a sensory field with a small part of its brain, leaving more brain to the important tasks, like fighting and sex. Why recursive? It has to be. If the sensory realm simply projected forward in the sense of a Cartesian theater, then it would require an Observer to complete the chain, but that leads inevitably to an infinite regress. The information has to act back on itself but not just in the sense of a feedback loop, as developed by Wiener in his work on cybernetics, more in the sense of the informational space operating upon itself.

Sensation, of course, is synthetic, it is the *illusion* of something: yellow does not exist outside the informational space generated by a suitably equipped entity. Can birds see yellow as I see yellow? I don't know, but they can certainly discriminate different yellows remarkably well. That doesn't count, of course, any spectrometer can do that. Can chimps see yellow? They have to; just as chimp hair is keratin, their hearts have a Bundle of His, their ears look like ours and their blood pigment is hemoglobin, they have to see yellow. These things did not arise de novo with *H. sapiens;* we did not, as it were, hit the ground running with all systems go. Everything we have came from something that went before, including language. Compared with ours, is the chimp visual system as rudimentary as their language system is next to ours? I doubt it, their visual cortex is large and their eyes are relatively bigger than ours. They pass every visual test as well or better than we do, so it seems most likely that when they look at something, they see it as distinct from "see" it. And that is about all I can offer on this intriguing and vitally important topic. All that remains is to fit emotion in with the sensations.

7.5. The Innate Cognitive System III: The Emotional Mind.

Emotion was defined in Chap. 5: "An emotion is one of a range of experiences occurring in inner subjective space; with an ineffable visceral quality that is entirely real to the subject but that cannot be communicated or shared in any way." The general principles of emotions as an output state were outlined in Chap. 6. As perceptions, the emotions have a great deal in common with the ordinary sensations. In a sense, they are like pains that we switch on ourselves, except they are generated in the brain rather than the periphery and are thus not localized An emotion is generated on demand by an instruction sent to certain dedicated brain structures whose activity then loops back to be perceived in much the same way as the sensations, i.e. as a real, vivid, wholly private and incommunicable experience. This formulation is totally opposed to the Freudian model, in which emotions are like liquids that are manufactured and can be stored under pressure deep in the brain until they burst free many years later to swamp the rational functions and drown the common sense. Or something like that.

In rough terms, the cognitive model says that an emotion is the result of an ordinary decision, rationally reached in accord with the various rules by which I run my life. I have a huge set of rules buried somewhere; something happens to me or around me; that information interacts almost instantly with the appropriate rules (how are they selected and activated?); a response is generated and dispatched to the effector organs. But in this case, the effector organs are a very complex system of subcortical structures whose efferent pathways return to the cortex. That is, there is a loop from the cortical, decision-making (executive) areas, down to the telencephalon and back again via thalamocortical fibers. Activity generated in the subcortical nuclei is routed back to the cortex where it is treated like a normal or even an unusual sensory experience.

All emotions are the result of a decision; not all decisions are taken in full awareness as they are too fast to apprehend or reverse. So the Freudians, who said emotions are generated unconsciously, were right, but the cognitivists, who said they were the result of a decision, were also right: they are caused by unconscious decisions. But alert readers will surely have noted that I never use the word 'conscious,' so what does it mean? It means that not all decisions can be introspected. Try the arm-raising experiment again. You can raise your arm until the cows come home but you will not be able to observe yourself in the act of making the actual decision itself. It is not that sort of decision. Decisions are too fast, just a momentary flicker of electrochemistry in a few cortical modules somewhere in the brain. We do not have to be aware at the moment of a decision for it to be ours. Emotions, however, are a little different in that we can often not detect the reasons even after the event.

In general, an emotion is an inner perception, generated in response to an observable event or a memory, that is private, vivid and incommunicable. Emotions function to impel and reinforce behavior; they contribute a powerful but primitive and unsubtle factor to the total causation of behavior. Again, there is every reason to believe that most higher animals have an emotional life. They have the perceptual apparatus to be aware of their surroundings, they have the subcortical centers that we believe are important in our own emotions, and they display behavior that seems a very close parallel of what we would call emotionality in ourselves. Perhaps they do, perhaps they don't, but if we act as though they do, we can safely predict their behavior just as we do for another human.

Why should we consider emotions again in a section devoted to the innate programs of the mind? Only to reinforce that they are primitive, unrefined and very powerful. We can usually justify our behavior by an effort of intellect but a very large part of what we do it is driven largely by an aspect of ourselves that has more in common with the chimps than it does with it does with any rational processes. Greed, dominance, possessiveness, sexual predation, power, lust, savagery, xenophobia, the blind fear of uncertainty, all the things that really mark us as humans are, with few exceptions, the products of the parts of the brain and our programs we have in common with our closest cousins, the great apes.

Perhaps this seems a little pessimistic, but would you give an angry ape a machine gun?

7.6. The Adaptive Cognitive System

In a sense, this section is unnecessary. I want to argue that humans have a considerable capacity to make rational decisions, but you may feel this is hardly a revelation. The computer I am using is the result of rational decisions. Agreed, the motivation for those decisions may not have been entirely rational but, like an ICBM, it could not have been built without true rationality. True rationality? The ability to devise and then function within a rule-abiding system; the ability to comply with a predetermined calculus in order to predict the outcome of events; the capacity to manipulate abstractions consistently, to draw valid conclusions from abstracted information, and so on. Within the decimal system of arithmetic, 1+1=2 is rational. 1+1=10 is also rational, but not in a decimal system, only in a binary arithmetic. Scientific research is supposed to be rational but often isn't; one way we keep it rational is by elevating the role of criticism in science to a compelling duty of all people involved. Another way is by insisting on transparency in the process of research; these are rational responses to the problem of irrationality in science.

I don't think I need to do more to prove we have a rational capacity. The questions that arise are: what is the nature of that capacity? Is it innate or acquired? How is it instantiated in the brain? How does information enter the process of rational manipulation and, more to the point, how can the answer return to the real world? We can try to answer some of these questions.

What is the nature of the rational capacity? It is a computational nature, the ability to reduce concepts to their elements and manipulate those elements, integrating information from a variety of sources and then reassembling it to yield a single outcome. We don't know what form these computations take; I am inclined to believe we may never know, just because reading the brain's codes may prove technically impossible, but that doesn't worry me. Our rational side is not such a problem. It is when rationality is kidnapped to serve the irrational that we should start to worry.

One question that does interest me relates to logic gates. If we can make logical decisions then, regardless of its form, we have some mechanism that functions as a logic gate. Maybe they are not the same as those devised by Shannon but that's not the point. The point is: are we limited in the logical processes we can undertake because of the nature of our innate logic gates, or are our logical processes free of such constraints? Most authors identify seven potential logic gates (and, or, not, not and, not or, exclusive or, exclusive not or) but, in daily use, most machines use only two, linking them in cascades to duplicate the functions of the remaining gates. How many do we have in our brains? It is probably inconsequential because we are able to make decisions *as though* we had them, and that is all that counts. If Intel can link two gates in sequence to mimic the rest, then so can evolution.

More importantly, how does information get to them and out again? The first part of that question is easy. When information from the outside world is converted into neuronal impulses at the level of the sensory transducers, it is able to enter the CNS and move around unhindered. Peripheral data can be freely shunted here and there to any center because it is already in the form of the 'common currency' of the CNS, information. If we say that the mind is an informational space generated by rapid switching of nerve impulses, then anything cast in the 'common currency' is able to enter that informational space without theoretical restriction. It is an undeniable empirical fact that afferent tracts carry information coded in nerve impulses; therefore, in this formulation, there is no conceptual barrier preventing information from the peripheries entering the neuronal tracts that form the computational brain, and participating in the processes of data manipulation. Information in the afferent peripheral conduits is of the same form and nature as all other information already within the computational system. In each case, the vehicle (spike potentials) is exactly the same; impulses from different neurons can communicate from one cell to the next because they use identical processes. That is, the informational content of afferent impulses needs only be transposed into the codes used in CNS processing, and the problem vanishes. Thus, on the afferent side at least, the conceptual brain-to-mind disjunction dissolves immediately: it doesn't exist, it never did, it was a pseudo-problem. So much for the easy bit.

You raise an immediate objection: "Hold it, that's too slick. You can't declare a problem non-existent just for your theoretical convenience." No, I haven't declared the problem of mind a non-event, I have said that if we redefine mind as an informational space, then information can enter it with no conceptual restriction. We are still left with the task of giving some substance to the concept of an informational space itself. In one sense, I don't have to as this computer is operating in an informational space.

Now we move forward one step, to the process of manipulation of the data. The actual mechanical process of data manipulation now represents no particular problem. We understand in considerable detail how networks of neurons function as switching devices, based in the standard view of neurons as conduits and relays. For the purposes of generating an informational space, it is what happens at inter-neuronal junctions that counts. Impulses are either projected forward or blocked, depending on the "setting" of the pre- and post-synaptic elements. The process is mechanical (actually electrochemical) but the function is semantic. The switches are switching information. They are not random, as their state is determined by a calculus so that the symbols which the impulses represent can be sorted according to the demands of the calculus and not of the material world.

Consider a small switching system with 1000 elements. If it were wholly a physical system then, by the statistical laws of thermodynamics, 500 would be open on average and 500 closed over the system's lifetime. If, however, the system is governed by a calculus, then one switch could be open and the rest closed for the lifetime of the system without breaking any laws, but it would cost energy. If there were no spare energy, then the calculus would break down and the system would "die." That is, in computation, the normal process of the neurons as tiny physical machines is taken over for another purpose, that purpose being to compute an outcome which, in the absence of the calculus, would be vanishingly unlikely. Computation costs energy, so each computation increases entropy faster than would otherwise occur; maintaining an informational space is not impossible but, over a period of time, it would just never happen by chance.

The question then arises: what determines the actual state of each switch? Answer: a prior calculation. Yes, that means an infinite regress but it started one day, probably prior to birth, and one day, it will end for all of us. The instructional set that determines the state of the switches that constitute the machinery that generates the informational space called mind is itself constantly modified and remodified by daily experience. It never stops. The brain is a ceaseless ferment of activity as the total instructional set modifies itself to deal with incoming data and calculate the maximal chances of survival (mainly the innate cognitive system) and of higher abstract purposes (the adaptive cognitive system).

This point is important: the brain never sleeps. True, the incoming data flow slows during sleep but it doesn't stop. Even during profound sleep, incoming information from the peripheries is processed and decisions made, albeit at a very low level, while the remaining modules or algorithms are only temporarily put to rest. Even before my eyes are fully open, they have data to process, the switching resumes and the mind comes to life, otherwise known as awakening. With luck, the mind is refreshed, but it is otherwise still the same mind as went to sleep the night before. It is the process of switching information that generates the space called mind, not the silent algorithms through which that information percolates. The rules are not the mind; they constitute an informational framework, they are part of the mechanics of mind but, without something to work on, they are silent. They just sit in the background, waiting for something to come their way, then they are activated and I become aware of something around me, some memory, some emotion or something I have to do.

The physical state of the brain's switching devices is, of course, a physical matter but that does not account for them. A statue is a material thing but there is more to a statue than the lumps of metal covered with bird poo. Why is the metal there, in just that garden, sitting on just that plinth, with just that pose and facing just that direction? These questions are not answered by the physical arrangement of metal and stone, which are only the efficient causes. The final cause is the *desire* of the burghers to *honor* and *commemorate* the *good* works of their *esteemed* colleague so that *coming* generations will be *suitably awed* and *respectful* of his *outstanding* achievements. All the words in italics are irreducibly mental in nature. We cannot escape this quandary. People say: "Because the emergent informational space depends on physical switches, then it is itself necessarily physical in *nature.*" This merely shifts that which requires explanation from one point of the causal chain to another. Yes, the neuronal circuits are physical entities, but what set them in just this state and not another? Mentality cannot be explained away by stealthy replacement of mentalist terms by physical terms, it simply pops up somewhere else. Mentality is a bit like debt: you can't borrow your way out of debt, all you do is shift it around the economy.

How are the neuronal switches reset? That is a routine matter of neurophysiology, of blocking and facilitating synaptic transmission. Why are they reset? Because an instruction arrived. Where does the instruction come from? Other neuronal switches. And what happens to the switches that have been reset? They, in turn, reset more blocks of switches. *Moto perpetuum,* the output of one set of switches becomes the program for the next, an endless recursive process of modifying and remodifying the physical basis of the informational space called mind, just as Turing predicted.

Now we are making progress. We have seen how information is extracted from the environment by the peripheral receptors and converted to data the nervous system can accept for transmission. It is then shunted to the part of the CNS that manipulates data for processing, prior to being dispatched via the efferent tracts to the various effector organs. So far, so physiologically unremarkable, but the last step is also unremarkable. There is nothing difficult about the processes by which skeletal muscles are activated by signals in the peripheral nerves. The motor endplate was one of the first forms of synaptic transmission to be described in detail. Anesthetists fool with motor endplates every day; they hold no mysteries. The autonomic system has also been subject to a massive research effort. Control of the various bodily functions is becoming clearer, and drugs to modify or rectify these functions are in daily use by billions around the world. Other hormonal systems are yielding their secrets as technology advances rapidly on all fronts. So where is the mystery?

We can summarize the position as it is now:

- Information enters the nervous system via the peripheral transducers in the form of nerve impulses. *This is not an ontological problem.*
- The information is then manipulated by means of switching its neuronal base. *There is no ontological problem in the processing of information by a suitable device.*
- That information is then sent to the effector organs via efferent nerves that mirror the input side. *There is no ontological problem in this sentence.*

Voilà. I conclude there is *no body-to-mind problem, no mind problem, and no mind-to-body problem.*

Be careful:

- I stand on my right leg. I do not fall over. I conclude that *my left leg does not support me.*
- I stand on my left leg. I do not fall over. I conclude that *my right leg does not support me.*
- Therefore, I conclude that *my legs do not support me.*

The success or failure of this model depends entirely on the validity of the concept of information. Is information a real thing? Can it be extracted from the natural world? Can it be manipulated, cut up, bundled and squirted down pipes? And when it gets to the end of the pipes, can it then act upon the material world to produce measurable changes? Let's see: Yes, yes, yes and yes. Just to be clear, is information insubstantial, unlocalized and colorless, odorless and tasteless to boot? Yes. But it can still act on the real world? Yes, provided the operator hasn't forgotten to bring the correct three pin plug. So what is the three pin plug in the case of *H. sapiens*? It is the exact point at which the individual neurons cease being elements in a set of logic devices, and convert back to their elemental function as conduits. In practice, that means a synapse. It is where the intracerebral connections (about 97% of cerebral neurons) contact the first stage of the efferent neurons, such as the pyramidal tracts or the brainstem nuclei of the cranial nerves, etc. When molecules of neurotransmitter from the last computational neuron cross the synaptic cleft to activate the first post-synaptic neuron, we are looking at the point of contact between mind and body.

7.7 Conclusion

Taking all this into account, is it fair to talk about a molecular resolution of the mind-body problem? In principle, I believe it is fair to do so. We have to think in terms of the molecular machinery of the neuron that allows it to be reset in a fraction of a millisecond, because if that is not available, there can be no switching of data and, hence, no mind. It is the peculiar architecture of the neuron which sets it apart from all other somatic cells. Normal cells are tiny, complex and very precise machines taking physical, chemical and energy inputs to process them using predetermined mechanisms, wholly for the purpose of turning those inputs into very specific physical, chemical and energy outputs. Normal cells function strictly according to the laws of the natural realm, including all laws of thermodynamics as we understand them, just for the work they do.

The neuron, on the other hand, has no function other than to function. It flicks on and off; on and off; that is all it does. It has no output. It consumes energy solely in order to acquit its function of restoring itself to *status quo ante* with no traces of what went before. In respect of its physical function, it increases entropy but it does no work in the physical realm. Its value lies in its capacity to underwrite the manipulation of data in order to reach decisions about how the matter-energy dispositions of the natural world should be altered. For that reason, it is unique in the body.

Part II:
Testing the Biocognitive Model of Mind for Psychiatry

"...when the paradigm is successful, the profession will have solved problems that its members could scarcely have imagined and would never have undertaken without commitment to the paradigm."

Thomas Kuhn

Testing the Biocognitive Model: Testosterone and the Challenge Hypothesis

"Why is propaganda so much more successful when it stirs up hatred than when it tries to stir up friendly feeling?"
—Bertrand Russell.

8.1. Introduction

So far, we have been developing a model of mind to provide psychiatry with the basis of a model of mental disorder. The biocognitive model of mind is a model of natural dualism, relying on the notion of information as a real but insubstantial matter, functioning as a virtual machine that accepts information from the real world, manipulates it and then sends it back to act on the world. At this stage, it is probably a good time to check the validity of the model by testing it against a real world event. The purpose is to see if it has sufficient explanatory power to make sense of something that seems so familiar that it is not a problem but, at its core, it is very puzzling indeed. If it can do that, then the biocognitive model is in a very strong position because it will have achieved something no other explanatory model in the history of psychiatry has even been able to do. If not, then at least it may make a more interesting story than the old "mental disease is brain disease" mantra.

This chapter will test the model against a phenomenon called the Challenge Hypothesis, a theoretical explanation of an almost universal behavioral syndrome relating testosterone and aggression. In males of many species, including humans, a surge of testosterone is seen immediately following a threat or challenge. High levels of testosterone are closely related to aggressive behavior, and aggressive behavior is needed to deal with the threat, so the hormone can be seen as readying the individual for defense. At the same time, a considerable part of psychiatric practice involves dealing with aggression or its effects. On every scale, aggression is a major public health issue for psychiatry, and for human society in general (remember Mutually Assured

Destruction?). Psychiatry, however, has no means of addressing the question of aggression, apart from labeling it a "chemical imbalance of the brain" (unless it is aggression by kings, presidents and prelates).

Even at its present level of development, the biocognitive model can integrate data from a wide variety of sources, including clinical practice, basic neurosciences, anthropology and ethology, and evolutionary theory, all the while remaining well within the limits set by the philosophy of science. Nonetheless, it is appropriate to test the new model to avoid the gloomy fates of psychoanalysis and of behaviorism. Supporters of those theories were convinced from the outset that their (mutually contradictory) approaches to mental disorder were 'scientific.' They were also notoriously antagonistic to criticism. Despite quite fanatical support among their followers, each theory failed because of flaws caused by fundamental breaches of the rules of science. It's of interest that, in both theories, the problems were well-known almost from the beginning but were firmly ignored by their practitioners.

The philosopher, Karl Popper, was of the view that any theory in science should be bold and unexpected, but it should be submitted to stringent testing to see if it has any validity [1]. If a theory fails the test, then we know for certain that it is not a general or universal rule. If it passes the test, then all it says is that the theory was right on that occasion. Refutation is therefore the only certainty available to us, and he saw this as the cut-off point or demarcation criterion separating science and non-science. Because of the discrepancy between the weight given to positive and to negative results, a scientific model with huge amounts of supportive evidence must be discarded if it cannot be refuted.

The biocognitive model for psychiatry is certainly bold and unexpected: as a dualist theory, it contradicts both the reductionism of biological psychiatry, and the monism of functionalism and other modern theories of mind. Using the challenge hypothesis, we will see whether the new theory can give a coherent account of phenomena such as social aggression, dominance and parenting. If it can offer a plausible explanatory account of how this important hormone functions, then it will be in a very much stronger position than any other explanatory model in psychiatry.

8.2. The Challenge Hypothesis of Testosterone

Since time immemorial, it has been known that the male gonads are essential to masculine behavior. Farmers have always castrated excess stock to pacify and fatten them while, for hundreds of years, boy sopranos were emasculated to preserve their ethereal voices (the practice was finally banned in Italy in 1870). The pure hormone essential for the male qualities was isolated in 1927 in Chicago and was first synthesized in Europe in 1935, for which the researchers (who also named it) were awarded the 1939 Nobel Prize in chemistry. During the post-war period, large scale manufacture began and the complexity of its biochemistry soon emerged. Testosterone is extremely widespread in nature, with practically the same hormone appearing in most vertebrates, including mammals, birds and reptiles. This suggests it appeared very early in the evolution of life on the planet. In mammals, its physiology is complex and its effects widespread.

In intrauterine life, testosterone is essential for masculinization of the brain. Neonatal boys show a high level of the hormone, roughly equivalent to pubertal boys, but this soon regresses and latency boys show more or less the same levels as girls. With the onset of puberty, secretion of testosterone rises rapidly, allowing full development of the body and reproductive capacity. Testosterone is responsible for primary sexual development (genitals and spermatogenesis) and secondary, including changes in the musculoskeletal system and in the skin and larynx, growth of body hair—and, of course, for behavior. The relationship between testosterone and male aggression, sexual and otherwise, leads to the concept of the Challenge Hypothesis [2, 3]

While the normal range of this hormone varies widely, it is not secreted uniformly and the peaks and troughs of secretion are significant on an individual basis. It has a basic diurnal surge and is also greatly influenced by activity, both sexual and physical. Beginning in about 1970, ornithologists realized that the various mating patterns exhibited by different species of birds were related to different levels of testosterone [2]. This was soon found to be the case in mammals [4], including humans [5, 6, 7]. Adult male birds show a basal level of secretion, sufficient to maintain the secondary characteristics but no more. At the start of the breeding season, the level rises to a point at which spermatogenesis can be initiated and maintained. Above this is higher level which supports the aggressive behavior needed to find a mate and defend a territory. However, once breeding is accomplished, some species show a sharp reduction in testosterone levels. These are the species whose males show typical parenting behavior. Other species, whose males are promiscuous or aggressively gather harems while taking no part in raising the offspring, show no reduction or even a further increase.

It is generally agreed that these strategies of masculinity are evolutionary responses to the demands of breeding. High levels of testosterone are physiologically demanding and also represent a 'high risk' behavioral strategy. A male animal can aggressively try to impregnate as many females as possible (e.g. elephant seals) but this will inevitably consume more energy and also increases the risk of injury or death. Alternatively, it can avoid conflict and expend its energy on increasing the survival chances of the few offspring that it has (e.g. most seabirds, notably penguins and albatross). The relative energy costs per viable offspring are about the same.

An animal with a high level of testosterone cannot avoid conflict. It is chemically driven, as it were, to respond to any and every perceived challenge with aggressive displays, including attacking the challenger and, if necessary, fighting to the death [3]. But there is a penalty: the act of perceiving and responding to a challenge causes a further surge of testosterone that is necessary to maintain the aggressive behavior itself. In turn, this reduces the chance of the animal ignoring challenges in order to avoid the biological expense of future conflicts. The more a breeding male is challenged, the higher his levels of testosterone, and the higher his levels, the more challenges he will perceive. The cycle can become self-perpetuating and is thereby laden with risk.

The "alpha male" is in constant danger of entering a state of excessively high arousal, as high levels of aggressive behavior must be maintained in a self-reinforcing cycle by high levels of testosterone. However, a defeated male that continues to attack will be injured of even killed, so the testosterone economy, as it were, has a safety mechanism: defeat causes a sudden drop in testosterone secretion. As a result, the hormonally-driven aggressive behavior quickly subsides, allowing the defeated male to slink away to lick his wounds and plan his comeback. In this respect, *Homo sapiens* shows the same patterns as the rest of the animal kingdom [5, 6], a matter of profound importance in human behavior.

Human males show the typical adolescent surge of testosterone that is responsible for the changes in body habitus from latency child to sexually capable young adult. The stable diurnal cycle of the hormone can be interrupted in a number of ways. Firstly, there is a group of normal variants. Most obviously, sexual activity itself causes a surge of testosterone, so the more the individual is sexually aroused, the more likely it is he will seek further stimulation. The opposite is also true: less activity leads to lower levels and thence to less interest. A wide range of normal physiological stressors, such as illness, malnutrition and pain will reduce testosterone levels, leading to a drop in sexual arousal and the aggressive or predatory behavior it generates. Psychological stressors, including anxiety and depression, are also major factors in suppressing daily and subdaily hormonal surges [7].

Second, and perhaps more significantly in humans, direct challenges to the individual's status lead to a surge of hormone [8]. If the challenge is successfully passed, the surge does not abate or even intensifies, so the successful individual is likely to seek more challenges (or fail to avoid them). Conversely, following a defeat, the level drops quite precipitously, minimizing the risks by ending the aggressive stance. Third, humans display the classic pattern of animals that share parenting, i.e. as the new father takes up his nurturing duties, his testosterone levels drop [3]. A new father is more likely to avoid conflict than a non-parenting male of the same age. Faced with a threat, fathers are more likely to snatch their children and run to safety than they are to respond aggressively. It should not be forgotten that these are general trends, not laws of behavior, as the mediating factor is a hormone whose secretion is governed by a wide range of highly diverse factors.

Since many other species show patterns of hormonal activity similar to the above, there is little of interest for psychiatry. We know that absolute levels of testosterone are a poor indicator of aggressive behavior; that established patterns of sexually antisocial behavior are often not much influenced by artificially reducing testosterone levels, and so on. However, humans show one feature that no other species displays: surges of testosterone in anticipation of an unseen challenge. For all other species, the defending male must have direct sensory evidence that a challenger is nearing his territory (including his females). He must see the intruder, hear him or smell him. What he cannot do is something we humans do all the time: he cannot book a contest for next week. When a sexually capable man knows a challenge of any sort will take place at a certain time, he demonstrates an anticipatory surge of testosterone. If he wins the contest, his surge intensifies and he struts around, looking for more challenges; if he loses, the surge fades away quicker than it arose [8] and his behavior becomes passive and submissive. That is, the knowledge that a competition will take place this afternoon is enough to produce a surge of hormone this morning. Similarly, merely handling a gun will produce a surge which can have measurable effects on behavior [6].

For a model of mind, the question now becomes: How can the knowledge of an impending competition translate into a hormonal surge? How can thinking of a competition cause a surge in the one hormone that is necessary for success in the competition? What is the relationship between a thought and the gene expression needed to flood the bloodstream with a hormone? Is it, we could say, a fact that, just by thinking, I can change my genes? The biocognitive model of mind says that this is in fact true, that thoughts can influence gene expression, and offers a model of the mechanisms involved.

The brain's various neurohumoral systems are of the same order as any other output state, i.e. on the basis of a range of informational inputs, high-speed decisions are made outside the reach of introspection, and the specific systems are activated according to the body's perceived needs. Some of the most important of these systems are entirely physical with no cognitive input (in any sense of the term), e.g. the TRF-TSH-T4 feedback system controlling thyroid function [9]. This type of system is wholly physical, a biological mechanism that is closed to introspection or access by any sort of will or intent. The processes governing the body's thyroid status are entirely biological in the everyday use of the word, in that they continue to operate when a person is asleep or even in a vegetative state from brain damage. The brain's informational content, meaning its acquired knowledge, has no influence upon this system whatsoever. However, this is not true of the reproductive hormones, especially of testosterone, which is powerfully influenced by the subject's informational state, i.e. by what he is seeing and doing, and what he believes.

8.3. Psychosomatic Interaction.

The concept of psychosomatic interaction is ancient. There is probably not a culture in the world that does not accept that, in some unfathomable way, the mind and body can influence each other, and not always for the benefit of the owner. Even our resolutely reductionist modern psychiatry still retains a group of diagnoses (Somatoform Disorders) where physical symptoms are "caused" by the mind. The classic Freudian idea of the hysterical conversion reaction soldiers on, impervious to political correctness, even though the lines of causation now seem a little tangled: a genetically-determined "chemical imbalance of the brain" causes a mental disturbance which then "causes" a raft of peculiar, bizarre or impossible symptoms, but not consciously because that's malingering. I must admit I prefer a simpler sort of theory. Can the biocognitive model give us a more parsimonious theory? I believe it can, but my goal in this chapter is to convince you, not myself.

The neurosecretory pathways and the biochemistry of FRH, FSH, LH and testosterone are available in any physiology text so we don't have to review them here. What counts is this: there is clear empirical evidence of a causative connection between the centers of the brain subserving the highest conceptual tasks, roughly the prefrontal cortex, and the initiating systems that activate testosterone surges. The problem is that 'conceptual tasks' are not the type of event that we normally associate with hormonal changes. A concept is a mental event, and orthodox psychiatry has no idea what mental events are, let alone how they cause brain changes. Worse still, the example I have chosen to test the biocognitive model, the Challenge Hypothesis, isn't even a disease state, it's normal, so psychiatry can't pull its usual rabbit out of the hat, the trusty old "chemical imbalance of the brain" excuse. Testosterone surges are not abnormal, they are not disease states; they are physiology doing what it's supposed to do to keep the species going. There's no quick way out of this; we have to deal with each empirical fact as we go.

Empirical fact No. 1: A male baboon on lookout duty sees a spotted shape gliding through the scrub toward his troop. Immediately, he gives a particular yelp and rushes toward where he saw it. All the males in the troop start to bark and run after him while the females grab their infants and, with the juveniles screeching in alarm, head for the nearest trees. We know that, in a few seconds, all the adult males will exhibit quite stereotyped behavior, prancing around, barking and baring their teeth in "threat" displays. Physiologically, they will also show a sudden surge in testosterone, and we know that the hormonal surge is necessary for the appearance of the threat displays. Leopards are traditional enemies of baboons but wise leopards will not stay around to argue the point with a bunch of angry male baboons. We need to explain how a particular sight can trigger the gene expression necessary for increased production of the hormone.

In technical terms, that's not difficult. Optical recognition systems are in daily use all over the world. Your cellphone has one built into it, every supermarket checkout has a dozen, practically every ticket we buy relies on one. The input sensor "recognizes" a specific pattern and sends instructions to the gate or whatever it is supposed to do. By recognize, we mean that the particular pattern of digitized impulses leaving the sensor triggers a programmed sequence whereas no other pattern can do it. This is simple, mechanical stuff that does not rely on any hidden mentalist concepts to complete its causal chain. There may be a direct, unmodified connection between the sensor and the effector, or the instructions may be routed through a further system which integrates them with other information. This is still only the very crudest data processing such as can be seen in robotic toys or calculators.

The phenomenon of innate pattern recognition, most commonly visual but also aural, olfactory etc, is extremely widespread in nature. In the main, these responses are stronger in early life when they serve to trigger avoidance behavior (fear reactions). Innate patterns of aggression do not normally appear until early adulthood, when they quickly become very powerful influences. There is convincing evidence that humans have a similar, innate capacity for pattern recognition which is most powerful in early life but slowly fades in significance during later childhood. One of the most powerful of all is the threat display, in which an animal perceives a threat and reacts in a stereotyped way. Cats arch their backs, fluff their fur and hiss. Goannas and many snakes turn to face the threat, inflate themselves, gape widely and hiss. Ducks put their heads down, fluff their feathers and run at the threat. Giant stick insects suddenly hang upside down, their abdomen facing the threat, and open their wings to display two large black dots and an orange gash that looks like a large, hostile face. Gorillas beat their chests and roar while human males stand upright, face the threat wide-eyed, straighten their shoulders and jab a finger at the offender. Practically all animals have a threat display in their innate behavioral repertoire, and practically all can recognize the threat and respond accordingly, either by countering with their own threat display or by withdrawal and submission.

If everything from stick insects to professors reacts to a threat in much the same way, we are not talking of what might be called a 'higher faculty' (even if it is regularly found in higher faculties). That is, there is no need to explain the perception of a threat in mentalist terms. Descartes would agree: he saw the human body as a "mere machine," of exactly the same order of nature as the bodies of all other animals. Animal behavior was, to him, just a matter of simple mechanics, or maybe fairly complex mechanics, but definitely not the result of anything that approximated what humans do when reasoning. In general, any behavioral phenomenon we share with animals doesn't require a special explanation. Of course, Descartes was an ascetic soul so he would have seen dispassionate intellectualism as more desirable than, say, fighting duels. In any event, the perception of threats is universal. Practically all species show some sort of threat display (i.e. a display triggered by a threat, in which they look threatening themselves), almost always more marked or more likely in males than females. The other response to a threat is, of course, the flight reaction; make yourself scarce or play dead.

In order to have a threat display, the animal must have a way of recognizing threats: there's not much point hissing at dead leaves. But if we say, "The dog recognized the snake was dangerous," we attribute to the dog some ability called 'recognition' and the perception of danger. Next, we have to say how and where it recognizes things, and whether recognition is a member of the same class of events as, say, digestion. That is, we are already treating recognition as a mental event, but if we allow dogs one mental event, where do we draw the line? We don't want to go down this path, so we need to provide a non-mentalist explanation of 'recognizing' that will account for the same phenomena without tying ourselves in knots. The concept of an automated pattern recognizer or filter will do just this.

We can start with a simple example, of a male bird that responds aggressively to the specific color of another male in its territory. We know the bird's eye has color detectors; all we need say is that the detectors for that particular color are stronger, or more common or have unique central connections and the conceptual problem is solved. Pattern recognition occurs at the level of the retina, which is certainly mindless. When the bird sees that color, impulses from those detectors are directed to the areas controlling aggressive responses, and so we have a non-mentalist explanation of all the elements previously covered by the mentalist word 'recognition.' Even in humans, for example, the olfactory detectors that respond selectively to pheromones do not become experiences in the sense of the smell of peppermint becoming an experience. They bypass whatever is involved in perceiving an odor and go straight to brainstem centers controlling sexual arousal. The subject doesn't know that is why he starts to become aroused, all he knows is that it feels good and he doesn't see much reason to object.

Visual pattern recognition is definitely more complicated than this. Many animals, including humans, respond selectively to the sight of a snake, and it appears that it is the pattern of small round objects (the scales) sliding past each other in a writhing pattern that is significant. Rhesus monkeys are not concerned when they see the pattern of a duck flying overhead, but when the pattern is reversed and the duck looks like a falcon, they respond with alarm. Humans are generally not concerned by a writhing movement overhead but if they see the same movement on the ground moving toward them, they react fearfully and withdraw.

When my daughter was 15 months old, I found a young bandicoot in the garden (about the size and shape of a rat) and took it inside to show her. She was very happy to see it, and reached out to pat it. A few weeks later, I found the first tree frog of the season and took it to show her. These are very pretty, brilliant green frogs but, to my surprise, she screamed and pulled away. My son liked the frogs as soon as he saw one, but she was frightened from first exposure—and still is. When he was two, my son found a blue-tongued lizard in the garden. While it wandered around looking for snails, he was happy to squat and watch it but it kept walking away so I decided to pick it up to show him. The way to do this is to wave a hand in front of their eyes. They respond with a threat display and it is easy to pick them up from behind the neck. As it suddenly jumped back, puffed itself up and gaped with a loud hiss, my son screamed and fell backwards. While it was ignoring him, he had no fear of it but its threat display directed at me provoked an immediate fear response in him. The same thing happened with a small python a few weeks later but when I picked it up and it settled on my arm, he showed no fear of it.

There is a clear implication of complex, multisystem innate fear responses in humans, well before the age at which significant mental concepts can form. The complexity of the stimuli and the integrated response implies central processing (i.e. not just at the level of the receptor organ) but, even in humans, it is automated. There is no need to invoke anything but mechanical information processing to account for the phenomenon. In the biocognitive model, we would say that the innate cognitive system can account for these observations without invoking any problematic mentalist concepts. I think we can account for a very large part of human behavior at this level, especially the part that gets us into trouble, but the task I set the model is not of the same conceptual order.

8.4. Psychosomatic Interaction and Testosterone

Testosterone is secreted in saliva, so it can be readily assayed. The salivary level equilibrates quite rapidly with the plasma level, providing a reliable measure of the sudden changes in plasma levels that follow various events such as challenges or defeats. For some reason, it has been studied more often in tennis players than other sports but we can assume the results are general. On the morning of a big match, a player's testosterone levels will begin to rise in anticipation. They peak during the match and decline when it is over. However, the loser's levels decline much faster and much further than the winner's. Very often, the winner's levels don't decline at all or may even rise, and the longer he is involved in victory celebrations, the longer they will remain high. Moreover, the attribution of victory or defeat is important. If members of a team lose, their levels of hormone drop. If they believe they were fairly beaten, there is a sharp drop but, if they believe they were cheated or they should not have lost, the drop isn't so precipitous. If they win, they have a surge of hormone; if they think they won because they were the better team, their levels will be higher than if they feel they won because the other team had a bad day, or the umpire made a mistake [3].

High levels of testosterone are intensely reinforcing, that is, they feel good. People will do all sorts of things to feel good, and things that make them feel good by means of a surge of testosterone are right at the top of things they do to feel good. Thus, if a group of men meet in a fairly unstructured social setting, they will very soon form themselves into teams and start a competition just because it feels better than hanging around doing nothing. If females are present, the competition quickly becomes serious. If the females are available, it can become nasty. It is well-known that, in groups of women, their menstrual cycles will synchronize, hence the name of the music that evolved in the brothels of New Orleans. If the girls were all menstruating, there was nothing the clients could do but sit and listen glumly to the piano player who played a bright, cheerful sort of music called, appropriately, *rag time*. In their own way, males are very similar.

In groups of men, such as armies or football teams, the strong sense of competition and the sense of belonging or kinship provokes a surge of testosterone. It feels good to be a man in a group, so they dress up in gorgeous uniforms that conceal their imperfections and stamp up and down in unison, puffed up and sexually aroused by their own glory. A victorious army or team goes on a sexual rampage while the losers hang their heads and slink away. During the early stages of the Nazi invasion of the Soviet Union in June, 1941, some 3.25 million Soviet soldiers were captured in the most catastrophic defeat ever suffered by an army. German army newsreels (available on Youtube) show long columns of dejected troops trudging listlessly into captivity while their captors prance around in a state of high excitement. Testosterone assays would have shown profound differences between the victors and the losers. As a footnote, some 97% of the Soviet soldiers captured during that few months were dead by the following January. It was probably the greatest single slaughter in our ghastly history, and all driven by testosterone.

In the absence of physical injury, defeat is a mental perception. A tennis player knows he is defeated when he looks at the score board, a soldier knows he is defeated when he sees his colors fall. A student knows he has failed when he reads his mark on a sheet of paper (if that still happens) and a businessman knows he is bankrupted when he looks at his bank balance. Yet the act of 'acknowledging defeat' causes a sudden, massive drop in a powerful hormone, even down to levels that would otherwise be considered pathological. This phenomenon absolutely negates the model of biological reductionism used in orthodox psychiatry these days. The standard biological model says that the brain controls the mind yet here we have the very clearest empirical evidence that the mind controls the brain. How does this come about? We can start with the second part of the process, the activation of the secretory processes governing testosterone release.

Unlike some other hormones, testosterone in post-puberty males is very much under cerebral control because the first elements in the process are neurons. Specifically, FRH-secretory neurons in the hypothalamus [10] are directly or indirectly under the active control of a number of different centers, including the prefrontal cortex, which is generally assumed to play a vital role in "executive decisions." From various sources, activating neural impulses arrive at the gonadotrophin-secreting neurons in the preoptic and suprachiasmatic regions of the hypothalamus. From this point on, the system represents no conceptual problems. In humans, the gene for GnRH, GNRH1, is located on chromosome 8. It is activated to its expressive state by a specific pattern of neuronal impulses impinging on the cell body via a G-protein receptor chain. Once activated, GNRH1 immediately causes production of the decapeptide releasing factor, which travels via the secretory neuron to the pituitary portal system and thence to the anterior pituitary. There, stored LH and FSH are released into the bloodstream to travel to their target, the testicular Leydig cells. By a similar process, testosterone is rapidly produced and secreted into the bloodstream, so that it can act upon its own target organs, one of which is the brain. The critical structure here is probably the amygdala, specific nuclei of which have long been implicated in aggressive behavior. All of this seems to take one or two minutes.

8.5. Cognitive Interaction and Testosterone

That part of the cycle is not problematical. The part that is problematical is the part between the player looking at the scoreboard and glumly saying "Looks like I'm out," and his testosterone level, which was high for the competition, starting to slide down the scale. What is the nature of 'defeat' that it can cause hormones to jump around? The nature of defeat is that it is a mental state, a cognitive content or item of information which is usually not put in words but, if it were, would be something like: "Whatever I wanted has now gone to somebody else and I am left with nothing. I have to give up that ambition and walk away, knowing people are not respecting me when I wanted to be respected, or they are angry that I let them down and will turn me away...etc." In effect, defeat is the inescapable knowledge that one has slipped down the social hierarchy, losing status and approval, probably losing territory (also known as money), social bonds, sexual partners and so on. It is the knowledge that one may never be able to recover, and the emotional reaction that that knowledge triggers. Knowing "I have lost" provokes a reaction of a similar form (but different content) to "There is a threat." A particular cognitive content provokes an emotional and somatic reaction which has measurable physical consequences.

What does it mean to say "a cognitive content"? There are two answers to this question. The first means the same thing as knowing that 1+1=2 (or, in this case, 1-1=0). It means being able to convey an item of knowledge to another person, to set up in him a facsimile of one's own mental state, because that's what communication is. Shannon put it thus: "The fundamental problem of communication is that of reproducing at one point either exactly or approximately a message selected at another point " [11]. This is not, however, the correct functional level as dogs can know they are defeated even though their arithmetic skills are not highly regarded. So there is another level to knowing defeat.

The second is the level of innate pattern recognition. Just as a male dog can recognize a familiar voice or that there is a stranger on his territory, so he can recognize he has been defeated. In the case of dogs, the defeat reaction is triggered by lying on his back with another dog standing straight above him so he looks up into its gaping and growling jaws. Quite often, the victorious dog will snap at the defeated animal's throat while making a rapid, high-pitched sound half-way between a bark and a growl (similar to a feeding growl), quickly moving from side to side but not causing any injury. That particular combination of stimuli is inhibitory of aggression in the defeated animal, i.e. it blocks further testosterone production and the aggressive behavior quickly fades away.

Humans can certainly experience defeat at that primitive or precognitive level, but we can also trigger the same response purely by an item of information. That is, the same knowledge that can be communicated to another person via the organs of communication also acts internally to activate the response known as defeat. I don't have to will myself to experience defeat; the knowledge is sufficient unto itself. If I have one apple in one hand and another in the other, and I conclude that I have two apples, nothing much happens. If, however, by the same processes of cognition, I conclude that his score is 50 and mine is 20, which means he will get the prize and I won't, then that knowledge in and of itself triggers the defeat response, with all that implies for my unhappy hormonal levels. Why does one item of knowledge leave me neutral while the other hurls me into despair? The question has two components, why (final cause) and why (efficient cause). The answer to the question of final cause is just this: that's what evolution bequeathed us. For a defeated animal, a sudden drop in testosterone level has higher survival value than if it stays elevated and causes the animal to keep fighting. Defeat and submission today means having another go tomorrow ("He who fights and runs away, lives to fight another day").

So it goes for humans because, as Descartes understood so well, we are also animals. The question Why (efficient cause) is currently beyond us as we have little idea of how abstract information is processed in the brain. We know that it is, we know that it is almost certainly digital and follows standard logical rules, but that's about it. However, that is not a problem. All we need to do is postulate that, by a natural process of computation, probably the same one as we use when calculating a bus fare, I can decide when I've lost and that information is able to active that innate systems of the body to do the rest. Our innate ability to perceive defeat is of the same order as the chimp's ability to perceive a stranger, or perhaps even peahens recognizing a peacock's tail. Information is processed at varying levels of complexity, decisions are made and instructions dispatched The only difference between humans and dogs is that we have another cognitive system, the adaptive cognitive system, that uses the same common currency of the CNS as the innate cognitive system and is therefore able to feed its decisions directly into the innate system, at which point it can no longer be introspected.

Of course, chimps, birds, snakes, insects and even jellyfish can respond to threats, the only differences being the levels of acuity with which those threats are perceived and the subtlety of the responses. Am I then taking this matter too far? Why should the human response to a threat be anything other than a strictly biological matter? The answer is that language alters the equation. Animals respond to threats as they perceive them. As the threat fades, so too does the arousal it has evoked. Humans, however, can be aroused solely by news of a threat ("The British are coming!") or the anticipation of an unseen challenge ("Meet me at dawn, sir!"). The information coded into a natural language can itself act as a sufficient stimulus, taking over the pathways which, in lower animals, can only be activated by direct sight, sound, scent, touch etc. Language is able to activate the highest cortical association areas into which each of the sensory modalities feeds. Information gained from a language (spoken or written) goes directly to the prefrontal areas which are presumed to subserve abstract thinking; it is a surrogate for actual experience. But from the instant the transmitted sound waves of the spoken language strike the cochlear, they are transduced into nerve impulses. In that form, they can interact with memory and other sensory inputs to activate the hormonal pathways outlined above and, in that form, they are no different from the volleys of impulses in the brain of a baboon after he sees a leopard slinking through the bush.

We can look at this again as a series of decisions leading to the stereotyped defeat reaction. In daily life, visual perceptions cause information coded in neuronal impulses to flow to systems and circuits where it is analyzed and decisions are reached. The decisions may be affect-neutral or they may be of a type that feeds directly to genetically-determined, stereotyped emotional, physiological and behavioral reactions. The adaptive cognitive system itself is affect-neutral in that its decisions do not automatically trigger intense reactions (e.g. 5 x 6 = 30). The innate cognitive system is very closely tied to the emotional and autonomic states, and most or all of its decisions do lead to intense reactions. However, decisions reached by the adaptive system can feed directly into the same systems as the innate system, either activating them directly ("50 to 30 means I'm done") or, perhaps not quite so effectively, modifying or even negating them ("OK, it wasn't so bad, I didn't really expect to win against such a big bloke and second prize is pretty good for a skinny jerk from the bush..."). The problem for humans is sorting out which is which: we are remarkably adept at convincing ourselves that our decisions are wise and dispassionate when they are, in fact, driven by motives that would not be out of place in a tribe of baboons squabbling on the veldt.

I fully accept that the primal level of threat perception is genetically-determined (as in the instantaneous decision "bigger than me," or "coming very fast," or "very loud roars," etc) but that is not central to the model. What is central is that this type of perception is itself the outcome of the manipulation of coded data inputs in the CNS, and is subsequently routed into specific brain tracts as a flow of neuronal impulses capable of activating their target brain nuclei by the standard processes of neuronal interaction. It is by this means that the mind-body problem is resolved: the output impulses of these prefrontal centers are in direct contact with the conducting neurons which transmit instructions to the effector organs. By this means, impulses arrive at the cell bodies of the nuclei of the hypothalamus and, by processes which are now fairly well-understood, activate the processes of gene expression, leading to hormone production, secretion and transmission.

To return to the Challenge Hypothesis, the suggested activating pathway is as follows: Perception of an external threat leads to physiological arousal, part of which consists of activating signals sent to the GnRH neurons of the preoptic hypothalamus. These cause secretion of the hormone into the portal system, which travels to the anterior pituitary and effects release of FSH and LH. In turn, these hormones travel to the testes where they stimulate secretion of testosterone, which then travels back to the brain and begins to prime parts of it for aggressive action, possibly after being metabolized to estradiol. It is not yet clear just what "priming" means, perhaps the neurons in the corticomedial amygdala nuclei are "reset" to a higher state of excitation, or an inhibitory block is removed, but the actual mechanism is not of great significance. What counts is that this particular nucleus becomes relatively overactive, and aggressive behavior increases. In his newly-aroused state, the alert male starts to scan the environment for evidence of further threats, and is more likely to respond aggressively to them than in the quiescent state associated with lower levels of testosterone. That is, once aroused, he is more likely to be directed to the 'fight' program of the 'fight or flight reaction.' Note that in order to act aggressively, he does not have to be sexually aroused, and vice versa: the two parameters are only contingently related. Aggression can be instrumental in achieving greater sexual success, but is not essential ('seduction by stealth' is a valid reproductive strategy, as every medical student knows). Sexual behavior and aggressive behavior overlap at many points, but they are still separate. A man in a desperate fight has high levels of testosterone but, even when he is winning, he is not thinking of sex. After he has won, then and only then will his mind turn to a different sport—of course, because his testosterone level is still very high and is slow to come down, so he needs to do something with it.

As described above, the testosterone surge prepares an individual male animal to face a challenge. If he wins, his surge intensifies; if he loses, it is inhibited at the molecular level and his aggression and his sexual drive soon die away. This is quite separate from the suppression of sexual interest by anxiety, but is probably very similar to that resulting from grief. It is by this means that we can offer rational explanations of certain clinical features of anxiety and depression. In the biocognitive model, these conditions, which were previously thought to be "chemical imbalances" of the brain, are not considered abnormal mental states. They are simply normal mental states activated inappropriately, i.e. they are biologically-determined, normal responses to standard life events. It means that the search for "the genes for" anxiety, depression etc. is misconstrued. To expand on this point, if a man with a broken leg lies down, avoids company, doesn't laugh, has little sexual drive and worries about his future, we would not regard that as abnormal: his brain is fine. It has just activated a predetermined response to the event of a broken leg. Similarly, what is called Depressive Disorder is a predetermined response to the perception of a loss. In this model, there is no suggestion that the brain of a depressed person is "diseased," any more than a grieving person or a person panicking after an earthquake is "diseased." Those reactions are just what happens when the mind perceives certain events and sends very precise instructions to the different parts of a healthy brain.

8.6. The Politics of Testosterone *Or* "This Is War, Woman. Stop Being Irrational."

We humans like to think we are very rational, halfway between the angels and the animals, as people used to say. We have, however, a great deal in common with the social apes but, at times unfortunately, our ape ancestry seems more effective in determining our social behavior. Like the apes, we are social and territorial creatures who form dominance hierarchies and, despite anything religions may have to say, these hierarchies govern our reproductive strategies. Competition for mates is perhaps the quintessential male attribute, and androgenic hormone secretion is critically important in male competitive behavior. Simply by perceiving a challenge, the requisite hormones are "switched on," which readies the individual for meeting the challenge, hence the term 'Challenge Hypothesis.' Since apes (and rats) readily perceive a challenge, the hypothesis is valid even without a generic explanation of challenges in mentalist terms. However, because of our capacity for language, the field or scope for our perceiving challenges is much broader than in other animals. For most species, a scent is required, or a particular roar, or a color or display pattern. In non-human species, there is no difficulty in seeing that this is entirely a biological phenomenon. For example, the nasal pheromone receptors may be connected fairly directly to the hypothalamic FRH-secretory neurons, and thence by the standard pathway to the amygdala or some similar mechanism. That is, for all other species, there is no thought involved in perceiving and responding to a challenge; it is a process we could easily mimic on a desktop computer with a few commercial transducers.

There is also no basic objection to the suggestion that the process by which the defeated animal perceives his defeat is biomechanical. When we lived in the bush outside Darwin, our yard was also home to pairs of orange-footed scrubfowl (*Megapodius reinwardt*), intensely territorial, mound-building, ground-dwelling fowls which form strong pair bonds for the breeding season. These birds arrive and immediately mark their territory by aggressive patrols and loud antiphonal duets at night. If another stray bird arrives, the resident pair will attack it until it flees across their border. A single intruder bird is invariably intimidated by two hostile resident birds. If, however, another pair arrives, there will be a battle for the territory that will continue until one or other pair flies away. Having a female partner causes the male to react aggressively, as does being on its home turf, but a bigger or older intruder can sometimes defeat a smaller resident. It is my impression that if the resident pair are defeated and forced out, they will separate. Defeat in battle and losing their territory seems to suppress their sexual bond.

Once again, we can explain this as a biological phenomenon without invoking mentalist concepts. Using simple data-processing concepts to explain "recognition of home territory," "territorial calls," "bonding," etc, we can account for the entirety of this behavior in biological terms. For example, a bird "knows" its own territory purely as a matter of memory (as it "knows" where the waterhole is); being on familiar territory permits a rise in testosterone whereas the anxiety of being on strange territory is inhibitory to the hormone; the sight or sound of another bird on its territory provokes a surge of testosterone; this leads to aggressive behavior which will continue until the intruder flees or the resident is injured, and fear and pain suppress its testosterone secretion, possibly via cortisol secretion [12]. After a successful defense, the resident bird's hormone levels continue to rise, so it stalks around its territory, calling loudly, and is likely to attack the resident cat that also thinks it has a claim on the territory (the cat, however, has been castrated and runs from such confrontations, but is still very aggressive in repelling feline intruders).

For humans, challenges such as "Meet me at dawn, sir," or "We'll wipe the floor with you tomorrow" have no biological equivalent. Without begging the question, we cannot translate the mentalist concept of a future threat into biological precepts. The biocognitive explanation is that the information contained in the language feeds directly into the same mechanisms governing physical threats, presumably the same as for the anthropoid apes. Depending on the proximity of the threat, there may also be a typical arousal response (increased heart rate, motor restlessness, sweating, etc.) but the main concern here is the process by which a thought ("I have just been threatened") is able to activate a hormonal system, i.e. the actual mechanism of a molecular solution to the mind-body problem. The answer is that the brain's many computational capacities, collectively called the mind, manipulate the information coded in its afferent input, and then direct flows of nerve impulses along predetermined efferent tracts to specific target organs. This is not supernatural but, at the same time, it is also not biological. The input is information in nerve tracts, the output is information in nerve tracts, and what takes place between is also a matter of information in nerve tracts.

If this formulation of the problem is correct, then we are in a very strong position to start to understand some ancient questions. Consider the phenomenon of mob excitement, such as the Roman games or modern football matches, political or religious meetings, rock concerts and the like. There is no doubt that this sort of activity is dangerous and often overflows into violence, or is deliberately used to foster violence. The biocognitive formulation of this phenomenon is quite simple: the audience goes along to the meeting with the express purpose of working themselves into a state of high arousal, because the arousal involves surges of testosterone and is inherently exciting—it feels good, as Skinner would never say. We cannot, of course, simply will ourselves to experience a hormonal surge (partly because we don't actually know that that is the cause) so we do it indirectly. If it is pure sexual arousal we desire, then fantasies suffice. In politics and football, we have to rely on other people, so it is a matter of utilizing some basic primate drives to achieve the same effect:

- Step 1: Form a social group (football club, political party).
- Step 2: Stake out a territory (including intellectual).

- Step 3: Identify an enemy (ordinary xenophobia, as displayed by baboons and birds).
- Step 4: Work each other up (battle cries, singing, displays of might, chasing stray enemies, etc).
- Step 5: Start a battle with the enemy (who have been busy doing the same on their territory).

Automatically, all members of the group will experience a hormonal surge, even those who are watching on TV, just because they see themselves as part of the fight. For laborers and clerks, for the unemployed or uneducated, for anybody who spends his week at the bottom of the social hierarchy, Saturday afternoon's wild excitement is as good as it gets. The real advantage of football games over sex is that the testosterone surge lasts much longer. And, of course, once the match is over, the last thing the supporters want is to ride the crowded, scruffy, smelly, dim train through the rain to their cramped homes, take off their scarves and silly hats and go back to being nobodies, so they try to prolong the excitement with alcohol and a street brawl. Football louts are certainly a nuisance, but it is in religion and politics that the true danger of our primate nature reveals itself.

The Nazis appealed to the dispossessed, the frightened and the insecure, promising them not just a powerful sense of belonging, but ready-made enemies (communists and Jews) to blame for all their problems and, most exciting of all, the power to hit back at the enemies. All this was done in a stage-managed atmosphere of high camp, with thumping bands and proudly strutting soldiers, with banners and torchlight parades under the gaze of adoring maidens. It was a direct appeal to primitive human nature, and it worked just because it gave the new members perhaps their first sense of belonging to something big and powerful. And with that came a huge and irresistible rush of hormone that they could not get anywhere else. None of the five steps above is unique to humans but, when it comes to organized slaughter, we have the inestimable advantage of an adaptive cognitive system.

For otherwise lonely young men, struggling with a sense of futility or meaninglessness, being welcomed into a group with an identity, a uniform, a goal and an enemy, cheered along the streets by pretty girls in an equal state of musth, is the highest excitement they will ever achieve, and it is all hormonal. We are talking of politics, so it has nothing to do with intellect. The excitement of marching together, singing together, eating and bunking together while forging ahead as part of a titanic struggle in the eye of history is mediated by the sexual hormones, but it is not thereby homosexual. It is a mutually-stimulating and reinforcing wave of self-indulgent arousal, an endlessly rising delirium which defines them as masculine and capable. This 'homosensuality,' or mutual delight in their shared manhood, overwhelms the isolation of civilian life because, for the first time, each of them knows exactly how the other feels. In their platoons and their companies, they have achieved one of the most fundamental goals of human life, to submerge into a common sense of belonging. In their comrades' eyes, they see the same sub-Olympian shades as they would were glowing in theirs (or perhaps they are but the reflections of the dancing firelight) and, inevitably, they are drawn to love each other fraternally. As long as they live, they will look back with yearning on their days under the colors. Suburbia is such a disappointment.

The same sense of belonging to "something big and powerful," of being at one with the power, is undoubtedly a factor in organized religion, and organized religion has not always been a force for good. It is easily perverted to profane ends, just because war and religion are equally thrilling to the unsophisticated. The doctrines and empires for which people are prepared to die are but the excuse, the gloss on what they wanted to do anyway, which is get excited to fever pitch. Unfortunately, people who regularly set their hormones flowing will soon want to do something with them. Religious devotion; the sublime thrill of music; armies; patriotism; the Olympic Games (sport *and* nationalism); money, power, control... These are all mediated by the innate cognitive system via its control over the testosterone economy.

In psychiatry, the close association between anxiety, mood disturbances and aggression is very well known [13]. In young men, sudden outbursts of aggression are a particular social problem. I suggest that the biocognitive formulation outlined above offers an explanation for these findings. The classic definition of an anxious personality is that the individual habitually responds to neutral events in the environment as though they were a threat. For them, becoming anxious is an immediate, unthinking or intuitive response: just like a baboon seeing a leopard, I don't have to think about danger to react to it (NB: DSM-IV does not recognize the anxious personality, attributing all anxiety disorders to Axis I mental disorders, meaning primary brain disturbances; See Chapter 16).

If we take a socially anxious young man who slips almost instantly into states of high agitation, there are only a few options available to him. He can either run and hide until he settles, get drunk or he can flip his agitation into aggression. This is done by a cognitive act, meaning a silent, high-speed decision based in his current perceptions and his memory. He does this because feeling threatened and deciding to stand and fight gives him something that running away can never do: it gives him a surge of testosterone, and that, as he learns very early in adolescence, feels very much better than running and hiding in shame. That is, the basis of a very large part of impulsive aggression (including the so-called Intermittent Explosive Disorder, 312.34 DSM-IV-TR) is not a mental disorder *qua* chemical imbalance of the brain, but is simply an unreasoned decision to give himself a sudden "charge" of hormone. Even if he is then knocked to the ground, at least he feels better about it and can be fairly sure his (few) friends won't shun him. An anxious, insecure youth with poor self-esteem who needs social approval will be more aggressive (especially in groups) than a self-secure young man who does not depend on group approval and is therefore able to laugh off insults.

Religion, politics, football and so on are not the causes of human violence but they make a very good excuse. The cause is inherent, blind to reality and works so much faster than rationality.

8.7. Conclusion

Humans are competitive; that much is part of our primate heritage. The struggle to win is wildly exciting in itself, and everybody loves a winner. The reason is simply that the hormonal surge pulsing through the winner is highly communicable, mutually reinforcing to women and to men. It is but a small step from the winning team being chaired off the field to the triumphant army sweeping bloodily across the countryside, destroying all in its path. The victors in a battle will always go on a rampage of some sort, just as the losers will want to hide their shame and misery. Competition, aggression, hierarchies and so on are phenomena of the same nature. We need to understand them because they represent a mortal danger to the species. The first step to studying them is to have a formal model that can account for the phenomena. The biocognitive model of mind is by no means complete, but I suggest that, as a model of mind-body integration, it provides a basis for understanding some of humanity's excesses.

This model suggests a mechanism of how a perceived threat, or the concept of an impending threat, are coded into the brain's activity to become part of the informational space called the mind. By this means, knowledge of an event that has not yet happened is able to activate the neurosecretory pathways subserving testosterone, the hormone that will be necessary to meet the threat. Unfortunately, the same hormone is instrumental in male aggression but the process is self-reinforcing: once started, it is preferable to continue rather than endure the sense of let-down that comes from deliberately switching it off. In this sense, testosterone is not terribly dissimilar to amphetamines. Humans like fighting, it is intrinsically more exciting that routine. They like to watch a fight and they like to join in a fight, so as long as we encourage people to get excited at football matches (with bands, alcohol and cheer squads) or at political rallies, we had better get used to the idea that, every now and then, one of these events is going to spill over into violence. The same goes for standing armies. As long as we insist on having large numbers of perfectly healthy, intelligent and well-trained young men standing around with weapons and other stimulants to hand, then, every now and then and despite all precautions, something is going to blow up, as they say. It's unavoidable, it must happen as surely as accidents will happen if children play with knives. It's just a matter of time, the ebb and flow of statistical drives will eventually win.

As for psychiatry, the so-called "chemical imbalance" concept of aggression is no better than an ideological catch-all that inhibits inquiry rather than stimulating it. The biocognitive model has considerable explanatory scope but it has the further advantage of blurring the boundary between normality and mental disorder without pretending to explain badness by incorporating it in madness. Humans do terrible things but it is a normal consequence of their primate physiology, not mental disorder. Idi Amin was not mad. He simply enjoyed murdering people, on the same level and for the same reasons as other people enjoy killing foxes by chasing them with dogs, shooting ducks or catching marlin that can't be eaten. It is inherently exciting. For the thrill of the chase, sober morality can never defeat the joy of wickedness.

If psychiatry persists in its crude, reductionist approach to mental disorder, then it will eventually be sidelined by other, more powerful models of explanation. You could say that psychiatrists have become the victims of their own myth of superiority, unable to accept that the idea they championed has been defeated because admitting you have lost is not as much fun as telling each other that you are still winners. As Kennedy noted: "The greatest enemy of the truth is very often not the lie—deliberate, contrived, and dishonest—but the myth, persistent, persuasive and unrealistic. Belief in the myth allows the comfort of opinion without the discomfort of thought."

So why is propaganda so much more successful when it stirs up hatred than when it tries to stir up friendly feeling? Because hating feels so good. Oh, the joy of a testosterone rush.

9
Testing the Biocognitive Model: The Iron Law of Oligarchy

"An autocratic system of coercion, in my opinion, soon degenerates. For force always attracts men of low morality, and I believe it to be an invariable rule that tyrants of genius are succeeded by scoundrels."

—Albert Einstein (1931)

9.1. Introduction

Among aviculturalists, it is common practice to put pairs of King Quail (*Coturnix chinensis*) in aviaries of larger birds to eat the spilled seed. King Quail are small ground-living birds, barely 10cm tall, but they are highly territorial. In the wild, if another King Quail enters their territory, they will attack it until it flies across the border. As soon as it is out of their territory, their attacking behavior ceases and they will start pecking energetically at the ground, as though "letting off the rest of the steam." In aviaries, however, the intruder immediately flies into the air and tries to escape, but it can't. It doesn't try to attack the resident pair itself. It doesn't try to hide because it has only one escape behavior in its repertoire, flight. It runs around frantically, beating itself against the wire as though incapable of acting aggressively in another territory. Thus trapped, the residents will keep attacking until they peck it to death. Now the interesting point is that they can't stop attacking, even after it is dead. As long as they see the pattern of another bird, they are in attack mode. Nature has equipped them with a means of repelling intruders but it hasn't given them the means of switching off the attack.

It is unfortunately the case that humans are almost exactly the same: we have inherent behavioral patterns which, for a variety of reasons, can be switched on but they do not switch themselves off again. They just keep running, on and on, until the original purpose has long been lost. Unless we learn to recognize and control these particular behaviors, they could be the end of us.

9.2. The Iron Law of Oligarchy

In his 1911 book, *Political Parties,* the German syndicalist sociologist, Robert Michels (1876-1936) described the well-known tendency of human organizations to form bureaucracies as an "iron law" of human behavior [1]. Regardless of their intentions at the beginning, he said, communities of people soon develop the familiar pattern where social, political, military and economic power concentrates in the hands of a small subgroup. Government by a small group, or oligarchy, inevitably emerges. Eventually, they take control of the larger group and divert it to their own advantage. He summarized his position in a few words: "Whoever speaks of organization, speaks oligarchy." Oligarchy, or government by the few, is just one form of government. It is opposed to monarchy (government by the one), democracy (by many), autocracy (by self-appointment), plutocracy (by the wealthy) or thearchy or theocracy (government by the divinity).

In principle, there is no reason why an oligarchy should not govern for the betterment of the many but, in practice, it has probably never turned out this way in history. Darcy Leach rendered Michel's thesis in a pithy aphorism: "Bureaucracy happens. If bureaucracy happens, power rises. Power corrupts." These authors followed the gloomy assessment of humans and power described by Lord Acton (1834-1902): "Power corrupts, and absolute power corrupts absolutely." Elsewhere, this erudite scholar noted: "And remember, where you have a concentration of power in a few hands, all too frequently, men with the mentality of gangsters get control."

We do not need to delve far into the history books to find horrifying examples of gangsters gaining control and perverting the state's industry and resources to their own ends. All too often, revolutions occur for noble aims but, within a few years, they turn on their own people and consume them. The Nazis came to power promising to deliver Germany from the suzerainty of Versailles; in twelve short years, they had brought down on this dazzling civilization of the German-speaking peoples the greatest catastrophe in their entire history. The Bolsheviks aimed to deliver the Russian people from the dead weight of three centuries of autocratic monarchy; in just three decades, they gave some forty-five million people the dead weight of the grave and most of the survivors a form of living death. Mao Zedong took power to give the Chinese people a new life but sixty million died in his murderous purges and in the chaos of his Great Leap Forward and his Cultural Revolution. In Cambodia, the Khmer Rouge fought as reforming zealots and governed as the institutionalized butchers of an historically gentle people. Closer to home (and orders of magnitude less destructive), the recent Republican administration in the US promised "compassionate conservatism," but brought military adventurism, unemployment and bankruptcy for the common people while the wealthy took home an ever-larger share of the national income.

Certain questions then arise. Why does power corrupt so surely? What social force compels the formation of bureaucratic structures? Once formed, what is there in the nature of bureaucracies that inevitably corrupts and perverts the original aims and intentions of the group?

Descriptive sociology can't answer that question because the answer is essentially a matter of human psychology at the level of the individual and of the group. So far, no theory of psychology has been able to do more than redescribe the phenomena to be explained in different terms. Behaviorists would say of Adolf Hitler that he was conditioned to act in a violently domineering way, but that seems most unlikely as his childhood was not especially awful for that time and place [2] and certainly not the worst in history. In addition, the striking feature of the acquisition and misuse of power by individuals is not the stereotypy of their behavior, but the apparently endless creativity and originality by which they take power and then pervert the goals of the group. Behaviorism may have explained the activities of laboratory rats but it contributed nothing to our understanding of this most central feature of human social behavior.

In the same vein, Freudian psychoanalysis had little of interest to say about autocracy. For all their grand theorizing, analysts were irrelevant to our understanding of the great dictatorships which blossomed so obscenely during the heyday of psychoanalysis. More recently, cognitive psychology describes but does not explain the apparently insatiable human drive for power. Finally, orthodox psychiatry does not address this issue because it has no theory of personality. Psychiatrists may be able to identify a personality disorder in a particular leader (not if he is clever and seductive) but has no explanation for it beyond the ideological catch-all of a "biochemical imbalance of the brain."

We are left with no formal psychological explanation for what would appear to be one of the most dangerous tendencies in the human behavioral repertoire. In fact, the discrepancy between the explanatory power of psychology and of the other, more typical sciences could not be greater than at this point: psychology is absolutely bankrupt. While we have the theories and technology to build thermonuclear weapons and the computers to program them, there has been no general explanation of the human attributes that drive us to build such infernal machines.

9.3. Human Nature in Biocognitive Terms.

In the biocognitive model, part of the informational content of the mind consists of the rules by which the incoming data is manipulated. The great bulk of these rules are acquired during the individual's early years. Some are acquired explicitly, i.e. by a process of direct experience or teaching, but some are implicit. Some are acquired verbally yet others, often very important rules, are acquired preverbally and the individual may not even be aware they exist. Some rules, however, are present from birth and appear to be independent of culture, the only possibility being that they are part of our genetic endowment. While they are not of the same order as, say, knowing when to serve sherry, knowing not to walk on a red signal or even knowing how to swim, these rules are still powerful shapers of human behavior. Because they appear to be innate and are more or less common to all other higher primates, some people prefer not to group them with the type of knowledge outlined above, i.e. rules in the ordinary sense of the word. Roughly speaking, they more or less equate with the concept of "human nature," the bundle of inclinations, dispositions or proclivities that are so important in our behavior but so hard to classify.

Because of the historical difficulties surrounding the concept of a "human nature," it is probably better to use the expression "higher primate nature." To an extent, this avoids the question of a metaphysical human nature by replacing it with an empirical construct built on field observations of our nearest relatives. We share many behaviors with the great apes and baboons, mostly innate tendencies and dispositions rather than absolutes. It may be the case that there will never be complete agreement over the full list of characteristics to be classed as "innate." Donald Brown [3] listed something like 460 "human universals" although many of the items on his list are derivative, rather than primary, as they depend on something higher in the list.

Nonetheless, we can arrive at quite a good list of primary innate behaviors by watching animals such as chimpanzees and baboons in the field. Just like these near-relatives, we are quite intensely social animals who form close affectionate bonds leading to the social stability that is essential for child-rearing. As part of this, we can display altruistic behavior but we are also territorial throughout the year (not related to breeding) and aggressively xenophobic. Outside the immediate demands of child-rearing, our social lives take the form of dominance hierarchies formed by competition between individuals, especially males. Like all animals, humans have the capacity for the "flight or fight" reaction in response to the perception of threats although, uniquely, we can anticipate unseen threats. Also uniquely, we have an enhanced capacity for communication, especially symbolic communication. Most people now accept that these innate inclinations are major factors in the survival and reproductive capacity of the individual, and thence of the tribe.

Other characteristics include an intense curiosity, humor, play behavior, of decoration of the body and the surroundings, and of stereotyped mourning when the social bonds are broken. There is also the odd combination of curiosity and a strong tendency to habitual or ritualized behavior, even when it serves no rational purpose. The combination of an intellectual awareness of death, curiosity as to what lies in the next valley and fear of what it might contain seems to drive the endless proliferation of theories of an afterlife. At the same time, combining the intellect with an opposable thumb gives the basis for the development and use of tools—and weapons.

It goes without saying that many of these characteristics are much influenced by the sex of the individual. Young adult males of all species are highly competitive and readily indulge in aggressive "horseplay" (i.e. that shown by colts) that quickly becomes the real thing. Males are more curious than females, more likely to explore the edges of their surroundings and much more likely to injure themselves in boisterous but unnecessary activities, especially of a competitive nature.

At this stage of our knowledge, we would tend to say that these behaviors are genetically-determined, or "hard-wired" in the modern idiom. They amount to rules, but not rules in the sense of the rules of tennis or of applying for a passport, i.e. something we can learn and teach in abstract. The innate drives are more "rule-like dispositions," and very few of us can verbalize them.

Different traits will appear and disappear at different stages of life or even different times of day. They can't all be in evidence at the same time. Their strength will probably vary from one individual to the next but they are never be far away. Their significance for human behavior lies in their enormous but largely unacknowledged influence in producing irrational and destructive behavior. For example, by any concept of rationality, warfare between human groups is shortsighted, wasteful and almost always results in the opposite of what its participants could possibly have hoped to achieve. Even though, by any dispassionate assessment, living in peace would be the rational choice, it is one of the most characteristic features of human society that we engage our intellects and our tool-making capacities to the pursuit of more and better means of slaughtering our neighbors, limited only by bringing down on our own heads whatever we had planned for our enemies.

It is difficult to know what proportion of our total behavior is driven by this innate system of rules but the inescapable point about all of them is that they are much more powerful than we would like to admit. Above all, the rules are easily activated but almost all of them have no innate means of self-termination. That is, once the aggressive drive is in play, it will act to control the individual's behavior (and thence the group's) until he or they can no longer fight. Territoriality, which includes the acquisition of possessions, spouses, etc., is the same: nobody ever stops. No king, no general, nor even a stamp collector or lover of cream cakes, has ever said "Enough is enough." Enough is never enough just because we always want more (sexual behavior is a little different because it has a goal and, once that is achieved, it is switched off—until tomorrow). It is possible to imagine that evolution did not bother to "equip" us with mechanisms for terminating these behaviors because there was no need. It is only in the relatively recent past (say eight thousand years) that humans have had the tools, the food and the numbers to start to run into the problem of innate behaviors becoming self-destructive. We have become like the King Quail in its cage: plenty of food and nowhere to run.

It should be understood that the innate elements are cognitive in the sense that they are rules, but they work through the emotions. We do not fight because it is intellectually a good idea; we fight because it is wildly exciting. In the first few months of World War I in all belligerents, hundreds of thousands of otherwise peaceable young men rushed to enlist because they thought the war would be over by Christmas and they didn't want to miss out. Most of them died. We do not collect gold or wives or snuff boxes because they are much use to us, we do it because it lifts us higher than our neighbors in the dominance hierarchy. For every emperor with a hundred concubines, there were 99 men who went without, so they either had to join the army to win their wives in battle, or accept a life of agricultural drudgery. For the soldiers, the choice between winning a wife or dying in the attempt was not so bad as to make it unreasonable. As well, there was always the choice of being a eunuch, either in royal service or in the church, and again, this did not strike poor and desperate young men as quite so unreasonable as it would seem today. It happened because the emperor needed to feel more important than his lords and was threatened when any of them took a new wife. Quite possibly, the emperor was not physically able to service his entire harem but it was enough to know that he could deny his inferiors something that they wanted: the perversity of power is its inutility.

My proposal is that Michel's Iron Law of Oligarchy results from the combination of the two aspects of human mind, the intellect and the innate or biologically-determined cognitive elements, commonly known as drives or instinctual behaviors. I believe this combination is dangerous in the extreme and we need to understand it better in order to counter it.

9.4. The Innate Need for Bureaucracy.

If humans band together for a common purpose, it will soon become clear to even the meanest intellect in the group that there is an easy or effective way of achieving their purpose, and many other ways that probably won't. Seeing this point is largely a question of intellectual ability. If the group is small and there is no particular sense of urgency, then they will be able to sit around and talk over the matter until they reach an agreement. However, as the group expands beyond a certain level, talking becomes counter-productive. It will be plain to all that the job isn't getting done. In order to achieve the goal, there has to be agreement that a small group will be given the responsibility of making the necessary decisions. That is, the group must form itself into a hierarchy, and this is something that humans also do naturally. Still in the cognitive realm, but separate from the intellect, we are driven to form pyramidal dominance hierarchies.

From studies of higher primates, we see that the purpose of dominance hierarchies is success in the mating game, but humans go one step further. From earliest times, we have recruited our innate tendency to form hierarchies into, say, building a village and, once that is done, into burning down the neighbors' village. So the group that cannot stop squabbling in order to form a tight-knit hierarchy will soon starve, or fall victim to the group that can. It is thus a simple matter of intellect ("common sense") that, in order to achieve the goals of satisfying say, the demands of food, shelter, safety, territory etc., individual humans cannot be as effective as a group. Immediately, we move into the problem of the arms race, because the group's neighbors will also have worked that out for themselves. That is, common sense is common to all humans.

This sets up the first requirement of Michel's law, that humans inevitably form themselves into bureaucracies. A bureaucracy is no more than the machinery which everybody recognizes as the most effective means of achieving a common goal. The bureaucracy functions like the veins of a leaf, sending instructions down a network to the distal extremities, and passing knowledge and products back up the channels of command so that the chief knows what the helots are doing "out there." Concentrating the power to make decisions facilitates and expedites the processes by which the group achieves its goals. However, it is what is called a "zero sum game" in that, for every person who gains a little power over the members of the group, there is one (or more) who surrenders it. A bureaucracy is the thinking head that controls the brute body following it.

In human terms, the veins of the network are lines of communication between privileged individuals, reaching directly to each other over the heads of their less-favored brethren. Perhaps they can read when the common soldiery can't; perhaps they are rich enough to have a dovecote or a mobile phone; perhaps they were born into or have earned the right to be anointed as members of a select cabal, the possibilities are endless but the principle is simple. The bureaucracy possesses knowledge, and has been given or has taken the authority to put that knowledge into effect so that the group may achieve its goal. When that is achieved, the group dissolves and everybody becomes equal again.

However, Michel's second point was that dissolution of the group never happens. Bureaucracies become all-powerful and, crucially, self-perpetuating. This is because the impetus that leads to them cannot be switched off. The intellectual wish to form a hierarchy to achieve a particular goal meshes perfectly with the human drive to dominate one's fellows. The intellectual need can be satisfied but the drive to dominate has no end. In the last chapter, I suggested that high levels of testosterone have a lot to do with this type of behavior. Nobody wants a low level of testosterone, life at the bottom is never so much fun as swinging at the top. The only means we know of terminating the drive to dominate are terror, because anxiety inhibits it, or death. Even castration doesn't work: the eunuchs of Byzantium were notorious for their intrigues.

Even though it may have been formed for rational reasons, humans cannot disband a bureaucracy because irrational reasons take over to hold it in place. Those who are profiting from it are driven endlessly to expand their power at the expense of their former peers just because they don't want anybody else to threaten their place in the dominance hierarchy. They want their peers to become their inferiors, indefinitely. In this respect, they can't help themselves because the need to dominate is an innate drive determined by evolution, not by intellect. Even religions, which talk about universal love and fellowship and all men being equal in god's eyes, necessarily and inevitably form vast machines of inequality to harvest power and influence from their dewy-eyed adherents. Despite their high ideals, they are impelled in this direction by millions of years of evolution. A pope, a patriarch or archbishop can no more flatten his church's hierarchy than the alpha male in a gorilla troop can watch a junior member of his group mate with one of his females, and for the same reason. This is the level at which the human lust for power originates. Churches and armies are just street gangs in grand costumes. Every attempt to get rid of a hierarchy ends up with a different sort of hierarchy. Is it because, in order to smash a hierarchy, we have to build one? Who knows, but the point is that lopping the head off a single hierarchy does not kill the species. We are the species.

How does anybody become the leader of the group? In the gorilla troop, the beta, gamma and all the other males are not the alpha male's peers just because they are not his peers: he can beat them in a fight. In the endless, seething competition that constitutes primate tribal life, and I include modern western society, not all are born equal or made equal by their experiences. At the very least, children are not the equals of their parents. Any rights they have are accorded them; their rights were not handed down on tablets of stone. At the same time, even before children have stopped wetting themselves, they are dominating others in their playgroup—or being dominated by them. As they grow older, the differences are magnified until one man holds more or less absolute power over his subjects.

Many people, if not most, are not much interested in exerting themselves to the extent of rising to the top; they will take what life hands them without arguing too much. Being second in charge of the workshop is often enough as it gives them time to indulge the things they believe are important, like fishing or football. So we see one pattern immediately: most people only want to be top at the things they think are important, but these are also competitive in their own right. Fishing is very competitive (just ask the fish) and football is war by another name. At Pope John Paul's funeral, President Bush was content to sit in the second row, no doubt reassured by Stalin's question about the number of divisions the prelates in the front row commanded (the Secret Service also had a part of the seating arrangements: a president seated behind a mullah is a smaller target than a president in the front row).

Left to their own devices, humans sort themselves into interest groups, then immediately form themselves into dominance hierarchies within those groups. Within the individual groups, they set up bureaucracies in order to achieve the group's goals effectively. So who floats to the top of the power structure? Only those who are excited by power, who need it for their own inner reasons or who are not scared of the burden. If there is a particularly high-spirited horse in the paddock, not every rider wants to mount it. If the biggest waves are out beyond the reef, most surfers will be found in the shallower water. Not everybody wants to climb Mt Everest, not everybody needs to find the source of the Nile, be first into space or become a millionaire. A few people will select themselves to head the bureaucracy just because they need to be in front, but then their agenda changes.

Once they have taken power, they stop looking forward at the goal and start looking back at their cheering supporters. Keeping their troops in line becomes more important than the goal itself, because the excitement of hearing the cheers here and now is always and inevitably more rewarding than whatever future goal the group entrusted them with. The fear of losing the applause comes to dominate. Stalin was probably the textbook example of this tendency. Entrusted with defending the USSR, he spent so much time and effort destroying his imagined internal enemies that he left the country wide open to invasion by an external enemy. Stalin trusted Hitler, or could we say Hitler did not set alarms ringing to the extent that, say, the handsome, popular and loyal Marshall Tukhachevsky did. So the first thing the bureaucracy does is set about eradicating other foci of attention, other sources of competition for the group's loyalty. Of course, they justify their purges by pointing to the need to maintain efficiency in the pursuit of the agreed goal but that is simply their means of keeping their followers in order. The thought that their followers may rush after another leader, or look for another goal, threatens them at the most primitive level, their biological need to dominate.

9.5. Taking Control

The process by which the leaders change from looking forward to looking over their shoulders is not acknowledged openly at any level in the group, except perhaps for those outsiders who also want power but do not want to share it with the current leaders. The *hoi polloi* may recognize it but will laugh it off so long as they feel they are getting their share of the original agreed goal, i.e. they can always be bought. The leaders may also recognize it and may acknowledge it to each other in private but will react savagely to anybody who dares to say it in public because that would threaten their hold on power. Power is its own reward, power is the aphrodisiac. Threats to power evoke the same savage, unreasoning onslaught of a King Quail that sees an intruder in its territory. Once aroused, neither the bird nor the human can stop attacking, even at the risk of losing the larger goal.

Once a person is promoted to a position of power within the group, he quickly incorporates the group in his territory. His followers become "his" just as his wife and children, and his horse and weapons are "his." They become a submissive part of him, required to do as they are told just as horses and wives and children and limbs must do as they are told, just as weapons must be where they were left for when they are next needed. This is regardless of the purpose or nature of the hierarchy, be it religion or politics, football, finance or whist drives: we are not talking about something reasoned or rational. We are talking of blind, unreasoning, genetically-determined drives which are not just analogous with baboon territorial or mating drives, but are precise homologies, transmitted by the same genetic means (and probably even the same genes) in humans as in bonobos. The only difference is that, in humans, the primitive drives are drawn in to supplement and, very often, take over, the original intellectual purpose behind the group. The fist of violent unreason slips easily inside the glove puppet of human rationality. Few can tell the moment it takes over, least of all the new dictator himself (who, of course, has most to lose if he does have that insight).

The more verbally proficient the leader is, the more easily he will be able to convince his followers that he is looking after their interests but, very often, he will simply be appealing to their own primitive drives with his clever wordplay. Hitler never once said "This is what you can do for me." Rather, he said over and over again: "This is what I will do for you, and this is what we can do for Germany." Indeed, he was seen as an ascetic, which reassured his people that his motives must be pure. The union of the intellectual goal and the primitive drive is a marriage of convenience that, once consummated, cannot be broken because to do so would threaten the basis of life as our evolutionary heritage determined it. The primitive drive breaks through the film of rationality to take over the intellectual goal because it is inherently more exciting. Intellect is cool but our primate heritage operates through wild emotion just because it is more fun.

So what do the followers get from the deal? They get whatever was in the original agreement, plus they get the intense excitement of being part of something bigger. They feel a sense of belonging, which is one of the most basic human drives: first and last, we are social animals. We need food because we are animals and we need affectionate bonds because we are social. In addition, they get the power of the mob and they like it. Being part of something very strong is thrilling, the normal rules are thrown aside and the mob bestrides the world as the new colossus. There is a further element which cannot be gainsaid. Just as groups of women will begin to menstruate together, so groups of men, intoxicated by their power and beauty, become sexually synchronized. The covert sexuality of armies, football teams, monasteries and academic ceremonies, of boots marching in unison and glorious uniforms, of stern visages and massed male voices demands only one resolution: domination.

Once a leader has determined that the followers are "his" in the sense that his dog is "his," then he cannot let them go any more than his dog will let another dog steal its bone. He cannot send his dog away if it ignores him, it must be punished, and the same goes for his followers. They cannot be allowed to wander at large, flaunting his authority; they must be punished as an example just because his authority is more important to him emotionally than any other potential goal. Works of intellect can never be as profoundly satisfying as crushing one's enemies, as Edgar Doctorow knew: "After all, why compose fiction when you could be devoting your life to your appetites? Why wrestle with a book when you could be amassing a fortune? Why write when you could be shooting someone?" [4].

9.6. Conclusion: To Control Our Base Instincts

So we see the value behind democracy. It is not so much that democracy allows us to elect the government we want, but it allows us to remove the government we don't want. The danger to human society will always be that what once seemed reasonable will turn into a nightmare, as the Nazis showed. Any person who thrusts himself forward as a leader has immediately declares his psychological unsuitability for the job. He has said: "My lust for power is stronger than anybody else's." Sure, he may be able to do the job but that is not what is driving him, it is but his excuse to take power. Ordinary humans fear social instability; dictators never do, it excites them wildly as they see it as their chance to snatch power whereas stability they loathe. It is by their immunity to the dread of instability that they name themselves.

The drives we humans inherited at the moment of conception compel us to oligarchy and thereby open the doors to unreason. Forget reason: oligarchy and blind unreason are our heritage. It is far better that we should know this than pretend otherwise.

10 | Testing the Biocognitive Model: Hylemorphic Dualism

> "No spell, however potent, can withstand for long the assault of a skeptical reflection. That is why it is the skeptic and not the believer who is in the end our savior."
>
> George Orwell, *Homage to Catalonia*.

10.1. Introduction

No, this isn't about a rare genetic disorder found in dizygotic twins. Of the many dualisms around, this is one of the oldest. It relates to the concept of the duality of matter and the principles that organize matter, as elaborated in the classical philosophy of Socrates, Plato and Aristotle, and continued through the Western Thomist tradition. Like all notions of duality, it is complex in its ramifications while offering few immediate solutions, to the point where twentieth century philosophy has largely ignored it. The general critique is that any duality simply replaces what monism sees as an obscure set of empirical questions with an insurmountable set of metaphysical problems. So difficult are these problems that, decades ago, Mario Bunge opined that dualism was not so much a doctrine as a cliff to push your opponents over. Dualists counter by arguing that redefining complex metaphysical issues as questions to be solved by the forward march of empirical science simply delays the inevitable: Chalmers was of the view that redefining the "really difficult questions" of matters of mind as a ham sandwich didn't advance matters at all.

Some of the earthier opinions have been summarized by a philosopher from Reading, in the UK, and I want to look more closely at his preferred model. In doing so, I feel considerably hampered by having no training in classical or Thomist philosophy. Psychiatrists, or even ordinary medical practitioners, with that sort of education are very few and far between. So, in what follows, readers will have to bear with my inadequacies: whatever strikes me as obvious is most likely to have occurred to somebody else over the past few millennial but I don't know of it.

10.2. Hylemorphic Dualism

David Oderberg argues in favor of hylemorphic dualism, which is certainly not the most popular intellectual position these days. First, he looked glumly at the position of dualism overall:

> "Dualism... persists in being more the object of ridicule than of serious rational engagement. It is held by the vast majority of philosophers be anything from (and not mutually exclusively) false, mysterious, and bizarre, to obscurantist, unintelligible, and/or dangerous to morals. Its adherents are assumed to be biased, scientifically ill-informed, motivated by prior theological dogma, cursed by metaphysical anachronism, and/or to have taken leave of their senses. Dualists who otherwise appear relatively sane in their philosophical writings are often treated with a certain benign, quasi-parental indulgence" [1].

Introducing his topic, he emphasized that dualism is more than just Descartes' classic "two substance" model. Others, which tend to be overlooked in the unruly shouting match include property dualism and event dualism. Property dualism takes the view that, while the mind may be material (as in "the mind is the brain"), it has mental properties such as consciousness which are not reducible to their cerebral substrate. Event dualism says that "...the correct distinction is between mental and physical events, such as thoughts on the one hand, which are irreducible to brain processes on the other." However, he added, for dualism's opponents, these variants are side shows to the main arena, in which substance dualism holds sway: "Cartesian dualism has clear and unassailable pride of place as the whipping post on which dualists are ritualistically flailed."

While Oderberg was of the view that Cartesian or substance dualism deserved a fair bit of the odium in which it is held, the dust from that ancient squabble tends to obscure other models of dualism deserving closer attention. He was not impressed by the notion of a natural dualism, preferred by Chalmers [2] (and the general approach followed in the biocognitive model), believing it was "...the biggest wrong turn in the recent history of the subject" [1, p73]. His preferred model has the following features:

1. All substances, in other words all self-subsisting entities that are the bearers of properties and attributes but are not themselves properties or attributes of anything, are compounds of matter (*hyle*) and form (*morphe*).
2. The form is substantial since it actualizes matter and gives the substance its very essence and identity.
3. The human person, being a substance, is also a compound of matter and substantial form.
4. Since a person is defined as an individual substance of a rational nature, the substantial form of the person is the rational nature of the person.

5. The exercise of rationality, however, is an essentially immaterial operation.
6. Hence, human nature itself is essentially immaterial.
7. But since it is immaterial, it does not depend for its existence on being united to matter.
8. So a person is capable of existing, by means of his rational nature, which is traditionally called the soul, independently of the existence of his body.
9. Hence, human beings are immortal; but their identity and individuality does require that they be united to a body at some time in their existence."

Put this way, it is not entirely surprising that monists at a dualist lecture should start smirking and nudging each other. Some of these terms are not self-evident, so we can work through them before moving on.

An entity can have properties and attributes. A property is a physical parameter of an entity (some feature that can be measured) that would still be there even if there were no sentient beings to measure it. Rocks had mass. and energy came from the sun, long before humans evolved, whereas attributes are features or descriptions granted or attributed to a thing by humans. Gold has the property of mass and the attribute of value.

Any entity we can nominate or touch is a substance. All substantial entities are compounds of two brute facts, each of two different orders of being, matter and form. Matter (including energy) means what you think it means, the raw material of the physical universe that is subject to the laws of physics, including thermodynamics, chemistry and so on. However, in classical philosophy, form does not mean what you may think. It is a metaphysical concept, specifically, whatever it is that organizes the matter into that particular entity and not another. It is something like a blueprint or plan, except it doesn't exist in the material world so we have no proof of its existence apart from the fact of a substance. Oderberg defines it later as: "The intrinsic incomplete constituent principle in a substance which actualizes the potencies of matter and, together with the matter, composes a definite material substance or natural body." Unlike the rock itself, the form of a rock is not a real thing of the sort we can pick up because it is not itself a compound with properties.

Point (2) says that, even though it doesn't fit in the same world as rocks and humans, form stands in an important relationship to matter, as it can act on matter to turn it into a substance, or entity, which then has essence (its essential nature as an example of whatever it is) and identity (such that we can distinguish it from other entities of the same essence). Form is not, for example, a kind of external mold into which magma is poured but it is the innate or intrinsic immaterial principle that made the elements into just that rock and not a fried egg. Therefore, despite it being wholly metaphysical in itself, form has a reality that cannot be denied. To rephrase that, since form can act on real matter, it must have a reality of sorts of its own, even though we don't know how form and matter interact. Yes, form is metaphysical in concept (so far) but no, it is not magical.

Closer to home (point 3), we humans are real entities compounded of matter pushed into place by a suitable form. A person is just one particular or uniquely identifiable example of a substance, but humans have a rational nature, and here it starts to get a bit tricky. A given heap of raw matter is converted into a person when acted upon by the form, but since humans are defined as having a rational nature (Point 4), then the form of a person and the rational nature of a person are one and the same thing. Wait: where did rationality spring from? Is it another brute fact or is it part of the form (blueprint) of humans? To avoid unnecessary proliferation of entities, we need to allow that rationality is part of the form of a human, just as hemoglobin is. The whole point of the human form is that it defines humans, and it would be a bit hard to define humans without mentioning rationality. But it still leaves us with this loose end, a nomological dangler, if you wish, that form can be used to define into the equation more or less anything the author wants, yet nobody can object. It seems that form is starting to acquire one of the crucial trappings of magical thinking, so we need to watch it closely.

But (4) goes further: "....the substantial form of the person is the rational nature of the person." This seems to be introducing unnecessary complications. All he need say is that the rational nature of the person is a subset of the form of a human (i.e. the form that converts the loose heap of matter into just that particular substance called a person). I don't see it as fair to equate the entirety of the human form with part of its job but we'll let that pass to see where this is going. There is also the difficulty of not knowing how far form goes. Is the form of a human generic or specific? He seems to be saying it has both properties, i.e. it organizes (actualizes) a heap of matter into a human form, but also gives each one of those forms sufficient individuality to identify him or her. Again, this point has to be watched.

Point 5 is also a bit worrying: "The exercise of rationality is an essentially immaterial operation." Again, be careful. This seems to be to be begging one of the critical questions dualism is meant to answer. Materialists (and monists are materialists) say there is nothing in the universe beyond matter and energy and their interactions. They would then say that the exercise of rationality is not and never can be immaterial, because the mere notion of immateriality has no meaning. Oderberg is assuming that it is meaningful, and it looks as though this assumption is going to be necessary for him to prove his case. I would say that this is a very important point: is the exercise of rationality an immaterial operation? By the way, what's an operation in a universe composed of matter and forms? Is an operation a property of matter or is an attribute of form, or vice versa? Difficult to say, but let's accept rationality as an immaterial operation just because you can't buy half a kilo of rationality (more's the pity, we could put it in the water supply).

The following step seems to be a giant leap into the void: "Hence, human nature itself is essentially immaterial." I don't know where this one came from and, as a committed dualist, it worries me. He has mentioned "the rational nature of the person" and seems to be implying that this is enough to define human nature. However, that seems rather risky, as many people would say that human nature, in its quotidian sense, doesn't have much to do with rationality, that they are concepts of a different, if not conflicting, nature. So once again, there seems to be yet another small but questionable step. If I disagree with it, I have to stop reading but if I want to read on, I have to agree, or at least suspend judgment.

This argument is turning into a good example of what is sometimes called an intuition pump, meaning that a first or superficial reading of a sentence leads to a conclusion that is not, in fact, supported by the literal content of the sentence. Moreover, he had already said that event dualism allows that a material thing (in this case, the mind) can have immaterial properties, so why can't we define human nature as a material thing with the immaterial property of rationality? That's not clear yet, maybe it will become clearer as we move on.

His next point (7) seems to be leading deeper into difficulties. Since it is immaterial, human nature therefore "does not depend for its existence on being united to matter." Oh dear. We now have the idea that human nature can exist independently of humans. So if humans die out, human nature will persist? Well, yes, because form is a brute fact, part of the fundamental duality of the universe. This is not entirely intuitive, but Point 8 causes my intuition pump to seize up: the rational nature of a human being, traditionally called the soul, is capable of existing independently of the existence of his body. Destroy the body, and the person will continue to exist because the exercise of his innate rationality is an essentially immaterial operation which cannot be affected by the loss of the body. Does this also mean that if he ceases exercising his rational capacity, he will cease to exist? What about people who lose their capacity for rational thought? None of this is encouraging to anybody trying to write a theory of mental disorder.

This argument now appears to depend wholly on the concept of disembodied information, which is a major epistemological worry. Go back to his Point 3: "The human person... is ... a compound of matter and substantial form." Can there be anything we could recognizably call a person if the matter fades away? I would say no. If the body dies, what happens to the form? It goes on and on. So where was it before birth? What is the form, we could say, of form itself? For anybody who is trying to widen acceptance of the concept of a natural dualism, these are not comfortable questions. Let's rush ahead and see where this ends. And it ends right here, Point 9: "Hence, human beings are immortal..."

This, as is now clear, is a *non sequitur*. He will say that a human minus his matter (which should only leave the form) is still a human being in some critical sense; and that vital bit is form; and now form is immortal. You can see his approach: if the form can survive death for one millisecond, then there is no logical reason why it shouldn't survive for ever. That wasn't in the game at all. I worried over this earlier: "But it still leaves us with this loose end, a nomological dangler, if you wish, that form can be used to define into the equation more or less anything the author wants, yet nobody can object... form is starting to acquire one of the crucial trappings of magical thinking..." For example, does the concept of form include all the information we have gathered during our lives? Does that survive death, too? And what about the capacity of thought itself? Does this continue in the absence of a brain? If not, there doesn't seem to be much about me as I understand myself that would be waiting around for eternity, or even much point in it: who would be bothered? As Popper said, "I find the thought of immortality quite terrifying."

To counter these (very reasonable) objections to Oderberg's formulation, I suggest there is no *a priori* reason why form should not itself drift in and out of existence, just as patterns in clouds drift in and out of existence, or perhaps like standing waves in a moving medium (time moving relentlessly forward?). That way, matter could transiently enter the standing wave form and, in the fullness of time, leave it to be recycled but this could lead to a justification for reincarnation, which I see as one of the sillier ideas around. Form is just an organizing principle. It seems to me that, by this approach, Oderberg could have made a case for a metaphysical account of birth and death: the child's parents may have tried to conceive but nothing happened until, one night, somewhere in a non-material universe, a baby's form drifted into existence and, hey presto, conception occurred. Timing is clearly an issue here but I own that immaterial worlds may do strange things with material time. Baby is born, grows up and, one day, his form just drifts apart and so he ceases to be. Given the basis of Oderberg's argument, I submit that is equally probable as immortality.

It now becomes clear why monists feel justified in smirking and nudging each other while dualists are speaking.

10.3. Applying the Biocognitive Model

For myself, I do not find Oderberg's case convincing but I will admit that may be a result of my stultifying scientific education. I find the proliferation of brute facts a worry, and immortality is not attractive: have any of these people an idea what it would be like to endure arthritis forever? Oderberg's general stance is Aristotelian but I would like to think we can do better with more modern approaches.

In a more recent paper, he has argued that: "Matter simply is not sufficient to support or explain the phenomenon of human conceptual thought" [2, p230]. His case is unexpected and, although I believe his conclusion is correct, I disagree with the evidence he uses. For example: "Nothing that is abstract, universal and unextended could be embodied, located or stored... in anything that is concrete, extended or particular. Therefore, the proper objects of intellectual activity can have no material embodiment or locus" [1, p89]. He must live in a different world. I have walls of books, cupboards of CDs, boxes of videos, a drawer of flash drives, not to mention half a dozen computers all stuffed full of abstract matters of intellectual activity that, if their physical format were destroyed (say, a fire), would all cease to be accessible. Aha, he would say, the flaw in your case is the word "accessible." They would still exist as form. Sure, I reply, but how would you prove that? I will accept that an undiscovered law of the physical universe (strictly, a relationship that depends on the properties of matter) can have some sort of existence (because it's actually working now), but a poem I wrote at school, which I can't remember and of which there were no other copies? My unwritten novel?

His case would be immeasurably stronger if he had asked: "*Is it true that* raw matter *alone* simply is not sufficient to ~~support or~~ explain the phenomenon of human conceptual thought?" Only the most flamboyantly devout reductionists would disagree, as the answer is surely something like this: 'Thought (and all abstract conceptual matters) depends on the availability of some physical medium as the base for inscribing its tokens, and then on some particular property or product of the way that medium is organized for the ability to manipulate those tokens.' (I distinguish between reaching an abstract or intellectual conclusion, and that conclusion existing as letters carved in stone). That is, if there is a physical mechanism by which the tokens can be switched, then abstract processing can take place. Thus, raw matter alone, dutifully obeying the laws of the physical universe, can certainly "...explain the phenomenon of human conceptual thought..." if and only if (1) the organization of the physical substrate allows it to co-opt the rules of logic for the purposes of semantic manipulation *and* (crucially) (2) the organization is such that the outcome of the semantic manipulation is able to direct the physical switches to open and close in non-random ways, i.e. to function, however briefly, contrary to the ordinary direction of the laws of thermodynamics. You will see that this definition excludes the possibility that human thought is random, or that it is predetermined.

Thus, we (and our computers) evade his Aristotelian strictures: "...hylemorphists take their primary cue from Aristotle, who asserts that the intellect has no bodily organ." That is sort of true, in that we can't find a bodily organ called intellect, but not even Aristotle could think without a healthy brain. Intellect emerges from the brain but it isn't itself the brain. I suggest Oderberg is making a common mistake: information exists as tokens inscribed in coded form on a physical medium; but the rules that allow us to decipher that code are themselves coded information, and constitute part of the mind; but minds are a "multi-step doing," not a single event, so whereas single events can be localized (as they depend on a specific physical machinery), a modular process cannot be localized; so minds have no physical location. It is true that the information the mind operates upon has a physical location (in the brain), but it is scattered diffusely through the brain substance, and its codes are a bit too small and a bit too complicated for us to read. He may have been better to use the argument from experience: if I see a blue sky, there is nothing blue in my head, but he had already ruled that out as a huge mistake in emphasis.

His claim for immortality of the soul depends very much on this notion of disembodied information; I say his claim is wrong, that there is no information without tokens, and a token is something inscribed on a physical medium. Thus, the concept of information without a physical medium is devoid of meaning, like a square circle or an Australian gentleman. Since disembodied information is not possible in this universe, immortality remains a matter of personal taste, perhaps "...motivated by prior theological dogma..."? In any event, my view is that immortality is not central to a concept of dualism and it just makes people angry so we should avoid it.

Let's go back to this convoluted concept of the form and see if we can improve on it. In Oderberg's approach, it is an ontological fact of life, beyond explanation. Everything that exists has its form, so every separate item has a separate form, which leads to unexpected conclusions: "...dead flesh is not a formally impoverished kind of living flesh: in dead (dog) flesh, from the moment death occurs, not only is the substantial organic canine form absent but it is replaced by the very form of a dead thing, in which new functions of decay and disintegration immediately begin to occur." This doesn't sit very easily with modern biology, which says that dead flesh is just flesh that is no longer capable of supporting the biochemistry that we call life. There is an absence, not a new presence. Putrefaction is not the result of a new form arriving on the scene that dictates ooze and stinks, but it is simply the laws of the physical universe re-exerting their primacy after a temporary hiatus. The processes of putrefaction are directly the result of the physicochemical properties of organic matter that no longer receives energy. Given the chemicals involved and their ambient environment, the only possible outcome is ooze and stinks. Not even Dr. Frankenstein could hold back the tide of the second law of thermodynamics. The concept of a new form to explain death becomes a casualty of Occam's razor: is the form of a dog dead for one hour different from one dead two hours, two days, a month, a year? Once started, this game has no end.

The temporary hiatus in the careers of a bunch of chemicals, otherwise known as life, was brought about, at a considerable cost in entropy, by the local suspension of the statistical laws of thermodynamics in order to achieve what looked like something incredibly powerful (a human or a giant tree) but that was, in fact, just briefly animated dust that could play tricks using the sun's bountifully supplied energy (which, in turn, came from the way the universe turned lumpy just after the Big Bang, don't ask me why but, if it hadn't, none of us would be here to wonder about it).

It needs to be recalled that the laws of thermodynamics are statistical. They apply across very large numbers (and Avogadro's number is very large) of particles at the atomic level, but not to individual molecules. It is possible to appear to suspend them for a while, but only at the cost of burning energy. Ultimately, like all debts, the entropy debt must be paid back (something the world's bankers don't seem to understand with the clarity we might have hoped).

By getting rid of forms *qua* dead bodies, we can dispense with a very large number of forms to arrive at a somewhat less cluttered universe. What looks like the form of a dead dog isn't, it's just the former residence of the form of a live dog. What looks like the form of a rock is just a crystalline structure resulting from the properties of particular molecules and energy flows over the millennia. There is no form for the inanimate, not for diamonds, not for galaxies. They are the way they are because that's how physics is; if it had been another way, if the spin of the electrons in hydrogen had been ever so slightly different, there would be no water and we would all be crystalline. But the electron spin can't be different; change that and everything above it in the universe changes until, maybe, the whole show ceases to exist.

We do not need vague metaphysics to explain what the laws of physics can explain parsimoniously, ranging from elementary particles to the level of the cosmos and with near-infinite predictive precision. Inanimate objects are determined by the physical properties of their constituents, not by any insubstantial metaphysical recipe whose existence is moot anyway. Rocks can't be other than rocky, unless they are very hot rocks, in which case they act like putty, but that is strictly physical, a product of the kinetic theory of heat, not of a new form buzzing in from... somewhere. Internally, rocks are formless, i.e. regardless of the direction you go, it's always the same. There is no direction in a "mere heap," no up or down, no form: imagine trying to find your way through a fog by looking for its grain.

Living things, however, are different. They do have a form. They are indeed *made* flesh just because some organizing principle acted upon raw matter, but it was not a metaphysical principle, it was the very natural but remarkable phenomenon of DNA. Crucially, DNA is not supernatural, nor does it reside across an ontological gap from the dull chemicals it turns into the minor miracles of a dog or a rose. DNA is very much in and of this world. I have argued that it does not represent information, in the sense of abstract thinking, but it is just "information," in the sense that a key "informs" a lock. The whole point of information is that it can be manipulated; the whole point of the "information" in DNA is that it can't be manipulated, its efficacy depends on it remaining the same in every cell of our bodies from the moment of conception to the instant of death. If it doesn't remain the same, if it turns cancerous, then the instant of death comes much closer.

Now it seems to my dull, biological-type eye that everything Oderberg wants his forms to do in the non-human world can be explained either by the ordinary laws of physics (including chemistry and so on) for the inanimate world, and by DNA in the case of the biological world. If you would like to become an expert on form in the inanimate part of the universe (including things like volcanoes and tropical cyclones), then enroll in the science department of your local university and memorize all the laws you can find. Knowing those laws will give you a full understanding of the form of the inanimate universe.

That still leaves the animate world. We should look more closely at the details of Oderberg's definition of form, and then at what it actually does. He offers this definition of form: "The intrinsic incomplete constituent principle in a substance which actualizes the potencies of matter and, together with the matter, composes a definite material substance or natural body" [1, p76]. Does this definition offer anything that DNA doesn't already do? Here is his account of what form does:

1. The form is substantial since it actualizes matter and gives the substance its very essence and identity.

As a start, that sounds just like the function of DNA: it is real, it turns raw chemicals into living things, and it determines just what species of living things they will be, and which particular individual. So far, so easy.

2. The human person, being a substance, is also a compound of matter and substantial form.

No arguments here; the physical structure of a human is determined by its DNA acting upon raw chemicals.

3. Since a person is defined as an individual substance of a rational nature, the substantial form of the person is the rational nature of the person.

Now a jump: we agree there is something about humans that makes us different from trees. For example, we can calculate when would be a good time to attack our neighbors. That is, something about our form/DNA gives us the capacity for rational, abstract thought. But abstract thought is not a thing that we can isolate or localize:

> 4. The exercise of rationality, however, is an essentially immaterial operation.

How does it happen that we have rationality when bricks don't? It is, he avers, beyond the laws of physics: "The features of the eye and ear that make them singularly unsuitable for intellectual operation apply equally to the brain, the nervous system, or any other proposed material locus" [1, p91].

> "The hylemorphic theory is dualistic with respect to the analysis of all material substances without exception, since it holds that they are all composites of primordial matter and substantial form. When it comes to persons, however, the theory has a special account. The soul of Fido, for instance, is wholly material—all of Fido's organic and mental operations are material, inasmuch as they have an analysis in wholly material terms. The soul of a person, on the other hand, is wholly immaterial..." [p86].

This is factually wrong. It is an empirical fact that humans and certain other animals have exactly the same brain machinery in areas known to subserve certain functions that we appear to have in common. It is not possible to say that those functions are material when they occur in animals and immaterial when they occur in humans. This is simply begging the question.

As it happens, that is only one of many errors in that section. Our nature as *H. sapiens* is determined by our DNA; our DNA gives us eyes and ears and brains; any cognitive activity that takes place in a human eye also takes place in a chimp's eye (and probably a dog's eye), so any difference between humans and chimps lies behind the eyes. Is there something about the brain that sets it apart from eyes, ears, gall bladders and bowels? Yes, there most certainly is. The brain has prodigious switching capacity, and that's *all* it has. In the human body, the brain is a unique organ in that it consumes a great deal of energy but it actually does no work. All other organs do work, that is how they earn their keep; if they don't, then evolution gives them the chop.

But brains are different; when we go to sleep, our brains are, except for a few pesky codes, exactly the same organs as when we awoke. A whole day's feverish activity, burning glucose and wasting heat, has achieved absolutely *nothing* that we can measure using the methods of physical science. What, then, is its role? Why do we and practically every other non-vegetable in the world have brains? The answer is simply what Oderberg said is impossible: brains are the organs of intellectual operations. That's what they do and, since intellectual operations are underwritten by the manipulation of codes, and the methods of physical science do not apply in the realm of codes, then physical science has nothing to tell us about what the brain actually does to justify its biological expense.

The methods of physical science cannot tell whether a person has spent the day writing a romantic novel or working on a doomsday machine. That is just because those activities, meaning rational or intellectual, do not take place in a realm to which the methods of physical science have access. They take place in an informational space generated by the brain; chimp brains generate an informational space; whatever takes place in that space has all the qualities of a human brain (but perhaps not the same subtlety in devising doomsday machines). "The exercise of rationality," said Oderberg, "is an essentially immaterial operation." Indeed, but what about the exercise of irrationality? Is that immaterial? Is it material to make a mistake? Or when animals do something perfectly rational, like move out of the hot sun, or lie in wait for breakfast? Even snakes are rational. Like the bank robber, they go to where the best pickings are.

The brain is an ultra-high-powered and ineffably sophisticated switching machine. Switching allows an informational input to be manipulated into a set of output instructions that can, with suitable plug-ins, lead to all sorts of interesting behaviors, such as designing thermonuclear weapons and reviewing philosophical papers. When Oderberg claims that, because eyes and ears are "singularly unsuitable for intellectual operation," so, for the same reason, is the brain, he is empirically wrong. Brains have an architecture that eyes and ears don't, one which gives them an exclusive patent on manufacturing and purveying abstract and dirty thoughts. If that architecture ceases to exist, or even malfunctions, then no thoughts are devised. The conclusion is that, when the brain dies, its informational content immediately lyses, the mind ceases to exist and immortality goes out the window. Also, chimps get some sort of second prize for being able to think at some level (at least at the level that means we should not use them as live subjects for napalm experiments), as do dolphins (using them to blow up warships), kangaroos (cutting their Achilles tendons for laughs) and children (burning them alive in Britain or cutting their throats in Syria, according to today's news).

"When the body my soul informs ceases to exist," said Oderberg, "as surely it does at some time, then the person I am dies but does not thereby cease to exist; hence, death and cessation of existence, for entities like us, are not the same event."

What does it mean to say "the person I am..."? Does it mean my form, which precludes my life experiences, or are they included as well? If the form is emptied of its acquired memories, could it garner some more matter and manufacture another human? That leads to endless discussions on reincarnation, which I prefer to avoid. Can post-mortem forms talk to each other? Will they recognize each other as the persons they were? It could be fascinating for genealogists, perhaps not so good for those who bred monsters (how ghastly for Frau Schickelgruber). What about unborn forms, or aborted forms; are they budded from some sort of hydra or are they carefully designed and planned by a Higher Form? I don't know, and nor does Mr. Oderberg because, in his list of moral and other crimes imputed to dualists ("...biased, scientifically ill-informed, motivated by prior theological dogma, cursed by metaphysical anachronism, and/or to have taken leave of their senses..." etc.), there is one he missed: that they are the sad and increasingly lonely victims of their own wishful thinking.

10.4. Conclusion

It is crystal clear that Oderberg was desperate to "prove" the existence of immortal souls. That led him to miss the simple truths of modern science: that we can account for the totality of the form of non-living things by boring physics, and of all living things by DNA. The notion of a metaphysical form is no longer necessary. Rational human intellectualism is steadily eroding the basis for even wanting to believe that we cannot understand ourselves.

By chasing immortality, Oderberg has overlooked that rationality isn't just a human faculty (if, cynics may say, we have it at all); that switching devices equipped with suitable codes do not operate in the physical universe but by separate, non-physical laws; that they thereby acquit rational functions by non-mysterious and totally predictable immaterial means; that the brain operates in a different realm from the rest of the body; that the concept of human nature is indistinguishable from the concept of higher primate nature since it is determined by part of the 98.5% of our DNA we have in common with our hairy arboreal cousins (much as they might like to pretend otherwise); that the concept of disembodied information is a contradiction; that human nature and rationality are most definitely not the same sort of thing; that putrefaction does not require a separate set of laws, only that one set be suspended allowing the more basic laws to take over again; and that immortality would be a total bore.

As a dualist, I have sympathy for Oderberg's stance; as a scientist, I think he's off the planet. He lost his footing in a tangle of words where the meaning of a word in one sentence isn't quite the meaning he assigns it in the next. His project started with a goal and he assembled his argument to reach it; in science, we do it the other way around. We start with empirical observations and see where they take us: "It is a capital mistake to theorize before one has data. Insensibly, one begins to twist facts to suit theories, instead of theories to suit the facts" (Sherlock Holmes, in *A scandal in Bohemia*).

I suggest the biocognitive model gives a far more convincing account of the dualist nature of human life than old Aristotle could do, 2,350 years ago. Everything Oderberg hoped his theory of forms could explain is explained better by the new model; everything he didn't want it to be is also eschewed by this model; and some of the things he shouldn't have asked of his model are rejected by the biocognitive model. And I am sure that, if Aristotle were alive today, he would be absolutely fascinated by the suggestion that elementary particles (called DNA) do everything that his forms were meant to do.

Finally, regardless of any strengths, the theory of forms fails one crucial test of a theory of mind: it cannot generate a theory of mental disorder. Perhaps I should rephrase that. Hylemorphic dualism has a simple answer for every appearance. It says that a person who is mentally-disturbed is that way just because his form dictates it. This implies a certain fatalism:

"Dr, is there anything you can do to help our son?"

"I'm afraid not, the fault lies in his form. He's just going to have to learn to live with it."

"But we're desperate, he's been talking of suicide."

"Oh dear, I don't think that would be a good idea. The human form is immortal, imagine being mentally disturbed for eternity. He should just hang on and delay the inevitable as long as possible. I mean, we're dead for an awful long time."

"Can't you give us any hope?"

"Hmm, not really. I'm only human, what can I do to interfere with the metaphysical realm? We can't give somebody a new form, you know. All our drugs are from the material universe. They can't jump the barrier to the other side."

"Do you think a priest would help?"

"I suppose it's worth a try. Probably won't do any damage, priests are the first to admit they're ineffectual. Not like us, of course."

"Of course. Perhaps we'll... just go home... Thank you, it's helped us to talk."

"Not at all. And don't forget, we're here because we care."

I don't believe Oderberg's case for hylemorphic dualism will convince anybody to abandon monism. More likely, it will be counter-productive: anybody raised in the modern materialist tradition who doubts its validity and is looking for alternatives will probably turn away from dualism in despair.

<table>
<tr><td>11</td><td>

Cells, Circuits, and Syndromes: The NIMH Research Domain Criteria Project

</td></tr>
</table>

"In order to be a perfect member of a flock of sheep, one has to be, foremost, a sheep."

—Albert Einstein (1953)

11.1 Introduction

In several strategically-placed editorials, the directors of the US National Institute of Mental Health have recently outlined their "vision for the future" of psychiatry [1-3]. There is also a non-technical review by the lead author, Dr. Thomas Insel, Director of the NIMH [4]. These papers are incredibly important as this plan commits psychiatry to a new research program lasting, we presume, well beyond the lifetimes of many of today's practitioners. Their program for psychiatry, the Research Domain Criteria (RDoC), is offered as the successor of the long-standing DSM diagnostic program. The modern DSM era began in 1972, with the publication of a set of Research Diagnostic Criteria (RDC). The lead author for the main paper was John P. Feighner, so the RDC were usually known as the Feighner Criteria. The concept later became the basis for DSM-III-IV and soon to be DSM-5 (after a long career, Dr. Feighner died of leukemia in 2006).

Now, 40 years later, "key opinion leaders" in psychiatry are turning away from RDC/DSM, quietly acknowledging that it hasn't gone as well as its architects hoped. This was not for lack of effort on behalf of its supporters, it is just that now, with the benefit of hindsight and the human genome project, it seems the goal of mapping the surface features of mental disorder to the genome was perhaps a slight case of overreach. They are, however, confident that the new program will succeed where the previous one didn't.

I will declare now that I don't share their optimism. My view is that the RDoC will do no more than shunt psychiatry on another decades-long hunt for the Holy Grail. The new program is based in a series of assumptions with no formal scientific standing. Essentially, it is no more than ideology masquerading as science, with no conceivable chance that it can achieve its stated goals. In this chapter, I will argue that the program will lead psychiatry into intellectually sterile areas because it is in fact the wrong research program for the present state of our knowledge. The problem is that, by the time a future Director of the NIMH finally admits the RDoC project has failed, psychiatry as a profession will probably have collapsed and its tasks distributed to other professional groups eager to feast on our collective corpse. For the poor "consumers," things will be worse, not better.

11.2. Outline of NIMH Program, *Or* Darkly Through a Fog

The whole goal of the RDC/DSM project was to write a basis for a classification of mental disorder as discrete, reliable categories of disturbance. I am not sure how clearly it was understood at the time (and I don't have access to 40yr old journals to find out) but the program only made sense in the context of a rigidly reductionist biological psychiatry. The unstated purpose was to map the individual conditions directly to the brain and thence to the genome (which was still long in the future). Without that, the whole project made no sense at all: why would anybody bother looking for separate categories of disorder, with no overlap between them, when Blind Freddy could see that there were, and never could be, discrete, individual, separate and non-confluent categories of anything human that might interest psychiatry? There is no conceivable measure or parameter of humanity that we psychiatrists could use that distributes categorically in the population. Everything, just everything, distributes according to the standard population statistics, essentially meaning the normal curve. So: height distributes normally, weight distributes normally, intelligence distributes normally, aggression distributes normally, fear and misery distribute normally, hallucinations distribute normally, even crazy beliefs distribute normally (unless you belong to a fanatical religious group).

The first step in the main paper we will look at [1], a commentary by a committee headed by the Director of NIMH, Dr. Thomas Insel, published in the *American Journal of Psychiatry*, is an acknowledgement that the current DSM program, initiated in the mid-1970s, has been a bit of a let-down:

> "Diagnostic categories based on clinical consensus fail to align with findings emerging from clinical neuroscience and genetics. The boundaries of these categories have not been predictive of treatment response... (they) ...may not capture fundamental underlying mechanisms of dysfunction."

You can almost hear them gritting their teeth: this is a very uncomfortable admission of defeat for their most important project of the preceding four decades. In ordinary language, it means that, even though they got all their friends to agree on the diagnoses, they could not line up the clinical syndromes with any sort of underlying brain mechanism. When it came to predicting treatment response, the categories were unreliable; two people with what seemed like the same disorder could react in totally different ways to the same treatment. Treatment, of course, meant chemicals. Their underlying principle was simple: "All mental disorder is brain disorder; identical brain disorders must produce identical clinical disorders; all brain disorders can be treated with chemicals; all patients with the same disorder should respond the same way to the same chemicals."

It didn't happen. Somebody forgot to tell the patients.

Still smarting, they continued: "One consequence has been to slow the development of new treatments targeted to underlying pathophysiological mechanisms." Accordingly, they believe: "...the question now becomes one of when and how to build a long-term framework for research that can yield classification based on discoveries in genomics and neuroscience... the time has arrived to begin moving (toward a)... Research Domain Criteria (RDoC) project to create a framework for research on pathophysiology, especially for genomics and neuroscience, which ultimately will inform future classification schemes." This is written in the special language that bureaucrats use when they are forced to admit they have wasted the taxpayer's money on projects that didn't have a chance in the first place so it will also need to be translated. Let's start again.

"One consequence has been to slow the development of new treatments targeted to underlying pathophysiological mechanisms." This means that, in the halcyon days of the early 1970s, when biological psychiatry was at last getting its hands on the patients that psychoanalysis had been messing up for years, it was fully expected that it was just a matter of a bit of research money and a little time before the Nobel Prizes started rolling in (not to mention the very big dollars from the drug companies). They believed that, with a bit of basic brain research (and neurophysiology was suddenly making huge progress because of new technology), all the mysteries of mental disorder would start to tumble before the juggernaut of biological psychiatry and new drugs would simply drop from the production line, or maybe even the trees. However, it didn't quite work out. Of course, it's not that the new drugs haven't actually arrived because they aren't coming, they are just a bit "slow."

So, rather than hang around waiting for them to be developed using the old methods (usually known as 'hit and miss' [5]), the NIMH and APA and their friends in the big drug companies felt they could jump the queue and dive headlong into basic research in order to find the classification that DSM hadn't given them: "...genomics and neuroscience... ultimately will inform future classification schemes." All this business of talking to patients and studying their symptoms and giving them nice questionnaires to complete had been the wrong move. Basic neurosciences will tell us all we need to know and, who knows, maybe one day it will be possible to diagnose a mental disorder without even talking to the patient.

The underlying assumptions are then rendered explicit: "First, the RDoC framework conceptualizes mental illnesses as brain disorders ... mental disorders can be addressed as disorders of brain circuits. Second, RDoC classification assumes that the dysfunction in neural circuits can be identified with the tools of clinical neuroscience, including electrophysiology, functional neuroimaging, and new methods for quantifying connections in vivo. Third, the RDoC framework assumes that data from genetics and clinical neuroscience will yield biosignatures that will augment clinical symptoms and signs for clinical management."

One again, a bit of translation is in order (you can see I spent 25 years in the public service, I speak their language fluently). Mental illness, they say, is brain illness. Simple. But not just any brain illness, it is now "disorders of brain circuits." This is important, because nobody really knows what this expression means. It leaves the whole program wide open to changes of interpretation and direction at any time, very helpful if you are a bureaucrat because, if things aren't going very well, you simply head off in another direction without explaining yourself. The expression "brain circuits" can be stretched to cover anything brains do, a program without limits with an inbuilt and endless excuse for failure.

"Second, the RDoC framework (they mean 'we' but this sounds more impressive) assumes (read that as 'we assume') that the dysfunction in neural circuits can be identified with the tools of clinical neuroscience..." Now it is crystal clear: don't bother talking to patients, scans and blood tests will do the job. The unspoken corollary is that laboratory tests will automatically overrule anything the patient says. "Third, (*we*) assume that data from genetics and clinical neuroscience will yield biosignatures that will augment clinical symptoms and signs for clinical management." This again confirms that their laboratory tests will overrule patients, but it is clouded in bureaucratic talk. Biosignatures means something the public can't dispute, as in: "Well, sir, you see your scan result..." Augment is a polite way of saying "push aside."

They warn, however, that: "... given the rudimentary nature of data relating measures of brain function to clinically relevant individual differences in genomics, pathophysiology, and behavior..." What they are proposing is "rudimentary" which means "exists only in our dreams." But we should let them speak for themselves: "In the near-term, RDoC may be most useful for researchers mapping brain-behavior relationships as well as genomic discoveries in human and non-human animal studies..." What we are planning, they are saying, will seem like a total mystery to the people we are supposed to be helping (patients and clinicians) but we haven't got a clue how long this will go on, so we don't want any silly carping from people who don't understand these things (that bit is actually a none-too-subtle warning to Congress to pay up and butt out). "RDoC are intended to ultimately provide a framework for classification based on empirical data from genetics and neuroscience" (ignore the split infinitive; grammar was never their strong suit). Forget your squishy clinical stuff, it says, we're going after the big game of neurosciences. Nonetheless, "Our expectation, based on experience in cancer, heart disease, and infectious diseases, is that identifying syndromes based on pathophysiology will eventually be able to improve outcomes." This worked for everybody else, so you better believe it's going to work for us, too, but it wasn't cheap for them so it won't be cheap for us, OK?

At this point, the authors indicate the nature of their research program: "The primary focus for RDoC is on neural circuitry, with levels of analysis progressing in one of two directions: upwards from measures of circuitry function to clinically relevant variation, or downwards to the genetic and molecular/cellular factors that ultimately influence such function. From this perspective, research for RDoC can be conceived as a matrix in which the rows represent various constructs grouped hierarchically into broad domains of function (e.g., negative emotionality, cognition). The columns of the matrix denote different levels of analysis, from genetic, molecular, and cellular levels, proceeding to the circuit-level (... the focal element of the RDoC organization), and on to the level of the individual, family environment, and social context. Importantly, all of these levels are seen as affecting both the biology and psychology of mental illness."

I have to translate this as, even though it sounds impressive, it really is quite mad. They are saying: "We will focus on neural circuits, whatever that may mean, and will build a program that throws a rope over everything we can think of, so there will be lots for our friends to do over the next thirty years or so, and we're going to build a sort of supercomputer that will relate your genes to your society and everything in between to everything else but don't worry, we'll be generous, we'll include anything that seems it might be involved because we don't actually have a model of mental disorder, or even a theory of mind to say what doesn't fit in, but we'll throw it all in together and stir it and something is bound to pop out. Isn't it? But rather than let anybody call it a hodgepodge or a mess, we're going to get in first and call it a matrix, even though matrices have nothing to do with minds that anybody knows of, but it sounds cool and should get us a bit of mileage, not to mention keeping Sen. Grassley off our case."

Now they provide a further warning: "... we recognize that there are many 'ifs' at this stage. We are still a long way from knowing if this approach will succeed." I think their accidental lapse into plain English should be self-explanatory but, just in case, it says: We haven't got a clue either, maybe it won't work but hey, think of the fun we'll have. Still, even without a clue where we're heading, how much it will cost or whether it will work when we get there (a bit like Columbus), things are happening fast: "APA, WHO, and NIMH met in July 2009 to map out common ground. These organizations have also articulated the importance of adding molecular and neurobiological parameters to future diagnostic systems ..." We had a meeting with our friends and guess what? They agreed. Isn't that heartwarming, and so unexpected too. So it must be true.

Now they wrap it up: "NIMH views RDoC as the beginning of a transformative effort that needs to succeed over the next decade and beyond to implement neuroscience-based psychiatric classification. We recognize that the creation of such a new approach is a daunting task, which will likely require several mid-course corrections and may ultimately fail to deliver the transformation we seek in clinical care. However, NIMH hopes that the scientific and clinical communities will recognize the importance of joining in constructive dialogue on efforts aiming to accelerate the pace of new clinical discoveries and improve clinical outcomes." This is actually an ominous warning that this is biological psychiatry's last-ditch effort to deliver the goods. Come what may, it *has* to succeed because there's nothing else. If we have to drop everything mid-course and start again, it won't be our fault, or even if it's a total disaster, it still won't be our fault because we've warned everybody so we don't want any shilly-shallying in the ranks, everybody should come on board and keep that money flowing because we're on a *Mission From God*. Or we're desperate, there's not much difference.

In the next section, I will try to be serious; one ought not to mock the less-fortunate.

11.3. More Fog

The second paper [2], which appeared in the prestigious journal *Schizophrenia Bulletin*, repeats what they said about the failure of the RDC/DSM process, with particular reference to the long-standing problems in the diagnosis of psychotic disorders. In brief, it acknowledges that the classic, Kräpelinian model of two functional psychoses has long been seen as failing in a number of respects:

> "Part of the problem is that the Kräpelinian assumptions have become embedded in the machinery of regulatory agencies, granting agencies and their review committees, and journal reviewers... the inertia of diagnostic orthodoxy exerts a powerful hegemony over any alternative approaches... How can we move beyond these impediments to support revolutionary findings for a new, biologically validated approach to diagnosis? Over the past two decades, NIMH and other funding agencies have supported research to understand mental disorders as brain disorders..."

Here, we have a remarkable admission. They are saying that the way they (ordinary psychiatrists) think about madness (schizophrenia and affective psychosis) is now controlling their ability to see the field objectively. We (clever people in NIMH) are trying to get everybody to see "mental disorders as brain disorders" but people just can't seem to get it through their thick heads ("...the inertia of diagnostic orthodoxy exerts a powerful hegemony...etc.") that nature doesn't carve up quite as cleanly as just two psychoses. So it will be necessary to take to psychiatry with a chain saw for a little delicate psychosurgery, and jam biology down everybody's throats because that's what we believe so everybody else better believe it, too. That is exactly what it says.

In fact, and from the advantage of being old and a long way off, I feel fairly confident in saying that the only people who are stuck in the grip of an inert diagnostic orthodoxy are not clinicians, but people sitting in ivory towers who don't actually see patients (like, oddly enough, the current director of NIMH, whose career has been in neurophysiology, and most of the big-name professors of psychiatry who are too busy jetting off to conferences). Those of us who do the dirty work of treating people in emergency departments, or isolated areas, or prisons, or busy suburban offices, have never bothered with the idea that you are either schizophrenic or bipolar. From long experience, we know that reality on the ground is never so neat and clean as it is from the eighth floor of NIMH in Bethesda, Maryland. However, it's nice of them to admit what we in the trenches have known for a lifetime: ordinary patients, untidy, ungrateful creatures that they are, rarely fit the neat DSM diagnostic criteria.

And now comes another remarkable admission: We (key opinion leaders) have spent decades (at $1.5billion a year) trying to hammer mental disorder into a biological mold. Why is this admission remarkable? Because, apart from academic psychiatrists, nobody in the world actually believes that mind can be given a biological explanation. Only psychiatrists still believe it. Moreover, their entire research program was conducted in the complete absence of anything that might amount to a theoretical justification of the direction they were taking. This may, just may, have had something to do with why their two-decade attempt had failed, but they were determined to make reality match their version of theory, so that's where the money goes.

Let's move on, still serious. This is, in fact, very serious.

Now, the authors outline goal 1.4 of the current NIMH Strategic Plan [6], which sets out the RDoC, indicating they will use a "consensus conference process" to redirect schizophrenia research to the matrix model outlined above. A consensus conference process, for those who have never been to one, means that the NIMH will organize a series of conferences and meetings, at government expense, to which will be invited all the people they think are likely to agree with them. The purpose of the meetings is so they can honestly say there was unanimous support for this new program. For the record, I too have never been invited to a "consensus conference process," mainly because critics are the last people they want at their carefully stage-managed exercises in spontaneous agreement.

Heading on, the new program will depart from the traditional model of psychiatry that describes categories of psychosis. Instead, it will attempt to look at dimensional commonalities among the psychoses and, if indicated, other serious mental disorders including patients who fall short of the full syndromes:

> "The overriding consideration, however, is that only by combining traditionally defined schizophrenia- and bipolar-spectrum patients in the same samples can we finally understand the relationships among genetics, neurobiology, symptoms, and functional capacity in these serious illnesses... The rationale for the RDoC approach is to facilitate translation of modern molecular biology, neuroscience, and behavioral approaches toward explicating the pathophysiology of disorders. By targeting circuit functioning and relevant behaviors, one particular goal is that this process will direct the search for treatment targets in various domains—including new molecular entities, neuroplasticity paradigms, psychosocial treatments, and other potential interventions."

This is just a tedious way of saying they are even prepared to dump one hundred years of research into the traditional diagnoses of schizophrenia and affective psychosis in their determination to force psychiatry into a biological model. If mental disorder as we presently understand it doesn't match the theories they have prepared for it, then they will also dump psychiatry and get on with their "modern molecular biology, neuroscience..." regardless of what the clinical evidence says. Or, as Sherlock Holmes said in *A Scandal in Bohemia:* "It is a capital mistake to theorize before one has data. Insensibly, one begins to twist facts to suit theories, instead of theories to suit the facts."

11.4 The Commitment

We can summarize this commitment by NIMH as follows:
1. Mental disorder is brain disorder;

2. Mental disorder is therefore properly investigated by those physical techniques already proven successful in animal studies and in physical medicine, such as "brain imaging, cellular and molecular analysis, genomic and genetic tests, and behavioral measurements" [3];

3. Molecular biology will reveal all there is to know about mental disorder, including treatment;

4. For mental disorder, the significant level of investigation is that of 'neuronal circuitry';

5. With the RDoC program, the goals are uncertain, the concepts are unstated, the methods are unproven and there is no guarantee of success. However, an "invitation only" conference agreed that this new direction is essential as the DSM project has underperformed and psychiatry currently has no direction.

The first four of these points represent a major ontological claim, i.e. we have a series of propositions about the nature of mental life and the proper means of investigating it. They are not minor claims in the sense of being of no great consequence in the empirical program outlined by NIMH. Readers with no background in analyzing complex claims may be tempted to skip over them as "mere preliminaries," a bit of intellectual skirmishing whose truth (or falsity) cannot influence the outcome of the RDoC program. This would be a very grave error, because the success or failure of the program depends entirely on these questions being explored to their limit, and shown to be correct in every conceivable detail. Just like a computer program, an error, no matter how small, can have catastrophic consequences once the program is underway. The same thing happened to the DSM program: it was directed at finding "genes" for mental disorder. None have ever been found, just because none exist. Human behavior is the outcome of a stupefyingly complex interplay of a myriad elements; the notion that there could be a gene or genes for, say, depression, is akin to claiming that there could be a gene or genes for politics, for sport or for art. That's not how genes work. You would think that researchers at an institution like NIMH would know that but apparently not.

Just for the record, each of points (1-4) listed above has, in fact, been examined in detail; and each of them has been shown to be wrong. The claim that mental disorder is a special case of brain disorder, variously attributed to Henry Maudsley or Benjamin Rush, but probably antedating either of them, depends on the success of one of two philosophical programs, mind-brain identity theory, or biological reductionism. Both of them have failed; we cannot explain human mental disorder in terms of brain disorders [7-9]. NIMH therefore has no rational basis in pursuing its first commitment. The second, that mental disorder can properly be investigated by the methods and principles of physical science, flows from biological reductionism; if reductionism is correct, then scans are the order of the day. As it happens, the case for biological reductionism is false; therefore, scans will not reveal the essence of mental disorder. I should point out that nobody at NIMH has written a theoretical justification of biological reductionism, it is just accepted as gospel by everybody there. That doesn't mean they have thought about it, it is simply the case that if you don't believe it, and show you believe it, you won't get a job there. It's a bit like the old Soviet Union: unless you joined the

Party and went to their meetings and said all the right things, then you couldn't get a decent job.

The material on which my conclusions are based is readily available, so why do the "key opinion leaders" of mainstream psychiatry not avail themselves of it before casting their votes? That is a fascinating and critical question about the nature of modern psychiatry, but it is a question of the sociology of academic psychiatry, and perhaps even a question of the individual psychology of the people who have risen in the profession to that level. More to the point, why did the director of NIMH not arrange for a critical voice, a devil's advocate, to be heard at his specially-convened conference? That may be a question of his persona but, more likely, it reflects on the sociology of institutional psychiatry, which is trying to have the trappings of science without doing the hard work of sorting out whether those trappings are appropriate. If, for example, the informational content of a human thought can never be decided by physical means (and we know for certain that nobody at that conference could answer that question), then "brain imaging, cellular and molecular analysis, genomic and genetic tests, and behavioral measurements" are a total waste of time and money.

In fact, we know why there were no devil's advocates at the NIMH meeting in July 2009: because none of the organizers was prepared to take the chance of being shown to be wrong.

My conclusion is that this commitment by the psychiatric world's premier funding agency is seriously misdirected because it amounts to nothing more than ideology masquerading as science. Their invitation to a "dialogue" is not to be taken seriously because their collective mind is well and truly made up: not one person at the (hugely expensive) meeting at NIMH HQ in July, 2009, questioned the central dogma that reductionist biologism will yield all answers to questions of mind and mental disorder. In fact, the chairman of the meeting is on record as dismissing the idea that psychology or "mental" factors may have anything to do with mental disorder [4]. We can be sure that when Dr. Insel called for "constructive dialogue," he meant a dialogue in which he called out the questions and everybody shouted "Yes." Disagreement would be deemed "non-constructive" and would not be heard. This is symptomatic of the insular and self-righteous attitudes that now control mainstream psychiatry.

11.5 Shining a Light through the Fog

My case is as follows:

11.5 (a). It is the case that the DSM project has failed, but it failed for logical reasons, not practical. Twenty years ago [10], I showed that reductionist biologism cannot yield a model of human mental disorder. Since then, this case has been expanded to the point where it is now beyond dispute that there can never be a non-mentalist (non-psychological) account of mental disorder. Biological reductionism, in all its shapes and forms, doesn't work. All conceptual models which might support the idea of a biological basis to mental disorder have either failed or are self-contradictory [7-9]. As of mid-2012, it is the case that not one of the world's funding bodies, nor any university or national or international group or assembly of specialist psychiatrists, can point to an articulated model of mental disorder to guide their daily practice, their teaching or their research. Because it lacks such a model, modern psychiatry is prescientific [11], and all commitments to a particular model (such as reductionist biologism) are therefore ideological, not rational. The claim that "mental illnesses are brain disorders" is pure ideology, i.e. an intense commitment to a particular view or belief system in the absence of a convincing rational case. Anybody who disagrees with this claim is free to present a model of biological reduction of mental disorder, but there isn't one available—nor will there ever be.

11.5 (b). Of the failed DSM project, "One consequence has been to slow the development of new treatments targeted to underlying pathophysiological mechanisms." *Post hoc, ergo propter hoc.* This is the classic error of assuming that if event A precedes event B, then A caused B. At this stage of our knowledge of mental disorder (i.e. in the absence of an articulated model), it is equally valid to assert that the reason new drugs "targeting underlying pathophysiological mechanisms" have not been forthcoming is that there are no such physiological errors. No biological psychiatrist in history has mounted a convincing, or even a vaguely interesting, argument in favor of the notion that mental disorder is necessarily biological in nature, or against the idea that it may be psychological. All we have ever seen is fervent hopes [4, 12, 13] but where there ought to be rational argument, there is only a vacuum.

11.5 (c). Specifically, there is nothing in the world's literature to suggest that the standard methods, procedures and principles of orthodox materialist science can rightly be applied to matters of mind, and that includes mental disorder. At this stage, before another penny is spent on the new RDoC project, the NIMH and its counterparts around the world are under an over-whelming ethical obligation to establish the truth of their claim that the methods of investigation that have been so successful in biology and general medicine can be applied in unmodified form to the subject matter of mental disorder. Until this is done, then any such attempt amounts to scientism, i.e. the inappropriate application of scientific methods, principles and procedures to questions of no empirical content. Is it the case that they can establish an intellectual matrix in which different conceptual levels,"... from genetic, molecular, and cellular levels, proceeding to the circuit-level ... and on to the level of the individual, family environment, and social context" can be investigated by the usual laboratory methods? If they can, then they are claiming they have solved the mind-body problem. There is, however, not a shred of evidence to suggest that they are even aware of the nature of this problem, let alone are in possession of a solution. Rather than offer a cogent proof, all they did was organize a group of like-minded people who arbitrarily agreed that biology trumps psychology, and that no further debate is needed. By acting in this peremptory manner, they are behaving more like members of a religious or political group than of a scientific community [11].

11.5 (d). The concept of "neuronal circuitry" is so broadly-defined that it can be used to justify any research on any topic for any length of time. However, a failure to produce results will be explained away as a lack of suitable technology, leading to demands for more money, rather than as a failure of their conceptual definition of the field. The DSM-III-IV project aimed to develop surface markers for underlying genetic defects; the failure of the human genome project to deliver such defects was predicted many years ago [10] but was ignored by the psychiatric establishment until it became unavoidable. It was then announced to the world of psychiatry as though it were an unpleasant truth that the researchers had stumbled over, and must reluctantly tell the clinicians who are bound to be disappointed. Rather than admit the project was misconceived, the massive machinery of institutionalized biological psychiatry, an industrial-academic-government complex, you could say, now plans to swing behind a new project. Unfortunately, by its very definition, their project cannot distinguish biological causes from psychological, just because it doesn't recognize psychological causes and therefore has no methodology for investigating them. Thus, the (inevitable) failure of the RDoC project will be explained as a lack of technology rather than the lack of clear thinking that it actually is, and its funding will therefore be guaranteed indefinitely. Essentially, the RDoC project cannot succeed, but it will never be allowed to fail because the people who have chosen it are also responsible for allocating research funding.

11.5 (e). By any definition, the term "neuronal circuits" includes everything we know about the cellular basis of memory [14-16]. This means the RDoC program will include the concept of memory as part of their research program. If they do this (and I don't see any possible way of avoiding it), then they should first declare their position on whether life experiences can cause mental disorder in a perfectly healthy brain, purely as a psychological reaction to adverse events. This is critically important because, as presently formulated, the concept of mental disorder as a psychologically-acquired dysfunction in a healthy brain would automatically be incorporated in the new NIMH policy. However, by their own definition, the RDoC program would have no means of identifying or investigating these disorders, just because it doesn't recognize them and has no methodology.

Prior to launching this program, the NIMH needs to prove that purely psychological mental disorders occurring in a healthy brain are impossible, otherwise they would be embarking on a search for the causes of mental disorder without any idea whether they are using the right conceptual tools. In my work, I have shown that the concept of psychological causation of mental disorder is not just possible, but is necessary, and have outlined a detailed mechanism of mind-body interaction which provides a model of psychologically-determined mental disorders. Before the first grants are authorized, NIMH officials are duty-bound to investigate this point, otherwise they would be committing public funds to a major research program they agree may not succeed, and despite powerful logical reasons to believe that failure is highly likely. We can, however, be fairly sure that this will not happen. NIMH will not be sponsoring a conference at which its board of directors will expose themselves to philosophical and sociological criticism, not because they are a cabal of conspirators, but because the inertia of biopsychiatry is now irresistible. I won't try to justify this claim because it would mean trying to convince eminent authorities that they are victims of forces larger than themselves, and they won't like that. In exactly this respect, Thomas Kuhn quoted no lesser an authority than Max Planck, who said you can't hope to convince your enemies of the error of their ways, you can only wait for them to die, and then a new generation will arise to look on the field with unbiased eyes [10, p151].

11.5 (f). At this stage of our knowledge of the brain, we assume that its switching circuits are of direct, causal significance in the appearance of behavior. I am not aware of anybody in the scientific world who would dispute this point: it is so basic to our understanding of the brain that it may well represent a truism. In his non-technical review, Insel stated: "Brain regions that function together to carry out normal mental operations can be thought of as analogous to electrical circuits." However, the NIMH program proposes to extend this to including *all* behavior in *all* mental disorder. Insel continued: "And the latest research shows that the malfunctioning of entire circuits may underlie many mental disorders." Bear in mind that the expression "the latest research" carries the same weight as "everybody knows," meaning it can be swapped to another opinion entirely as it suits the speaker, but I certainly haven't seen that bit of hot news he's talking about.

I suggest that this goal represents a profound misapprehension of brain function: while switching circuits certainly can malfunction, the NIMH has overlooked the most fundamental point of switching circuits as they exist anywhere in the universe: that they actually switch something, and that something is information. That is, assuming our understanding of the brain as a vastly complex switching organ is correct, then there is another layer of function not accessed by "brain imaging, cellular and molecular analysis, genomic and genetic tests, and behavioral measurements." This level is the abstracted level of the informational content of the brain, as distinct from the physical level of the machinery that manipulates the information. To quote Norbert Wiener's 1948 book, *Cybernetics* (i.e. three years before Dr. Insel was born): "The mechanical brain does not secrete thought 'as the liver does bile,' as the earlier materialists claimed, nor does it put it out in the form of energy, as the muscle puts out its activity. Information is information, not matter or energy. No materialism which does not admit this can survive at the present day" [17]. Over sixty years later, Insel's NIMH is trying to deny just this point.

But have a closer look at that: Information is information, not matter or energy. What this means is that any method of investigation that relies on matter and energy (meaning, all of them mentioned by NIMH) cannot access anything in a circuit that isn't matter and energy. What is there in a circuit that isn't matter and energy? Information, the very thing that circuits exist for. The NIMH RDoC program embodies the notion that analyzing the "mere circuits" of the brain as a matter-energy machine, while ignoring the content of the information that the circuits are manipulating, will tell us all we need to know about the whole human. That's like weighing a computer to see if it is faulty. This is a profound misapprehension of the nature of information, they could not be further from the truth if they had tried to write a comedy skit on psychiatric research.

However, let's assume that the clever scans and molecular analysis allowed us to build a complete model of the brain's switching systems. Even if we had that, we would still be left staring dumbly at the myriad blinking switches, aware that they were switching something, but completely ignorant of what it was they were switching. We might, for example, be fairly sure that a person is angry, or frightened, but we could not know what he is angry about, or what frightens him. Similarly, we could know that he was speaking, but we would not know the language or the content of his speech. As formulated, the new NIMH program represents an inappropriate application of scientific methods and principles to questions they are not designed to answer. It is scientism, but it is not and never can be science.

11.5 (g). So far, the NIMH case is more a reflection on the sociology of science than on how science should actually be conducted. The position is that, having gained control of the opinion-making process in psychiatry, a group of like-minded individuals are attempting to impose their inchoate views of the science of mental disorder by fiat alone. On this point, there is no question: not one of the people who attended the July 2009 meeting at NIMH can put up a case that the methods of ordinary biological science can explain mental disorder, let alone such frankly mentalist concepts as values, ethics, morality and etc (and I don't even know who was there). That is, their vision of a science of mental life is a hollow reductionist parody of what ordinary people, and philosophers, would regard as the minimum notion of humans as rational, sentient beings.

While the director of NIMH, Dr. Thomas Insel, has declared that the organization he leads "...hopes that the scientific and clinical communities will recognize the importance of joining in constructive dialogue on efforts aiming to accelerate the pace of new clinical discoveries and improve clinical outcomes," we can be sure that he does not have in mind anything like a critical dialogue. When he uses it, 'constructive' means 'agrees with us.' Any disagreement would be blocked as non-constructive. As biopsychiatrists conceive it, there is no role within the profession for criticism of their model, the one they have basically made up, yet criticism of the *status quo* is the driving force of scientific progress. Absent criticism, we are left with just a shell of a science, a hollow but vastly expensive edifice which lends itself to being suborned by vested interests.

Conclusion

In a rather hyperbolic conclusion to his non-technical review, Insel claimed: "From the scientific standpoint, it is difficult to find a precedent in medicine for what is beginning to happen in psychiatry. The intellectual basis of this field is shifting from one discipline, based on subjective 'mental' phenomena, to another, neuroscience. Indeed, today's developing science-based understanding of mental illness very likely will revolutionize prevention and treatment and bring real and lasting relief to millions of people worldwide."

Who said "Those who cannot remember the past are condemned to repeat it"? Santayana, as I recall. There are plenty of precedents in medicine for projects that went nowhere. I can think of a dozen without any effort at all. In psychiatry, there are hundreds. In 1977, just for fun, I sat down in our small medical library and dredged through the old *Index Medicus* to find as many theories of schizophrenia as I could. There were eleven. Do you remember the idea that schizophrenic serum had a toxin in it, sort of endogenous LSD?

Somebody fed the blood to spiders and their webs became messy. Probably their legs were stuck together with dried blood. Somebody else decided it was due to epileptiform discharges deep in the hypothalamus. He proved this by shoving recording needles through the maxilla into the telencephalon—while the patients were awake. If that didn't induce something, I don't know what would. My favorite was the lovechild of a British psychiatrist, Dr. Ian Skottowe. In about 1938, he published an article in which he said that the cause of schizophrenia was an inability of the frontal cortex to get enough insulin. How did he know this? Because insulin coma therapy was very good for schizophrenia. You see that the problem of extrapolating backwards from drug effects is not new, nor is the problem of making disastrous mistakes by extrapolating backwards from drug effects. Insulin coma and subcoma therapy were, in fact, absolutely useless. They were pure placebo.

So I have to disagree: there are plenty of precedents in the history of medicine and psychiatry for the type of folly proposed by Insel's NIMH. A "science-based understanding of mental illness" will not work, if all it means is avoiding the hard work of talking to patients to find out what is troubling them. Because that's all this entire program is about: how to stop people complaining about their damned problems without getting too (ugh!) close to them.

You read this here: I believe the RDoC program which the NIMH hopes to inflict upon the profession of psychiatry, and upon our patients, will fail, just because the NIMH and equivalent bodies throughout the world have failed to articulate a model of mental disorder to justify and guide their research program. Moreover, their adamantine refusal to consider they may be pursuing the wrong goal is the antithesis of the scientific method. It is unfortunately true that "...the inertia of diagnostic orthodoxy exerts a powerful hegemony over any alternative approaches," but so too does the "inertia of theoretical orthodoxy." Committing the world of psychiatry to an uncharted research program is the worst sort of pseudoscience. The mentally-ill of the world, and their families, deserve better.

12 A Critical Review of Thomas Szasz: I. The Major Claims

> "The simplification of anything is always sensational."
> —G.K. Chesterton

This is the first of two chapters to examine the status of the claims made by the psychiatrist, Thomas Szasz, with regard to the concept of mental disorder, and how the question should be approached. The first chapter isolates the six major themes that run through his most influential books. These are established by quoting directly from his writings, the purpose being to clarify the propositions that identify his work as unique. It is, however, the case that everything Szasz writes is liberally peppered with rhetorical and polemical devices so I comment on these in order to separate his very characteristic style of presentation from the actual content of the material he is presenting.

Editor's Note: the death of Dr. Szasz was reported just as this book went to press in late 2012.

12.1. Introduction.

In a paper delivered to a recent conference, a speaker outlined the model of "autonomous psychotherapy" advocated by the "antipsychiatrist," Thomas Szasz (a label he now disputes strongly). Szaszian therapy follows what may be called the "extreme libertarian" approach, i.e. the notion that human freedom trumps all other considerations at all times and is to be restricted only by the reasonable laws of the land. When applied to psychiatry and psychotherapy, this model leads to Szasz's well-known position that therapy can only be a voluntary, contractual exchange between two adults of equal standing, in which one person purchases information (*sic*) from the other. He excludes children from participating in any form of psychotherapy. Because the engagement between therapist and client must be voluntary and free of compulsion, it follows that no person can be treated against his will, regardless of his condition, so that suicidal patients are at liberty to end their lives as they see fit. Similarly, people nominated as psychotic by the larger society are free to roam the streets in any condition and engage in any behavior so long as they obey the law, and there should be no restrictions on drug use. In essence, Szasz advocates giving people what they like for any reason they like, as long as they take the consequences themselves. This applies to all forms of psychiatric treatment, as well as other matters such as drugs, pornography and guns.

The form of the therapy flows from Szasz's widely-publicized argument that there is no such thing as mental illness. This concept, he argues, is meaningless, so that conventional psychiatrists and their patients who profess to be engaged in treatment of mental illnesses are in fact joint conspirators in a game of deception. By nature, this game is necessarily paternalistic, deceitful and destructive. These views are readily recognized as lying outside the mainstream. Since they were first published in 1961, as *The Myth of Mental Illness: Foundations of a Theory of Personal Conduct* [1], Szasz has attracted close and often passionate attention. A revised version was published in 1974 and today, Szasz maintains an enviably brisk publishing schedule: in the twenty or so years since he turned seventy in 1990, he has published some seventeen original volumes, as well as numerous papers and lectures, and has revised about seven earlier works.

Szasz is unquestionably a controversialist whose combative style of writing has not endeared him to the psychiatric establishment. My concern in these chapters is to determine the basis for Szasz's claims: is he justified in advocating what, at first glance, is a fairly tough and unyielding, perhaps even heartless, approach to the question of human distress? What is his theoretical framework, and how does this bear on the practice of psychiatry in general and of psychotherapy in particular? Essentially, this is an epistemological analysis of the work of Thomas Szasz, to determine how seriously we should take his ideas: what does Szasz claim to know, what can he justify, what are the explicit and implicit beliefs that are shaping his claims, etc?

In this chapter, I extract the general statements or claims on which his work is based. We will also look at his style of communication and what this means for the uncommitted reader. The next chapter examines his claims against the general principles of the philosophy of science and of psychology, which allows us to draw conclusions as to the validity of his work. Because he is such a prolific writer, and his more recent works do not add to his basic themes, I have chosen five volumes, written and published over a period of nearly thirty years which, it seems to me, encapsulate his major claims. These are:

- *The Myth of Mental Illness: Foundations of a Theory of Personal Conduct* (1961; my copy is the revised edition, 1974) [1] (abbreviated as *MMI*).
- *The Manufacture of Madness: a Comparative Study of the Inquisition and the Mental Health Movement* (1970; my copy 1977) [2] (*MMad*).
- *The Theology of Medicine: the Political-Philosophical Foundations of Medical Ethics* (1977) [3] (*TMed*)
- *The Myth of Psychotherapy* (1979) [4] (*MPsy*)

- *Insanity: the Idea and its Consequences* (1987) [5] (*Ins*)

As noted, his public profile began with the publication of his seminal work, *The Myth of Mental Illness,* in 1961. All of his subsequent volumes refer back to it while it, in turn, does not refer to any of his later works. Intellectually, it is the starting point of what amounts to his life's work. I have heard that he has said the revised edition was published more to satisfy his publishers than his audience but I have chosen to use it because it gave him the opportunity to correct any oversights (which, regrettably, creep into every written work). In these two chapters, all emphasis in quotes is in the original.

It may be asked why, when Szasz himself has written so much, and others have written so much about him, anybody would bother thinking that there could be anything new to say. However, the problem with Szasz lies in the general prolixity surrounding him: there is so much material to cover. As noted above, he has achieved a prodigious output and there is a huge secondary literature of some 2,000 books and papers. The question then arises whether the rewards would justify the effort. Does he genuinely have something original and valid to say, or is he just another polemicist whose influence will hardly survive his passing? That is, should the budding psychiatrist, psychologist or psychotherapist make room for Szasz in her reading list, or should she pass on to more worthwhile authors? My own position is that I attended the lecture in 2010 as a novice. It was simply scheduled as a keynote address at a conference I was attending but I had no idea what it would be about. My previous exposure to the ideas of Thomas Szasz consisted only of a lecture he gave in Perth, Western Australia, in July 1977, and reading part of *The Myth of Mental Illness* later that year. While I well remember his behavior during the lecture, I can't recall a word he said. For whatever reason, I never finished his book but somewhere, I retained a sympathy for his ideas.

As it happens, most modern medical students and trainees in psychiatry have never read any of his work, and this is also true of many young psychologists, social workers and psychiatric nurses. For somebody who claims to have original and powerful views on such a large social institution as the mental disorder industry, being ignored is the most bitter fate of all. The question then arises: has he been isolated by his enemies, or is his work no longer relevant? Indeed, has he been rendered irrelevant by his own efforts? It seemed to me that, as a vaguely sympathetic person with a proven record of criticism, I could examine the most influential of his work from the point of view of how reliable it is. The papers that follow will not convince a committed Szaszian, but they are not my target audience: committed people will never allow themselves to be convinced.

12.2. Basic Stance

Szasz's major claims are repeated with great frequency throughout his work but they first appear as a series of propositions in the prefaces to the first and second editions of *MMI*. From the beginning, he states that the concept of mental illness is "scientifically worthless and socially harmful" (p. xiii), nothing more than a "metaphor" serving moral and political aims. Psychiatry is a "pseudo-medical enterprise" which needs to be torn down in order to construct a new "science of man." He sees no difference between involuntary psychiatric treatment and religious beliefs imposed by force (p. xi). He further develops these notions in the *Introduction to MMI* by defining psychiatry "...as a theoretical science, as consisting of the study of personal conduct. Its concerns are therefore to describe, clarify, and explain the kinds of games people play with each other and with themselves; how they learned these games; why they like to play them..." (p8).

What he calls "language games" are "...one of the central areas of interest for psychiatry." Theories of psychiatry seek to explain human behavior, and forms of psychotherapy seek to change it. However, much of what is deemed to be abnormal behavior is essentially moral in nature because it relates to social goals. Given the moral basis of behavior, he argues that viewing abnormal behavior as "illness" necessarily breaches the most fundamental rules of moral and ethical conduct, hence his claim that psychiatry is immoral, repressive and destructive of basic human rights. He refers repeatedly to involuntary detention in mental hospitals, involuntary medication, ECT and psychosurgery as clear examples of immoral behavior inflicted on defenseless people by the psychiatric establishment.

In the Introduction to *MMI*, he noted that modern psychiatry was then about a hundred years old (i.e. now 150yrs old): "How," he asked, "did the study of so-called mental illnesses begin and develop?" What social, economic and other forces, including medicine, shaped it as "mental illness"? Throughout this book, he uses the diagnosis of hysteria to illustrate and develop his case. He views hysteria as "...a form of non-verbal communication ... a system of rule-following behavior ... and an interpersonal game (relying on) strategies of deceit to achieve the goal of domination and control" (p10). He then claims that his "...interpretation of hysteria... pertains fully... to all so-called mental illnesses, and... to personal conduct generally. The... differences between hysteria, depression, paranoia, schizophrenia (etc. are) analogous to the manifest diversity among languages." So-called mental illnesses are just attempts at communication using "iconic signs."

But, he asks, how were these private languages classed as "mental illnesses" in the first place? Illness, as everybody knows, consists of characteristic anatomico-physiological changes in the body that can be identified by the normal methods of physical science. In the case of mental disturbances, there are no such changes; thus, the history of psychiatry shows a protracted process over many years during which conditions which had previously been deemed to be cheating or malingering were reclassified as diseases on the basis of no evidence whatsoever: "...in modern medicine, diseases were *discovered*, in modern psychiatry they were *invented*."

MMI consists of fifteen chapters divided in two parts. The first part outlines the basis of his claim that mental illness is a myth while the second generalizes his claims to form the "foundations of a theory of personal conduct." Starting with the great French neurologist, Jean-Martin Charcot (1825-1893), Szasz examines the history of the concept of hysteria, arguing that Charcot used his prestige to shift the diagnosis of hysteria from what might be called 'disreputable antics by malingerers' (i.e. where the bizarre conduct of Anton Mesmer had left it) to that of a valid disease entity. Charcot did this, Szasz says, for entirely personal reasons of manipulating and dehumanizing his patients "...to gain certain social ends." Essentially, these were to extend his feudal control over the huge numbers of poor and dispossessed patients in his world-renowned hospital: "Charcot must have known that he was deceiving himself when he believed that hysteria was a disease of the nervous system." Increasingly as the influence of psychoanalysis spread, malingering (fraudulent assumption of the behavior of illness) was reclassified as hysteria, and only later was hysteria redefined as a formal brain illness. Further, as governments and insurers intruded on the therapeutic relationship, patients turned to psychiatrists as the mediators of their "best interests": "...the social function of psychotherapy is similar ... (to) religion... alcohol, tobacco, cosmetics and various recreational activities" (p59).

The great bulk of Szasz's reasoning about hysteria is based on Freud's work and is therefore largely *terra incognita* to contemporary students of psychiatry. He argues at considerable length that hysteria is just an attempt by the patient to give vent to powerful pressures in his life; that he is not sick in any sense of the term; and he is therefore acting to deceive his audience. The psychiatrist, on the other hand, also knows the patient is not sick but goes along with the deception for reasons of power, prestige, money and personal need. Szasz does not agree with the Freudian notion of the unconscious repression of affect. Instead, he believes the symptoms should be seen as a language of sorts that can be correctly translated, except that doctor and patient have a powerful vested interest in making sure that it is not. From this, Szasz generalizes to argue that all mental disorder is pretence, so that treating it as illness entirely misses the point of the patient's behavior and damns him to a second-rate life. What is called mental illness is a metaphor for life problems. These can be managed within the context of a psychotherapeutic relationship, where the psychiatrist is a teacher, interpreter and guide, sharing his knowledge in a contracted relationship, so that the patient may change his life if he is so inclined.

In Part Two of *MMI*, Szasz outlines his concept of a theory of personal conduct. Continuing with the example of hysteria, he argues that it is a form of communication by means of complaints about the body and bodily signs. The goal of this behavior is to make life easier for the sufferer through activating the social rule under which the healthy assist the ailing (p145). However, "...laws... also create and encourage propensities to engage in the very behaviors which they prohibit" (p157), so society tends to treat these dependent people badly. The agent of social control of these "deviants" is, of course, the psychiatrist who, acting within his pseudo-medical framework, dreams up a multitude of ways of punishing the people who are falsely claiming to be ill, all the while pretending he is there to help them. Life is a series of games, and mental illness is to be seen within the context of the family game and the religious game. This, however, can be very dangerous as the religious game has always involved scapegoating of various defenseless sections of the community, as the medieval witch hunts amply demonstrated.

In this respect, Szasz claims, psychiatry fulfils the traditional role of the witch-hunter, by discovering and punishing deviants who fail to play their part fully in the great social game of life. The obstreperous, the elderly, the ugly and deformed will take refuge in playing "sick" and will go to very great lengths "...to be authenticated as 'sick' in the particular ways in which they want to be seen, or see themselves as being, sick." Mental illness, with all its symptoms, is to be seen as a convoluted game between patient and psychiatrist, as part of the family game and the larger society game, but it is a game of deception and malfeasance, not of honesty and personal growth. This, he avers, is true of all mental disorder and all psychiatry (in which, from time to time, he includes psychology).

His view of humans emerges as this part unfolds, but it is a little gloomy: "I have long considered lying as one of the most important phenomena in psychiatry... The patients, like children, lie to the doctor. And the physicians, like parents, lie to the patients" (p223). This is not, however, the clearest of his work as he does not distinguish sharply between normality and abnormality, if (in keeping with his analytic background) he sees much difference at all. He sees humans as game-players *par excellence*, and society as an aggregate of these games. It follows that the explanation of human behavior is largely based in learning theories, but not the restricted theories of the behaviorists because he accords a central part to religion as a source of hope and zest in life. Thus, he ends this section with a faintly optimistic lilt.

Over decades, he has elaborated on these basic ideas. One of the most influential of his later books was entitled *The Manufacture of Madness: a Comparative Study of the Inquisition and the Mental Health Movement* [2]. This is a lengthy and very much stronger development of his thesis that "... the concept of mental illness has the same logical and empirical status as the concept of witchcraft... mental illness serves the same social function in the modern world as did the concept of witchcraft in the late Middle Ages... (mental illness and witchcraft) have the same moral implications and political consequences..." In the modern world, we have "... the substitution of a medical mass-movement for a religious one, the persecution of mental patients replacing the persecution of heretics" [2 p. xix-xx]. It is not, however, a matter of all psychiatry being bad, just institutional psychiatry, because it uses the power of the law to oppress its victims: "Indeed, just as the Inquisition was the characteristic abuse of Christianity, so Institutional Psychiatry is the characteristic abuse of Medicine... Institutional Psychiatry is... designed to protect and uplift the group (the family, the State), by persecuting and degrading the individual (as insane or ill)" (p. xxv). In each case, the institution scapegoats its victims "...to justify their social control, oppression, persecution, or even complete destruction... Institutional Psychiatry fulfils a basic human need—to validate the Self as good (normal), by invalidating the Other as evil (mentally ill)."

The great bulk of the book consists of a lengthy historical account of the development of the witch hunts throughout late Medieval Europe. From it arises his view of how the conjoint roles of the mental patient and his psychiatrist are the modern avatars of the ancient duo of the witch and her religious persecutor and executioner: "...both the medieval witch and the modern mental patient are the scapegoats of society. By sacrificing some of its members, the community seeks to 'purify' itself and thus maintain its integrity and survival" (p260). However, large parts of this volume are cast in the intensely metaphysical type of language used by psychoanalysts and are thus a little opaque to the modern reader.

His subsequent books develop the elements of his basic thesis. *The Theology of Medicine: the Political-Philosophical Foundations of Medical Ethics* from 1977 [3] is a collection of essays, mostly written in the 1970s and published in non-medical journals. These are unabashedly moralistic in tone, in which Szasz gives full rein to his radical ideas of freedom. Very often, he argues, by attempting to improve somebody's life, we make it worse, his clear conclusion being that we should not try. Starting with an extreme libertarian stance, he tackles a number of vexed question, such as drugs of addiction (he favors their free availability, even if children get them), suicide ("...preventing people from killing themselves is like preventing people from leaving their homeland" p 85; long-term prisoners should have access to poisons to end their lives if they wish) and other problematic areas. That is, he sees compulsion and restriction of freedom of choice of the adult as utterly immoral and unjustifiable under any circumstances except the criminal.

In the last essay, he nominates the concept of "...individual self-determination or freedom, in a political sense" (p145) as his over-riding moral-political value. He explicitly identifies the then extant communist parties and the western "bureaucratic... paternalistic... therapeutic state..." as the coequal enemies of personal freedom. In the west, he sees the alliance of medicine in the service of the state as dangerous in the extreme, a wholly moral stance masquerading as objective science and thus all the more insidious and destructive:

> "...in modern industrial societies, medicine is actually a part of the state—it is a sort of *state religion*... forcing taxpayers to buy abortions for poor women is like forcing taxpayers to buy alcohol or cigarettes for poor men. What mischievous nonsense."

He is aware that some people will not be able to manage the freedoms he proposes as the minimum: "...I would let the individual suffer the consequences rather than punish the whole society by prohibiting the 'abused' substance" (p155). A great deal of this volume consists of his cheerful, almost gleeful, celebration of the myriad inconsistencies of the welfare state and how, in the guise of helping its citizens, it manages to restrict their freedom and diminish their responsibility.

In *The Myth of Psychotherapy* (1979) [4], he outlined the history of psychotherapy as he saw it, starting with the amusingly scandalous Anton Mesmer and continuing through the arcane and largely subterranean twists and turns of Freudian psychoanalysis. Without exception, he excoriates the larger-than-life characters that populate this book as rogues and scoundrels: "Sigmund Freud's claims about psychoanalysis were fundamentally false and fraudulent" (p103). Psychiatry willfully confuses and conceals its moral content because it is, at base, totally dishonest, a *pas de deux* between the confabulating patient and the deceptive doctor. Unfortunately, his case loses a measure of its impact by his use of now-forgotten talking therapies such as that of the pharmacist Emile Coué. However, if his claims were true when he made them, they are still true as nothing much has changed in the world of psychotherapy (except a few more have come and gone).

The object of *Insanity: the Idea and its Consequences*, from 1987 [5], is "...to present a critical exposition of the idea of mental illness and its consequences." This explores the relationships between physical illness of the brain (neurology), so-called mental illness, imitation and fraud, the sick role and crime. He sees the defining element of any illness as anatomico-physiological derangements or disturbances that can be identified by the usual methods of physical science. All other conditions or states that are now commonly called illness, including objectionable, antisocial, eccentric, weird, wicked, silly or self-destructive behavior, are not illnesses in any meaningful sense of the word. Searching for "causes" for these behaviors is pointless: "...the belief that crazy people who do crazy things suffer from a lesion of the central nervous system rests on nothing more than a leap of faith" (p15). This leads to a lengthy and more detailed exposition of his basic themes: that mental illness is a metaphor; that people only act crazy; that psychiatrists are power-, money- and fame-hungry cheats whose role in modern society is the exact homology of that of the witch-hunters in the Medieval; that society selects certain people to persecute as the scapegoats for its own manifold failings and sends them to the psychiatrists to be brutalized; that any restriction of personal freedom is reprehensible; and that psychiatry is leading the charge in the war against personal responsibility.

12.3. Summary of Szasz's Basic Position.

We can summaries these points using quotes from these works:

12.3 (a): "...mental illness is a non-existent or fictitious condition" [5, p107]. That is, there is no objective physical basis to the types of behaviors termed psychiatric diseases: "...mental illnesses are not *bona fide* diseases... they are personal problems in living... I simply prefer not to place deviance in the category of disease" [5, p162].

12.3 (b): People who claim to be mentally ill, or who act in such a way as to attract the sobriquet, are acting fraudulently and with full conscious intent to deceive: "...Mesmer's practice, like that of all psychotherapists before and since him, was devoted exclusively to persons who pretended to be ill" [4, p49]. There are dozens of points in this book where he explicitly states that patients are only pretending: "...their patients who pretend to be ill... persons with pretended illnesses..." (p55); "...both had hysterical—that is, pretended—illnesses..." "What was wrong with these 'nervous patients'? ...the patients pretended they were ill, because they malingered or faked illness" (p96). "I have described elsewhere the pretences of neurotics and psychotics claiming to be patients..." (p196). "...patients with ...most so-called mental illnesses do not make 'appropriate efforts' to get well. Indeed, they usually make no such efforts at all, and try, instead, to be authenticated as 'sick'..." (p197). He repeats this claim many times in his other works.

12.3 (c): All of what is now called mental illness, disease or disorder, etc, is simply problems of living compounded by frank deceit and should be dealt with accordingly. Crime must not be attributed to or excused by mental disorder because that is the worst form of dishonesty. Soldiers with "so-called war neuroses" are simply acting crazy or sick to escape their duty [4, p90-91].

12.3 (d): Psychiatrists who diagnose or treat people as mentally ill are party to a conspiracy to defraud. There are so many supportive references that one can almost open any of his books at any page and find comments to this effect. For example: "All this (psychiatry) is fakery and pretence whose purpose is to 'medicalize' certain aspects of the study and control of human behavior" [1, p4]. Except for a very restricted form of psychotherapy, all psychiatric treatment is either a money-grubbing sham or state-sanctioned brutalization of society's scapegoats: "...doctors have invented two different kinds of such non-existent diseases, bodily and mental... mythical disorders of the uterus and ovaries... mythical ailments of the liver... examples of the (mental) are all of the mental diseases... the various anxiety and stress disorders today... as the medical profession and the public have redefined the rules of the medical game, (telling the truth) has ceased to be an option altogether" [5, p36].

12.3 (e): Psychiatrists in public practice are complicit agents of the repressive consumerist society, deceitfully denoting various people as deviants in order to keep themselves in jobs and society free of nuisances. All psychiatric treatment other than "autonomous psychotherapy" of fee-paying adults is fraudulent and brutalizing.

12.3 (f): Treatment of mental problems should be by voluntary pecuniary contract between coequal adults with absolutely no coercion whatsoever. Third party payments are not permissible: "...in autonomous psychotherapy, the relationship between the therapist and the patient is like that between an architect and the workmen who actually build a house" [3, p61].

12.4. The Style of Thomas Szasz

Szasz's style of presentation is a rather unusual combination of the analytic and the polemic. His general approach is what is called ordinary language philosophy, and appears to be modeled closely on that of the British philosopher, Gilbert Ryle (1900-1976). Following the publication of his major work, *The Concept of Mind*, in 1949 [6], Ryle exerted a lasting influence on philosophy, especially philosophy of mind. In a carefully detailed dissection of the ideas behind the term 'mind,' Ryle advanced a common sense version that has often been seen as the logical basis of behaviorism. For himself, Ryle was not much interested in behaviorism as such but his main goal was to assail the inherently contradictory notion of the Cartesian "ghost in the machine." He did this by a protracted, even tedious, process of exploring all possible nuances and ramifications of ideas of mind in common use, showing that, in the final analysis, they were nonsensical. In place of the idea of a soul piloting the body, he advocated what are now the standard materialist views of the concept of mind. These have been highly influential and will remain so for many years.

In the five books listed above, Szasz appears to have referred to Ryle twice, and only in passing (he rarely refers to philosophers). One was a brief mention in *MMI* [1] of Ryle's antidualism while the other referred to his well-known use of the term 'category error' in *Insanity* [5]. Szasz has not, however, made further use of Ryle's work, especially the very convincing case that Ryle mounted against what is now called cognitive psychology. This is significant as the model of mind that Szasz develops in these works is a thorough-going example of a fairly simple cognitive psychology.

The polemical approach in his output is much more overt and has frequently tended to obscure his message. He disdains the modern approach to scientific writing, the "objective impersonal," adopting instead a passionate rhetorical style to convey his message. While this may have made his ideas accessible to the general public, it has probably also worked against him in arousing quite vehement opposition among what should be his main audience, his psychiatric colleagues. He uses many rhetorical devices, some of which will be described here but firstly, he makes no attempt to approach his topic dispassionately. Each book launches into a violent onslaught almost from page one. The problem is that, by the end of page one, this has sorted the readers into two groups, those who freely accept what he is saying, and those who aren't so easily swayed. For the latter, reading Szasz can be excruciating because of the torrent of tendentious devices and dubious philosophy, and most just give up. Consequently, Szasz has spent fifty years preaching to the converted, while mainstream psychiatry has continued on its course, entirely oblivious to any truths he may have had on offer. My experience has been that this has tended to increase, rather than decrease, orthodox psychiatry's defensiveness.

Second, Szasz appears to have no awareness of the possibility that people who hold opposing views may, in fact, have looked at the same set of empirical facts as he has and simply reached different conclusions. Without a moment's break, he accuses his opponents of the worst forms of duplicity, apparently unaware that their perceptions stem from a scientific model which he just doesn't share. For example, as in the reference to Charcot above: "Charcot must have known that he was deceiving himself..." In fact, Charcot explicitly stated that hysteria was due to a "hereditary degeneration of the brain," i.e. a disease, in every formal sense of the term. There was no self-deception: history has shown that he just happened to be wrong. However, Szasz's judgment of Charcot's honesty is based on his own opinion that hysterics are necessarily lying, so it follows in his system that anybody who supports hysterics is also a liar. This is one possible explanation among many, but is certainly not established fact. Charcot's patients may have been fooling him but that does not imply that Charcot was "deceiving himself."

Thirdly, Szasz makes many errors of fact that would be known to psychiatrists but, crucially, not to non-psychiatrists. For example, he has essentially built his case on the example of "hysteria." What he doesn't say is that the word had at least four very distinct meanings at different times in the past century, often at the same time. It is precisely because of this endless confusion that it has been dropped by all modern nosologies. First, there was the sense in which Charcot used it, of dramatic but fleeting and inconsistent neurological signs (such as glove-and-stocking anesthesia, bizarre seizures, etc.), often accompanied by intense agitation and subsequent exhaustion. The second was to describe multiple physical pains and symptoms for which no cause could be found. This approximates the notion of Briquet's Hysteria, roughly the equivalent of DSM Somatization Disorder. Szasz also uses it to include cases of undiagnosed, isolated pain, as in atypical facial pain (a well-known syndrome), whereas these are specifically excluded by this category.

Fourthly, there was Freud's notion of painless loss of a neurological function, to which he assigned the etiological name of Conversion Reaction (now Disorder). In the Freudian formulation, the notion of "hysterical pain" was self-contradictory. Finally, it was used to nominate a particular personality type, the Hysterical Personality (now Histrionic Personality Disorder), which is the sense in which Harry Stack Sullivan used it, as quoted extensively in Chap. 12 of Szasz's *MMI*, "Hysteria as a Game" [1]. Knowing that Sullivan was using the term differently from everybody else (which he usually did; Sullivan was an inveterate neologizer) completely alters the impact of the chapter in the overall context of Szasz's argument that hysteria is a fraud. Szasz, of course, will say it doesn't alter anything as they were all examples of duplicity but that begs the question, i.e. he assumes the truth of that which requires proof.

Some of his rhetorical devices include actual rhetorical questions, meaning highly tendentious questions that must be answered in a certain way or the whole section becomes nonsensical. These lead the reader to a fixed conclusion that either has to be accepted, or stop reading. Szasz was aware of this: "Much of this may seem obvious. It is, indeed, obvious to me... And it may be obvious to the reader—especially after he has read this far" [5, p195]. Needless to say, any reader to whom it was not "obvious" (i.e. not accepted whole-heartedly) would already have given up.

He frequently prefixes terms, whose validity needs to be established, with the expression "so-called," indicating that he has no intention of defining them. There are many examples of terms such as "so-called psychosis," "so-called neurasthenia," "so-called mental disorder," etc. These expressions lead the reader away from a crucial point: that the words in question actually mean something to the person who uses them. Thus, a person who says that another man is psychotic is saying something about him *which must be explained*. Saying that he is a "so-called psychotic" merely announces that no attempt will be made to explain the observations to which the label attaches. Eventually, this becomes silly: Szasz refers to the "so-called idle rich" and to "so-called organized gangsters." The clear implication is that none of these things exist whereas, manifestly, they do, even some cases of idle, rich, organized gangsters. The needs of his rhetoric had taken control of his language.

Another oddity is his frequent use of inversions, unusual juxtapositions of opposites which function in the role of what Daniel Dennett has called an "intuition pump" [7]. This means that a first or superficial reading of a sentence leads to a conclusion which is not, in fact, supported by careful consideration of the facts contained in the sentence: "...people who work might be said to be 'playing' the work-game, whereas the so-called idle rich 'work' at playing" [1, p255]. That is just silly and detracts from his claim to be explicating the "game-playing model of human behavior" [1, p250]. Finally, he frequently indulges in the classic error found in Skinner's *Beyond Freedom and Dignity* [8], that of mistaking redescription in a different jargon for explanation (for details, see [9] Chap. 3). The example above is a case in point:

"…people who work might be said to be 'playing' the work-game…" They may, but, equally, they may not: they may, in fact, be working and not playing any sort of game at all. He gives no evidence that digging ditches in the full heat of summer, or catching fish on an icy trawler in the depths of winter, not to mention cleaning diarrhea on Christmas Day or operating through the night constitute a game in any meaningful or convincing sense of the word. The point has to be proven, not insinuated as a suggestion then subsequently treated as an established fact. As in this example, he uses what are called "scare quotes" to introduce a contentious topic, as though using it advisedly, then later uses it without the quotation marks, as though it had been fully explained when, in fact, it hadn't. This simply allows him to import the meaning that needed to be proven, such as the highly questionable notion that work is just a game. Anybody for whom it is not entirely obvious that humans are nothing but games players (i.e. anybody who isn't easily convinced by glib reductionism) will be one of the many who hasn't read that far.

If everybody is playing a game, what game is Thomas Szasz playing? Or is he the only genuine person in history? The name of his game will be revealed at the end of the next chapter.

12.5. Conclusion

All of these literary features add up to a corpus of work that lies uneasily on the borderland between a serious contribution to the conceptually difficult and socially problematic concept of mental disorder-cum-aberrant behavior, and self-serving, inflammatory, moralistic propaganda with no scientific content. The point of serving notice on these types of devices is to alert the reader to their presence. Does Szasz have an important message to tell, or is his life's work just verbal pyrotechnics? The first step in answering this is to recognize the polemical material and strip it away from any underlying facts or justified opinions. It would appear that he thoroughly enjoys (and has profited handsomely from) his self-appointed role as scourge of the psychiatric orthodoxy; my concern in the next paper is to establish the logical validity of the claims listed above, independently of the passion with which Szasz clouds and obscures them.

13

A Critical Review of Thomas Szasz: II. The Clash of Morality and Empirical Science

"There is no great harm in the theorist who makes up a new theory to fit a new event. But the theorist who starts with a false theory and then sees everything as making it come true is the most dangerous enemy of human reason."

—G.K. Chesterton

13.1. Introduction

In the last chapter, based on five of his most important works, we identified a number of major themes in the work of Thomas Szasz. We can briefly summaries them as follows:

a) "Mental illness is a myth."

b) "So-called mentally-disordered people are deceivers. Their so-called mental illness is a game."

c) "So-called mental illnesses are problems of living."

d) "Psychiatrists are party to a conspiracy to defraud."

e) "Psychiatrists in public practice are agents of the repressive society."

f) "Treatment in psychiatry must be a voluntary, pecuniary contract between coequal adults."

These lead to a significant question: "Has Szasz made a serious contribution to the conceptually difficult and socially problematic concept of mental disorder-cum-aberrant behavior, or is his output just self-serving, inflammatory, moralistic propaganda for an ultra-libertarian political ideology?" In order to begin to answer this question, I suggested that it is necessary to strip away his many polemical and rhetorical devices to examine his claims independently of the passion he brings to bear on his subject. Having cleared the scene, we can now consider his claims from the point of view of the philosophy of science.

13.2. "Mental Illness Is a Myth"

Szasz defines illness as anatomico-physiological disturbances of the body, i.e. he stands very firmly in the modern, materialist-reductionist tradition. If it doesn't have a biological basis then, whatever else it may be, it isn't illness. As a synthetic truth, there is no objection to this point. Those who claimed that the whole of mental disorder is of a biological nature are duty-bound to prove their point whereas, in fact, they have never tried [1-3], meaning Szasz may gain this point by default. However, while he may win the debating point, he may also be wrong. He has never established that point: he simply defines illness as "anatomico-physiological disturbances of the body." That is to say, he begs the question, i.e. he assumes the truth of that which requires proof.

When Szasz started psychiatry in the 1940s, he trained in psychoanalysis, as was the norm for American psychiatrists of that era. Based on a very limited knowledge of the brain (e.g. before the electron microscope was invented and well before the era of molecular biology), he appears to have decided that all claims for a biological basis for mental disorder were fraudulent. Indeed, as an autobiographical chapter makes explicit, he had actually made up his mind years before he began his medical training, while he was still at school [4] and probably no more than age 16yrs. Whether he had ever met any mentally disordered people is not revealed in his autobiography, but it seems most unlikely. At the time, he had absolutely no education or experience of the subject of mental disorder, and no evidence for his notion; his later training in analytic psychiatry did not address this point; yet he has held it fervently ever since, without demonstrating further knowledge of brain function. This was bold in the extreme and it was his good fortune that it turned out (so far) to be correct, but it wasn't science and he cannot justify his opinion. This is partly because absence of proof (of a biological cause for mental disorder) is not proof of absence, and partly because he has never attempted an *a priori* proof of the proposition that mental disorder cannot be biological in nature.

This, of course, has nothing to do with the broader question, of what the clinical phenomena we take as "evidence of mental disorder" amount to. It is one thing to agree, as he does, that "these behavioral phenomena exist," something else again to pronounce *ex vacuo* that they are not due to biological disturbances in brain function. Mental disorder (as brain disease) may be a myth but what about the phenomena? They don't disappear just because they are not biological. To quote one of Szasz's favorite philosophers, Gilbert Ryle: "A myth is not a fairy story. It is the presentation of facts belonging to one category in the idioms of another. To explode a myth is not to deny the facts but to reallocate them" [2]. Szasz recognizes only two classes of non-criminal abnormal behavior, namely, brain disease and deceit. By decree, he reallocates these phenomena to the category of pure deceit. However, in our present state of knowledge, this is a metaphysical claim that must be argued from first principles. He has never attempted that task. In fact, he shows no awareness that there could be a third class of abnormal behavior, something categorically different from either brain disease or deceit.

His claim that mental illness is a myth rests on his personal definition of illness and, thus, it has no scientific merit. As it stands, it is pure ideology, meaning orthodox psychiatry, which claims to operate in the scientific arena, occupies a different semantic context with, essentially, no overlap with Szasz's analysis of human behavior. A conversation between a committed Szaszian and an orthodox psychiatrist will not lead to communication as they speak different languages. This arises because Szasz failed his primary duty as a scientist: to question his own beliefs and opinions. He accepts without question that whatever he believes is necessarily true, just by virtue of the fact that he, Thomas Szasz, believes it. He does not entertain the possibility that he may be wrong.

13.3 "So-Called Mentally-Ill People are Liars and Cheats"

In general, he is saying that, because mental illness is a myth, all mental patients are acting with full conscious intent to deceive. With full conscious awareness, they play a social game called "mental illness" with the clearly-defined goal of deceiving their social surroundings and thereby gaining certain benefits for themselves.

It is evident fact that certain people exhibit, either intermittently or permanently, behavior that lies outside the statistical norm. For example, some people exhibit signs of terror for no good reason; others cry all the time and may try to kill themselves; others claim to believe irrational things or to have sensory experiences that nobody else can discern. These peculiarities have long been of concern to the ordinary citizenry, especially to the families and friends of those showing the particular behaviors, and so society attempts to explain what, for most people, is inexplicable.

Throughout recorded history, various explanations have been proffered for this behavior. Two of the oldest include the ideas that people act in unusual ways because of some physical change in their bodies, or because of some metaphysical change in their souls. There is probably nothing in the physical environment that has not, at some stage or other, been offered as the unique cause of "crazy" behavior. These include all manner of chemical substances that can be added to or subtracted from the diet, and a huge range of other physico-chemical insults, injuries, allergies or infections. Modern biological psychiatry claims that the chemical disturbances are inherent or genetic. The rational basis of these ideas is the ontological claim that, by a formal process of explanatory reduction, mental disorder can be reduced to a matter of brain disorder [1, 2].

Opposed to this view is the equally widespread and ancient notion that aberrant behavior is caused by some malign supernatural influence. This may be something as simple as the alignment of the planets at the moment of the odd one's conception, birth or whatever, or it may be that another person has caused the unfortunate's misbehavior by malign magic. The ultimate, of course, is that the mind of the disturbed person has been taken over or possessed by some supernatural entity, a state which can only be redressed by supernatural means.

These are "external" causes of disturbance, in that all of them are external to the afflicted mind. It is conceptually possible to explain the disturbance as internal to the mind itself, that is, there is a primary and intrinsic derangement or disturbance of the individual's mental function that is both necessary and sufficient for the appearance of the abnormal behavior. That is, the mental/behavioral disturbance has nothing to do with the state of the brain. Learning theory (behaviorism) took the view that the individual had simply learned the wrong things to survive in the larger world. Simple cognitive theory says that he has wrong beliefs which conflict with reality. Freudian theory says that the disturbances are in the subject's mind but are buried in parts of the mind to which he has no direct access. If we line up these twists and turns in the theory of mental disorder, we could perhaps see them as a matter of bringing responsibility closer and closer to the individual, until, finally, we have Szasz's view, in which responsibility is pinned to the person himself, i.e. he chose it, he brought it on himself and, until he chooses to do something about it, he should suffer, just as the alcoholic must suffer from his self-inflicted hangovers.

So how does the student choose from the range of theories on offer? What would compel a newcomer to say: "Aha, the case for possession is overwhelming, I shall train to be an exorcist," or "Biology is clearly all there is to the human condition, so hand me the brain scanner." What would amount to a convincing case that all the behavior my grandmother saw as "madness" should be seen, in Szaszian style, as simple cheating and pretence? That is, what empirical evidence is there that Szasz is correct? There is, of course, no empirical evidence that can be brought to bear on this question, as it is a metaphysical question, a question about the ultimate, unseen nature of things.

In his historical study, *The Manufacture of Madness* (MMad) [6], Szasz spent considerable time elaborating how it was impossible for anybody charged with witchcraft to prove her innocence. If she confessed, she was a witch and was sent to the stake; if, even after protracted torture, she protested her innocence, she was *ipso facto* a very naughty witch and was sent to the stake. There was no escape from the charge of witchcraft just because the social power structure needed to get rid of certain people and, once having made the accusation, had no intention of relenting. This is one of the hallmarks of the paranoid stance: it cannot be proven wrong, just because the belief precedes the evidence used to support it.

Thomas Szasz explicitly believes that all apparently mentally-disturbed people are lying and cheating. There is absolutely no possibility whatsoever that anyone could claim to be a Szaszian psychotherapist and not also believe that all one's clients are inveterate liars and cheats. This gives rise to a problem, not dissimilar to that faced by an alleged "witch" in medieval times: how to convince her accusers that she was not treating with the devil. Once the Inquisition believed she was, there was no escape. From the moment it started, the ritual had only one possible outcome.

There is a similar problem for anybody who sees Dr. Szasz for mental trouble: how can he (the patient) convince the psychotherapist (Szasz) that he is not lying? According to Szasz, there is no conceivable way the patient can establish his *bona fides*. He is a cheat and a liar who is only pretending to be troubled, and that is all there is to that. The very behavior that leads the patient's family to believe he is mentally ill is, for Szasz, simply a fraud and a charade; the man is not ill in any interesting sense of the term so, in the absence of brain disease, that leaves only pretence as the cause of his problems. Problem solved. It would not be possible for a "so-called mental patient" to prove to the satisfaction of Dr. Szasz that he (the patient) is not lying: Szasz's belief in the fundamental dishonesty of each and every mental patient, without exception, long preceded any contact he may have had with them. On his own statement, he is impervious to facts. So Szasz must therefore answer the same question he sets his opponents: What is the evidence that would compel him to abandon his belief that all "so-called mental patients" are liars and pretenders? If he replies that there is no evidence, that he cannot possibly be wrong, then his claim is ideological, not rational, and need not be taken seriously.

In fact, Szasz has painted himself into a corner over this point. Quite apart from his historical analogies, he cannot prove his claim that all complaints of mental disorder are charades and dissimulation. Moreover, he knows that.

Szasz knows perfectly well that he has no knock-out fact that will leave him master of the arena, just because he has never used it. His whole case is polemical, a half-century tirade which rests only on a Rylean analysis of language. Fortunately for him, right at the beginning of his career, he chose fairly safe ground. Unlike his close contemporaries, such as Eric Kandel [7], Szasz was not greatly impressed by Freudian theory [4]. He had already decided that the idea of a biological cause of mental disorder was false. He clearly didn't think much of behaviorism (I suspect he came to behaviorism much later) and he was trained as a physician, so he obviously wouldn't have held with magic spells and potions. What else was there? Nothing. And nothing is what he has bequeathed us. He has not left to posterity a theory of mental disorder, i.e. an attempt to explain the observable phenomena; all he has left is a theory of non-mental disorder. It is not a theory of mental disorder because it is an attempt to explain the "observable phenomena" (his words) away. He does not offer an explanation of how the features arose because he wants us to stop believing in them: those very features are all lies, deceit and imposture. Thus, there is nothing to explain, any more than I have to explain to you how Tinkerbelle's fairy dust worked. For a Szaszian, it follows, then, that all attempts to explain mental disorder are just "explanations," meaning fictions, falsehoods and fantasies.

The observable behavioral phenomena which grandmothers and neighbors call "lunacy" are, he says, pure fiction. Displaying them is a matter of taste; they are no more to be explained than wearing costumes at Mardi Gras or eating sheep eyes need to be explained. In Szasz's impressively clear-cut world, the "so-called mental patients" weighed up the risks and benefits and decided what to do with their lives. Some people make money, others write sonnets or rap songs, others make war while others pretend to be crazy and inveigle themselves into a position of dependency from which they cheerfully manipulate the world. "End of discussion," Szasz laughs, "so where is the difficult question that everybody else can't answer?"

Except it isn't the end of the discussion. It's only the beginning, because he has stumbled over an important point: that an explanation of *disordered* (abnormal) behavior depends wholly upon an explanation of *ordered* (normal) behavior. That is, a theory of the disturbed mind should flow directly from a theory of the normal mind, otherwise known as the philosophy of mind. Szasz understood intuitively that all the psychiatrists who claimed to know the correct explanation of mental disorder (be they Freudians, biological psychiatrists or behaviorists) were talking rubbish because a theory of mental disorder cannot be written in the absence of a theory of mind. And no psychiatrist has a theory of mind (remembering that he had already decided, as had many other people, that psychoanalysis was bunkum). Psychiatric claims to know the basis of mental disorder are themselves no more than ideological claims because not one of these people has ever made any attempt to answer the quintessential metaphysical questions in which the claim is nested [3]. However, nor did Thomas Szasz. Throughout history, the vast majority of psychiatrists have been guilty of pretending that an ideology of mental disorder amounts to a science of mental disorder. Szasz is also guilty of the same logical error.

Does Szasz know this? In fairness, I doubt that he can tell the difference between a fact and something he believes: to Szasz, they are one and the same thing. If he believes something, it is a fact so that anybody who disagrees with him is therefore guilty of denying the obvious. On the crucial point of knowing the difference between truth and falsity, he evinces an adamantine certainty. Therefore, the only way anybody can disagree with him is by lying. Thomas Szasz does not live in a world where well-meaning people have looked at the same evidence as he has and reached different conclusions; like the committed witch-hunters of yesteryear, he is surrounded only by fools, scoundrels and liars. His cosmology does not admit of other categories.

It is psychiatry's misfortune that, over the years, there have been enough fools, scoundrels and liars in and around the profession to have given Szasz the ammunition to sustain half a century of contempt. Nonetheless, this still does not prove his claim that all mental patients are actors, just because there can be no proof. It isn't an empirical claim. It is purely and inevitably an ideological claim, of precisely the same nature as the alternative claim, that all mental disorder is biological in nature.

13.4. "All True Mental Problems are Due to Problems of Living"

We can look at this claim from several points of view. First, it is an empirical fact that problems of living vary in severity from trivial to crushing. It is also a fact that the equipment each person brings to bear on his particular problems of living varies dramatically: intellect, prior experiences, social status, emotional resilience, physical health, subcultural influences, etc., not to forget that essential social lubricant, money. It is also undeniable that part of the person's equipment could be self-destructive, e.g. a culture which says that real men must never complain of distress but should use alcohol in good times and bad. It is also perfectly feasible that the individual's life experiences could lead to a compelling reluctance to enlist help, such as an intense fear or suspicion of authority, or of white men, etc.

Given these factors, it is perfectly feasible to assume that, even if assistance is available, a person could enter a state of distress that becomes self-reinforcing with no socially-acceptable means of asking for help. I once worked in a prison where, each morning, the officers called out: "All inmates with mental problems come forward now." Szasz would say to any unhappy prisoners hiding in the ranks: "Fine, if you don't want help, you are responsible for what happens to you." Others might take the view that it is important to try to make contact with the sufferer without triggering his fear or hostility just because, if nothing is done, he is likely to reach a point of no return without knowing how he got there. Not all humans are so blessed with insight as the psychiatrist. Making the attempt to reach out to the terrified is purely a moral decision by the therapist. Szasz cannot say that his moral views (of very explicitly not reaching out) must take priority over another person's, any more than he could say that taking sugar in your tea is immoral.

In the second place, the claim has no merit because the critical question here is: "What is the nature of the unseen processes that drive a person to claim to be mentally ill or to act in a way other people call disturbed?" Szasz replies: "The unseen processes are simply moral processes and need no more explanation than whether you take sugar in your tea." Again, this is a pre-emptive decision, one directed at blocking discussion rather than facilitating it. He claims that the behavioral manifestations on which we make the decision "He is crazy" are the predictable outcome of the subject's fully conscious decision to act crazy, a decision of exactly the same nature as choosing which sport to play. If a person appears in hockey gear, we can assume that he has already decided to play hockey (we will overlook the difference between playing hockey and "playing hockey" which Szasz regards as so important but does not explain). But this doesn't make any sort of sense in the context of mental disorder. If you see a young thug snatch an old lady's purse, do you "choose" to feel angry, are you "playing angry," or do you just get angry? If your mother dies, do you choose to play the grieving game, or are you genuinely gripped by intense and painful emotions that you could no more turn off than you can turn back the clock to see her smiles again? He does not attempt to answer these questions.

The same point arises as before: Szasz has tripped over an ancient problem in philosophy, but without realizing that it is old territory. First, he needs a theory of mind that allows us to understand the nature of any decision, so that we can be sure of our grasp of *moral* decisions. In fact, he doesn't have a theory of mind at all. Second, his theory must be able to clarify the difference between primary and secondary emotions, so that we can immediately tell the difference between genuine emotions and spurious (assuming he sees anything as genuine, which is not at all clear from his work).

The final point is that here, and at many other points in his work, Szasz shows an unhealthy tendency to arrive at universal rules for all humans by generalizing solely from his private experience. It is clear that Szasz has had a fortunate life (his own family life in pre-war Budapest sounds idyllic, even at the height of the Depression); yet, having just read several thousand pages of his work, I find he betrays no inkling whatsoever of what happens to ordinary people during their lives. I believe it is fair to say that if ordinary people could will themselves out of mental trouble, they would do so, and they would do so without any gratuitous advice from university professors. The fact that ordinary people—workers, soldiers and peasants, men and women, good and bad—can reach the point where life is too burdensome to endure says that there is something unseen happening which we clever, educated people must explain. Telling speechless soldiers that they are just trying to evade their duty misses some incredibly important point about the nature of their personal experience. Saying to weeping young mothers that infanticide is a perfectly valid option but she should prepare for prison overlooks some vital point about the human condition. Telling a teenager, who has just carved a swastika on his chest because he hears God telling him to be the new Führer, that he is just acting crazy to get his parents' attention seems, in some vitally important sense, to trivialize his experience.

In short, Szasz has written a moral account of mental disorder that is based upon one point only: that of denying the reality of mental pain by blaming the victim. He does not attempt to explain mental disorder because he is intent upon explaining it away. He cannot explain the bizarre sense of going out of one's mind (not least because he has no personal experience of it and therefore doesn't believe it exists), so he turns it on its head and puts the responsibility on the individual who feels powerless to halt the slide in his life. Szasz may never have been gripped by overwhelming terror, but that is his good fortune. However, his personal good fortune is no basis on which to propound a general theory of mind for the whole of *Homo sapiens*.

13.5. "Psychiatrists Who Diagnose or Treat People as Mentally III are Party to a Conspiracy to Persecute them and Defraud Society"

Szasz is in no doubt that, as a group, psychiatrists stand in a long line of religious maniacs, political crooks, charlatans, scoundrels and liars who fraudulently imprison and torture people for fun and profit but, that apart, they are probably quite nice people. As with all sweeping allegations of this type, which attempt to label a whole class of people, most of whom the claimant has never met, there is a grain of truth somewhere in the tirade. The unhappy grain of truth in Szasz's allegations of cosmic dishonesty in the world's quarter of a million psychiatrists who speak different languages, who trained in different countries, who don't travel much and who mostly try to work fairly hard, is that they are bereft of a formal theory of what they are supposed to be doing [3]. Psychiatry is indeed engaged in a cosmic conspiracy; unfortunately, it just isn't the one Szasz thought he had discovered. The modern institution of psychiatry is a walking, talking and hugely expensive example of what Thomas Kuhn called a protoscience [8].

As has been shown in chilling detail by the journalist, Robert Whitaker [9, 10], psychiatry lurches from one dreadful cure to another. However, as I have shown [1-3], the reason for this therapeutic desperation is just that psychiatry has never followed the path of medical orthodoxy by developing an articulated model of its subject matter, mental disorder. Orthodox medicine has its reductionist biological model of disease; psychiatry just has fads. Nonetheless, and despite their myriad shortcomings, these fads have a major advantage over Szasz's life work: they attempt to explain the phenomena in hand without dismissing them as fabrications.

Everything hinges on this one point: if mental disorder is a reality, if ordinary people can become trapped in overwhelming distress from which they can see no escape, then all Szaszian allegations of psychiatric dishonesty collapse. There may be incompetent psychiatrists, poorly-educated, lazy or insecure psychiatrists with the full gamut of human weaknesses and foibles (avarice, grandiosity, insincerity, etc.) but they are all committed to the idea that they are working within the only model they know to do something to keep their patients in some sort of equilibrium. This is quite separate from the notion of whether they have a theory, or their treatments work, or anything so practical. What it says is that psychiatrists may be intellectually naive, but they are not thereby dishonest.

Once again, if Szasz claims that all psychiatrists are party to a conspiracy to defraud, he has to nominate the evidence that would compel him to recant. If he cannot do this, his claim is ideological. My reading of him is that he would sooner die than admit that his case remains unproven but I suspect he would say, with a contemptuous laugh, that it doesn't need proof, that it is so blindingly obvious that only a fool could fail to see it. If that is the case, then he is simply playing the weaver in *The Emperor's New Clothes*, selling a new suit that stupid people won't be able to see. Needless to say, he doesn't have any proof because he has never found any. He believes in this vast, world-wide conspiracy and he therefore expects that any person with an ounce of brains will also believe it.

The goal of a theory of mental disorder is to *explain* human distress, not dismiss it as fantastic lies. Szasz does not understand this elementary point. He doesn't have a theory of mental disorder because he doesn't have a theory of mind. His reflex dismissal of the logical possibility of overwhelming, self-sustaining human distress is not a theory of mental disorder; it is an ideology of contempt for those who do not measure up to his standards of mental stability. On this point, he differs from all the other psychiatrists in the world, solemnly swallowing the non-science dished up by Freudians, Skinnerians, Pavlovians or biological reductionists like Eric Kandel: they, at least, try to extend their understanding of the human state by looking beyond the immediately obvious. At the age of sixteen, some 75 years ago, and in utter ignorance of the entire field of what are now called the cognitive sciences, Szasz decided that mental illness is a myth. It is clear that there is no evidence from any area that could budge him from his protracted adolescent opinion. That is the absolute antithesis of the scientific attitude.

As it happens, I have several ounces of brains but I don't believe in Szasz's vast, world-wide conspiracy. If that makes me a fool, then I shall have to live with it.

13.6. "Psychiatrists in Public Practice are Complicit Agents of the Repressive, Paternalistic Consumerist Welfare State Etc."

This is not a scientific fact, it is an opinion, and he can hold it if he wishes: *de gustibus, non est disputandam.* Szasz leaves no doubt that he believes that everybody who isn't on his side is at least immoral, and probably a fool to boot. If he wishes to make this particular claim as a scientific fact, it is empirically wrong but, if he intends it simply as rhetoric, it is fatuous and he cannot complain if people do not take him seriously. More pertinently, Szasz cannot define the notion of universal psychiatric complicity in crimes against humanity in such a way as to include his enemies while excluding himself without, at the same time, sliding into either self-contradiction or inanity.

13.7. "Ethical Treatment in Psychiatry Consists of Autonomous Psychotherapy Between Coequal Adults Etc."

For the behaviors that concern psychiatrists, the question of what constitutes the correct model of treatment cannot be decided by fiat. In any complex system (and I include humans), rectification of dysfunction should be rational, where rationality is determined by the rules of the system in question. Thus, in a strictly physical system such as a mousetrap, a nuclear power station or a kidney, the controlling rules are determined by its structure and function within the context of the laws of the material universe (the time-space continuum, including the laws of thermodynamics, etc.).

For more complex systems, in which the material elements are governed by internal informational systems, the controlling rules are those of the system's particular logic. Informational systems do not follow the laws of thermo-dynamics (see *World of Warcraft*, which cheerfully and profitably ignores them all). In the event of an output failure in an informational system, then the first step is to look at the instruction set and its accompanying data files. It is the case that any informational system can experience a primary malfunction, i.e. for strictly non-physical reasons, it can fail to compute as anticipated. There are many possibilities: the instruction set can degrade, the data can contain faulty items, the instruction set may be self-contradictory, the data flow can overwhelm the computational system, etc.

Szasz's model of humans is essentially that of rational decision-makers. He calls it the "game-playing model of human behavior" [6, p250], meaning he endorses a cognitive-rational model of mind. He does not define games and leaves it to readers to reach their own conclusions. In a Szaszian world, people gather information and use it to make choices. Those choices determine how they get by in the hurly-burly of daily life. Further, young people learn which games to play (p 253), the context implying learning in both the classic (Pavlovian) behaviorist sense and of Wundtian folk psychology. Therefore, if Szasz accepts that human behavior is governed by their innate informational capacity (which he cannot possibly deny), he must then accept that errors can creep into that informational system. We are not all rational all the time, i.e. for non-physical reasons, we can fail to compute as anticipated: even Szasz makes mistakes (actually, quite a lot of them). The moment he admits the possibility that humans can err, he has opened the floodgate: he cannot, for ideological reasons, restrict the nature of the errors he will accept as valid. So: on the same page, he says: "...speaking a language with a foreign accent is one of the most striking examples of transference." Just for the record, this is wrong. The definition of transference is: "the transfer of powerful repressed emotions from unresolved conflicts in the past to a figure in the present." Freudian transference has everything to do with emotions and nothing to do with motor memory.

More to the point, his example immediately admits the possibility of unconscious determination, meaning he cannot exclude the possibility that people's emotions (and not just their verbal behavior) can be determined by factors (learned or otherwise) lying outside full awareness. That is, he admits by default that people are not rational decision-makers at all, meaning his concept of humans as the knowing architects of all their pretend-distress is faulty. He cannot deny that his inchoate model of mind permits unconscious determination, so that his model of rational psychotherapy cannot be universal. At best, his "autonomous psychotherapy" is a very restricted approach that may be helpful to some intelligent, psychologically-minded, well-behaved people who are on the brink of sufficient self-knowledge to resolve their problems. For the bulk of the human race (including, I dare say, you and me), it would just be an expensive waste of time. The question of what we should do for suicidal teenagers is not addressed in any of his major works.

Before anybody partakes of Szaszian "autonomous psychotherapy," either as a customer or as an intending student, it would be appropriate for the therapist to explain why it is not just a case of "blaming the victim." I would be fascinated to hear the explanation, because it won't come from Szasz himself.

13.8. A Note on Psychiatrists as Witch-Hunters

Szasz holds very strongly to the idea that psychiatrists have inherited from the Church the mantle of persecutors and executioners of deviants. For hundreds of years in many parts of Europe, odd, difficult and otherwise innocent people were labeled as witches, then tortured and murdered, whereas we now agree that witchcraft was a myth. Starting from the viewpoint that mental disorder is a myth, Szasz has concluded that psychiatrists are persecuting people for mythical reasons. Specifically, he claims that psychiatrists are the modern heirs and successors of the witch-hunters, holding part of the population to ransom for the purpose of maintaining peace and decorum while enriching themselves, and thereby occupying the same social role as the Dominicans who facilitated the Inquisition.

His case appears to be of this form:

1. People nominated as witches were persecuted by the religious state.
2. Witchcraft was a myth.
3. Mental disorder is a myth.
4. Therefore, psychiatrists are persecuting people nominated as mentally-ill on behalf of the therapeutic state.

Set out this way, it is not immediately convincing, so where does the problem lie? We do not take exception to points (1) and (2) but point (3) is problematic. If this proposition fails for any reason, then his case collapses. In S.12.2 above, I have argued that it definitely fails. Look again at Gilbert Ryle's aphorism: "A myth is not a fairy story. It is the presentation of facts belonging to one category in the idioms of another. To explode a myth is not to deny the facts but to reallocate them." Szasz criticizes mainstream psychiatrists for presenting the facts of behavioral disturbance in the idiom of biological medicine. Seventy-five years ago, as a schoolboy with no knowledge of psychiatry or psychiatrists, he decided he knew more than anybody about the nature of mental disorder (recall what Garrison Keillor said about teenagers and self-certainty). By nothing more than chance, Szasz got it right (many other bright young Jewish boys in Central Europe at the same decided that it was real and biological, or real but psychological, or religious etc.). Having decided that all mental disorder is fraud, he then allocates psychiatrists to the category of dishonest persons but, as noted, this is just another of his many ideological claims. It is ideology because he makes no attempt to explain the "observable phenomena" (of mental disorder) in rational terms, only to explain the whole thing away as dishonesty. What shifts him from being just another psychiatrist with some quirky views to a fanatical ideologue is the fact that there is nothing the patient or the psychiatrist can say or do to convince Szasz otherwise. Like the good bishops sitting on the Inquisition, Szasz is unmoved by mere denials of wrong-doing by the weeping wretches at his feet, be they patients or psychiatrists.

Having made a major claim about the form and nature of the structure of modern society, he offers no evidence whatsoever to support his claim. In fact, there are large differences between the roles of the Inquisition and the role of institutional psychiatry. Witches, for a start, almost never nominated themselves, whereas the great bulk of mentally-disordered people do. Psychiatrists, according to Szasz, do not believe their patients are mentally disturbed, they are only pretending. The Dominicans, however, were not pretending: they most definitely believed their victims were the real article. These roles are therefore not sociological homologies.

Thus far, his claim that psychiatry is the legal heir and successor of the Inquisition cannot be accepted. However, there is more to it, as psychiatry has a morbid record of treating mentally-disturbed people badly, as detailed in Whitaker's studiously low-key histories [9, 10]. But what impels monstrosities like the lobotomy, cardiazol shock therapy, and now massive drugging of a large and growing part of the population? Is it just the same lust to persecute that the early Church, Hitler, Stalin and all the rest showed? I don't believe so. I have argued at length that the fault in modern psychiatry is not the blood lust of its practitioners, or even their venality, but their failure to develop a formal model of mental disorder. When they see certain behavioral facts, facts that Szasz also sees, they are moved to "do something" so they can "get those unfortunates better." Because they have no model of mental disorder, they grasp blindly at therapeutic straws and then, full of good intentions, all stampede down that well-known road to damnation. The effect is the same, i.e. patients are dreadfully mistreated, but the motive is different. Szasz denies that any psychiatrist other than himself wants to get patients better and that he is the only honest psychiatrist in history. These could only be described as rather bold claims. It would help his case if he provided some empirical evidence to support his case but he can't—and won't.

Accordingly, we can conclude that Szasz's historical case fails on the basis that any parallels between institutional psychiatry and the Inquisition are serendipitous. He has never shown that the medieval church and modern psychiatry occupied similar structural roles in a theory of sociology. Indeed, he doesn't even offer a theory of society beyond a mass of undefined games. He has offered a mildly interesting historical analogy with no predictive value, but it is not a convincing homology.

13.9. The Origins of the Exceptional Ideas of Thomas Szasz...

The ideas of Thomas Szasz are indeed exceptional. Stripped of his many errors, his conspiracy theories, his extremist political views, his polemics and his endless rhetorical devices, there really isn't much left beyond blaming the victim and abusing everybody who doesn't agree with him. Where does this come from? I think the answer is perfectly clear: all is revealed in the astounding autobiographical chapter he contributed to the volume edited by his assiduous acolyte, the psychologist, Jeffrey Schaler. It is astounding, as much for what it leaves out as for the breath-taking insightlessness of what it says. But Szasz is an exceedingly clever wordsmith and the omissions are not always readily apparent.

Szasz was born in Budapest in the immediate aftermath of the collapse of the Dual Monarchy. In the tumultuous transition to a republic, there was a short-lived communist government which unleashed a period of "red terror," an invasion by Rumania and vast dislocation as the country lost most of its territory and a third of its population. After extensive, vicious street fighting, a fascist regime under Admiral Horthy took control and exacted bloody revenge, including pogroms against Bolshevik Jews. A few years later, the Great Depression brought the struggling country to the edge of collapse. None of this touched young Thomas Szasz, who was born into a well-connected, wealthy, upper middle class, secular Jewish family. Szasz *père et mère* adored their two sons and indulged them endlessly. Their second son, Thomas, was believed to be rather sickly so he was not allowed to mix with the other boys or join in their games or sports. Eighty-five years later, Prof. Szasz states without a shadow of concern that, from a very early age, he learned that if he wanted something or didn't want to do something else, he had only to pretend to be sick and his wish became his parents' command. They never doubted him and he freely admits that he cheated them mercilessly for many years. When he was thought to be upstairs sick in bed, he was usually playing ferocious games of table tennis (ping pong) with his brother.

Moreover, in the absence of any real friendships with boys of his age, he spent much of his free time with his mother. Together, they took long walks along the river in their ancient and cultured city, deep in conversation on his favorite subjects, religion, politics, philosophy, the arts, etc. This is apparently how he spent many afternoons as a teenager. He did not play sport, did not have any real outdoor activities, no military or other interests and was not involved in religious activities to any great extent. One day at about this time, while walking to school, he decided that mental illness is a fraud. While this clearly indicates the level and scope of his interests, it is *ipso facto* the clearest evidence of how far he was removed from the life of an ordinary teenage boy.

By the time he was eighteen and ready to begin university, the future was looking very grim so the family decided to leave Hungary to join his paternal uncle, a professor of mathematics who was already in the US. It was, of course, almost impossible for Jews to leave Europe but by an amazing stroke of luck, they managed to obtain visas. Szasz migrated and continued studying. He decided to study medicine but not for any interest in helping his fellow humans, only because he was curious as to what went on inside them. After some initial difficulties due largely to having a Jewish background and pointedly refusing to play this down, he entered the university where his uncle was teaching and began his medical training. He was not conscripted because he was studying, then the war ended and he was able to complete his education.

Next, he decided to study psychiatry but again, makes it quite clear that he really had no interest in humans *per se*. In those days, as Kandel [7] emphasizes, psychiatric training was not onerous but the younger Szasz seemed to have a remarkable ability to cause friction, largely by what appears to be an intensely self-righteous attitude with no ability to compromise. Soon after he qualified, during the Korean War, he was conscripted so he enlisted in the US Navy and had a very gentle war as a specialist officer in the main naval hospital in Bethesda, Maryland. While in uniform, he read a great deal but didn't appear to have done much work. There is no evidence in this chapter that he paid any attention to the large numbers of disturbed men who were returning from Korea.

On discharge, he moved around several times until he found a position in the university department of psychiatry in Syracuse, upstate New York. He is quite open as to why he went there: he wanted a quiet job in a pleasant rural setting where he could spend his time reading and writing on his favorite subjects, philosophy, religion and politics. After some friction with various authorities over his singular ideas, he settled in and will shortly clock his fifty years as a tenured professor at that institution.

13.10. ...And What They Mean

Based on the detail he gave in this chapter and his main work, there are certain conclusions we can draw. Firstly, Szasz is a highly intelligent and verbally proficient polyglot with all the advantages of a classic *Mitteleuropa* education in a loving family: not for him a poverty-stricken upbringing in the backwoods, a few years of inept schooling and then working in the fields or in a coal mine. There were no drunken family brawls and no incest; he was never abandoned; there was not even a cruel, repressive father or a wicked stepmother. It would seem he was never hit in his life. Quite remarkably, he was not teased or bullied at school, he had no lecherous sport or music teachers nor was he torn apart by adolescent guilt heaped on his head by priests. His was an idyllic existence but he clearly does not realize just how rare that is. From birth, he enjoyed the inestimable advantage of a life surrounded by supportive and mostly adoring people, a life unclouded by doubt, especially self-doubt. There are no shades of gray in the spectrum of his life, all edges are crystal-hard and razor-sharp, all notions are of such pellucid clarity that uncertainty or doubt becomes a moral failure.

Next, for ninety-two unbroken years, he has been phenomenally lucky, enjoying a truly charmed life in which everything appears to have fallen into his lap. From grossly indulgent and gullible parents to slipping out of the looming disaster of wartime Europe, greatly facilitated by having the ready cash to pay the many fares, taxes, imposts and bribes (which most of his countrymen didn't, thus sealing their fates); from having an influential uncle to his sinecure in the Navy and then an indulgent employer in the form of the State University of New York, Szasz has coasted through life with hardly a hiccup, all the while believing his good fortune (literal and metaphorical) has been due to his stellar brilliance and his superior moral equipment. His minor run-in with the New York state mental health commissioner, which he has tried to turn it into a latter-day Dreyfus Affair, was trivial but he quickly made it worse by his inflammatory attitude (I have survived a dozen such incidents, mostly worse, with none of the help he had). That is to say, this near-delusionally self-righteous person with a biting contempt for lesser mortals (all of us) believes that anybody who hasn't had such an easy life as he has must be a fool, a cheat and a liar. Using his exceptional life as his starting point, Szasz has attempted to inflate the politics of contempt to the level of a universal theory of mind.

His cast-iron principles, which led to the conflict in Syracuse among much more, appear to have hardened with age; he did not object when he was conscripted, which was fortunate because he could have been imprisoned and deported, and being deported to Stalinist Hungary in 1954 was not such a good idea.

As a psychiatrist, Thomas Szasz has spent the greater part of his long career talking, reading, writing and travelling; anything but practicing psychiatry. His clinical experience is extremely limited (how many poor, black drug addicts did he see?) and was doubly or even trebly handicapped by the prejudices he took to work each day. He sees only what he wants to see, and facts that contradict his ideas are quickly turned into evidence of everybody else's duplicity. He evinces absolutely no capacity for self-criticism or self-analysis, and dismisses all criticism with utter contempt. He hears nothing anybody says unless it is adulatory but, if his fawning disciples start to show doubts, he rejects them with not a moment's regret. Thomas Szasz is an outstanding example of the aphorism that it is a short-sighted man who takes the limits of his own field of vision for the natural limits of the world.

Outstanding? No, that is the wrong word entirely. Thomas Szasz is a frightening example of the dangers of trying to generalize from one's own personality disorder to reach a universal statement of the truth of the human condition. In my opinion, his writings show he is a mean-minded and pernicious extremist who uses his prodigious intellect to conceal the fact that he has absolutely no understanding of or empathy for the human condition. He never makes the slightest attempt to see the world from another person's point of view. This is partly because he thinks they are cheats, liars and fools (it is worth reiterating that he says he cheated and lied to his parents and teachers for decades) so there is no point in identifying with their misery, and partly because compassion, empathy, care, consideration and so on are completely outside his experience, so he conceals his deficiencies with contempt. Human distress is alien to him and leaves him utterly bewildered but that, of course, is not his fault. It is the fault of the other seven billion humans who, with precious few exceptions, have failed to benefit themselves from their good fortune in sharing the world with a genius of his stature, instead perversely deluding themselves that affectations such as love, kindness, care and consideration are worth more than telling your neighbors where they have gone wrong.

In short, in the absence of suitable life experience (like yours and mine), Thomas Szasz doesn't "get" mental disorder, it is a closed book to him, but he mistakes his transcendent good fortune for a universal insight. Worse, he holds his opinions with a fixity and immutability indistinguishable from, say, the Nazis who murdered so many of his compatriots on the basis of their (so-called) racial inferiority. Without having conducted a survey, I am sure that the vast majority of psychiatrists who teach medical students and psychiatric trainees see no reason to teach fixed and immutable beliefs. Thus, they would pass him over. There is indeed a conspiracy to ignore Thomas Szasz, but it is the soft conspiracy of the like-minded. One by one, teachers of psychiatry look at the evidence Szasz himself provides, and individually decide it is not worth wasting limited time on his vicious ideology. After all, why should psychiatrists teach their students to blame the victim?

As for modern students, would they not avidly read an anti-establishment figure as part of their adolescent drive to break free of societal control? Apparently not. I can only suggest social reasons for this. Firstly, and despite his belated efforts, Szasz is firmly identified with the age of hippies, meaning the age of their parents and grandparents. Second, he is seen as an ideologue by a generation that disdains ideology. You could say that modern students prefer iPads to iDeologies. In addition, medical students are shocked by the overt heartlessness of Szasz's approach. My experience of modern medical students is that, while evading ideology, they are not heartless. Finally and, to my mind, most damagingly, my conversations with students suggest they see him as simply wrong. In his comfortably Manichean world, Szasz sees only formal brain disorders, or dishonesty (somewhere, there are also problems of living but medical students are interested in serious stuff and leave problems of living to psychologists and social workers). However, anybody born since the dawn of the age of personal computing (sometimes taken as the Apple I in 1977, or the IBM 5150 in 1981) will see things differently.

Without hesitation, the modern generation accepts the idea that, in a complex machine governed by information processing, output can fail in the total absence of any physical fault in the machine. That is, they understand and accept the notion of a "software" fault. The idea that there has to be a biological basis for all mental disturbance strikes them as just plain silly: everybody knows about software glitches, so why should mental disorder be any different? Why could it not arise as a result of an erroneous or self-contradictory informational state? This is what modern students understand intuitively, and it is also why biological psychiatry does not appeal to them. In fact, there is no *a priori* reason why this should not be the case, so Szasz's major claim fails at once. That is, his precocious, or should I say precious, intuition at the tender age of sixteen, over 75 years ago, has been overtaken by the march of history. Like Freud, like Skinner and so many other historical characters, he simply backed the wrong horse. Well, folks, that's science but no hard feelings.

It is for these reasons that professors do not need to conspire together to censor or suppress the work of Thomas Szasz: forcing students to read his work would soon kill his reputation as a person with something valid to say.

13.11 Conclusion: Thomas Szasz, Man of the Past

In summary, the work of Thomas Szasz derives from his unique and idiosyncratic ideological stance which appeals to a very small part of the population, specifically intelligent and excessively intellectualized people with restricted emotional lives who are looking for a ready-made excuse not to probe their failings too deeply, or people who are comfortable with persecutory conspiracies as a universal explanation (or both). People who are swayed by simplistic adolescent moralizing and historical revisionism might choose to be swayed by him while the rest of us, who prefer a more nuanced and humane approach to life, move restlessly on. He has not proven mental disorder is a myth, he has not demonstrated any understanding of the phenomena in question, and he has not advanced human knowledge. However, he uses his inability to understand as a license to attack anybody who doesn't agree with him, even when they are making some sort of honest attempt to find out what it means to be losing your mind.

In the conclusion to the previous chapter, I indicated that it is necessary to recognize the polemical material in Szasz's work so we can strip it away from any underlying facts or justified opinions, the goal being to see any underlying errors and unjustified opinions. The purpose was to establish the logical validity of his claims, independently of the passion with which Szasz delivers them. Having stripped his passion and polemics, his rhetorical devices, his juvenilia, his politics masquerading as philosophy and his generally poor reasoning, I am forced to conclude that, from a rational point of view, there is nothing left on which to construct his "theory of personal conduct." Specifically, he does not have a model of mind, he does not have a model of disturbed mind (just because he doesn't accept it exists), and he therefore has no basis to criticize any other psychiatrist on epistemological grounds. He can criticize them for any number of perfectly valid empirical reasons, but he cannot claim that his approach is ontologically superior. Finally, he has no demonstrated justification for his claims about the nature of psychotherapy and how it should be conducted. A theory of psychotherapy should proceed from a theory of mind but he doesn't have one, so he has inserted moralizing into the gap where a theory of psychotherapy ought to be.

To return to the previous chapter: "The question then arises: has he been isolated by his enemies, or is his work no longer relevant? Indeed, has he been rendered irrelevant by his own efforts?"

There is practically no chance of a modern medical student or trainee in psychiatry being taught the principles outlined by Szasz. He is not on the curriculum of any of the major psychiatric training schemes that I have ever seen. Effectively, he is completely ignored by the one profession he needed to influence. I have no doubt that his influence will rapidly fade within a few years of his passing. His dwindling band of ageing supporters will not be able to halt the progress of history brought about by the information revolution. This was not the result of an ordinary conspiracy, partly because psychiatrists can't organize much at all, but mostly it was because they didn't have to. Psychiatrists of my generation started to read Szasz, put the book down and never went back, just as I did, probably because it was tiresome: "I have long considered lying as one of the most important phenomena in psychiatry... The patients, like children, lie to the doctor. And the physicians, like parents, lie to the patients." This may be the experience of Thomas Szasz, but it is not mine and I see no reason to defer to a person with such limited experience and no theory of mind.

My psychiatric experience, in mental and general hospitals, in prisons and army barracks, in cities and remote areas, in private and public practice with dozens of races and religions, young and old, male and female, clever and not clever, educated and illiterate, rich and desperately poor, in a highly developed western country with its own Third World subculture, and in poor parts of Asia, vastly exceeds his and has led me to totally different conclusions: when I look at mental patients, I do not see liars and scoundrels skulking before me. I am sure this is also true of the overwhelming majority of psychiatrists. Szasz's irrefutable claim, based on no conceivable evidence, that all patients and all psychiatrists are part of a huge conspiracy to lie all the time, is not an empirical claim. In one word, it is paranoid. Any psychiatrist who wants to see the "observable phenomena" we call mental disorder from a scientific point of view is obliged to discard any Szaszian ideas about the nature and correct management of those phenomena.

Part III:
Clinical Syndromes
as a Test of the
Biocognitive Model for Psychiatry

"The member of a mature scientific community is, like the typical character of Orwell's *1984*, the victim of a history rewritten by the powers that be."

—Thomas Kuhn

<table>
<tr><td>14</td><td>

Testing the Biocognitive Model:
Clinical Syndromes (1)

</td></tr>
</table>

"This impression of scientific certitude in the midst of substantial and potentially crippling problems is a tribute to the ability of psychologists and the psychiatric profession to acquire and wield power."

—Eric T. Dean

14.1. Introduction

In one sense, writing this chapter is a waste of time. I want to show that it is intellectually feasible, as well as beneficial for our patients, to look at some of the major clinical syndromes from the vantage point this theory offers. I am, however, acutely mindful of certain impediments to this goal. The first problem is the vast mental health industry that aims to prove the exact opposite of anything a theory of this type may say. This industry is composed of an intellectually insecure academia, an avaricious Big Pharma and a venal, corporatized mental health bureaucracy, ably supported by a well-meaning but completely suborned public or "grass roots" movement. Note that I did not specify psychiatry: the mental health industry has a number of subsidiaries who are all working to the same goal, including nursing unions, the burgeoning psychology and social work industries and the most recent starters, the relentlessly growing rivers of unqualified people who draw salaries as Personal Care Assistants, Mental Health Rehabilitation Trainers, Personal Growth Workers, Mental Health Mentors, Transition Facilitators and so on. All this is predicated upon the uselessness of those whom PC dictates we shall know as "mental health consumers," if not customers. The mental health industry has a powerful vested interest in making sure that its customers remain useless in perpetuity. It is not in their interest to encourage alternative points of view, so they don't. It could even be said that they not averse to preventing challenges.

The second problem is that anybody wishing to mount a challenge to the establishment is bound to do so in terms of rules the establishment itself has written. This means that if, for example, I wanted to show that, say, the concept of the antisocial personality disorder is wrong, I would need to undertake an exhaustive review of the literature, with a large epidemiological study to support any views that may emerge. Needless to say, the people who control the funds for such activities are just those who stand to lose most from the success of the review and the survey. Moreover, the same people control the psychiatric publishing industry, which is not predicated upon providing a forum for challenges to the establishment [1]. Its purpose is to reinforce whatever beliefs the establishment may hold by patiently assembling an entirely biased corpus of literature and preventing any alternative points of view seeing the light of day. Anybody who doubts this need only dip into the work of, say, psychiatrists Peter Breggin or David Healy to find how the publishing industry has actively suppressed results that were unfavorable to the stance adopted by their patrons in the mental health industry.

Needless to say, I don't have access to funds so I can't conduct a survey. And even if I could overcome these small hazards, it would not be published. The psychiatric publishing industry does not exist to print criticism of those who control it for their own benefit (very largely academics) or those who pay for it (the drug industry). Challenges will not come from within the establishment, as David Healy describes so clearly in the case of the dangerous psychiatric side effects of the antidepressant, paroxetine [2]. Challenges come from without, exactly as Thomas Kuhn predicted. Whitaker was once congratulated by a psychiatrist for his brave efforts in exposing the historical crimes of psychiatry [3, 4], to which he replied: "So why didn't you guys do it yourselves?" One part of the answer is very simple: the material in his books would never have been published by the psychiatric publishing industry, such as the publishing arm of the American Psychiatric Association, APA Publishing. The industry does, however, regularly publish criticism of his work [5].

Thus, this chapter will not meet the standards set by the establishment for criticism of their views; this does not greatly concern me, as we all know that nothing meets their standards for criticism of their views. How do we know this? Because, in gross breach of scientific ethics, no worthwhile criticism of their views is ever published. *Res ipso loquitur* (and don't say it isn't submitted because I certainly do).

14.2. The New Plague

The most devastating disease since the Black Death is surely what we call now Bipolar Disorder. In barely forty years, it has come from nowhere (0.2% of the population with low rates of continuing morbidity) to one of the most devastating conditions known. In four decades, it has grown to afflict as much as 6.4% of the population (i.e. 3,200% increase) with rates of permanent disability approaching 50% (or 90%, depending on whose survey you read). In children over the past twenty years, the rate of diagnosis of pediatric bipolar (PBAD) has exploded by some 4,000% in the US, while Australians, never to be outdone by their rowdy cousins across the Pacific, proudly boast an increase of not less than 8,000% in PBAD in the same period. In terms of total loss of productive life, this condition greatly exceeds that other modern epidemic, HIV/AIDS.

In 1974, when I began my training in psychiatry, manic-depressive psychosis was rare. Not only was it rare but if you had to have a serious mental disorder, this was the one to have. Schizophrenia was a life sentence: in and out of hospital, lots of drugs and perhaps ECT, then a slow recovery and very gradual return to a restricted sort of life punctuated by further admissions over the years. For years, I lived opposite a psychiatric hostel in suburban Perth. I knew most of the twenty-five residents from my time in Mental Health Services or I got to know them over the fence. Each of them had a diagnosis of schizophrenia and I don't doubt that each of them would be given that diagnosis today.

In those days, having a neurotic disorder was a pain but not dangerous. Neurotics could be jollied along and most of them made lives of sorts for themselves but rarely ended up in hospital for more than brief periods. The really bad diagnosis, of course, was a severe personality disorder, with psychopathic personality the jackpot. There was no treatment, hospitals wouldn't let you in and all the staff hated you, anyway. If your fates had decreed a terrible life, this was it (in about June, 1977, a patient I knew who was a bit difficult and overbearing but otherwise manageable was turned away from Graylands Hospital, Perth, WA, just on the basis of the formal diagnosis "Explosive Personality." Later that day, he stole some dynamite, went to King's Park in the city and blew himself up).

Manic-depressives, on the other hand, knew that, come what may, they would get over it. They had jobs, homes, families, friends, hobbies and sports waiting for them; they came into hospital, they stayed a while then they went home and we didn't see them until next time which could be years later or, quite often, not at all. Many of them were never seen again, unless it was in the suburban shopping center, when they would always want to talk about how they were getting along.

The picture today couldn't be more different. Renamed as Bipolar Affective Disorder (BAD), what was once seen as a rather amusing affliction of the artistic fringe is now a major public health problem, with costs and a disability burden to match. The diagnosis of schizophrenia remains a touch under 1% of the population, but residential care is increasingly dominated by sufferers of BAD. Worse still, their lives are blighted. They are in and out of hospital, not infrequently half a dozen times or more a year. They are prescribed (and mostly take) quantities of drugs which, in the Bad Old Days, would have been seen as simply dangerous practice (one of my early consultants, a roguishly cheerful, deaf old Irish psychiatrist, said that if patients needed more than three drugs, the diagnosis was wrong; he also said "A clever manic lightens my day"). Today, the same patients don't work or study, they lose their families, their friends, their interests, their health and, increasingly, their lives. People with a diagnosis of psychotic disorder die as much as twenty years younger than their birth cohort. But the worst part is surely the quality of life. Their lives become an endless treadmill of appointments, counseling, drugs, day centers, admissions to hospital, more drugs, drug complications—

total dependency, in other words, as dire and demoralizing as life in the back wards of one of the asylums of yesteryear.

Clinically, manic-depressive psychosis as it used to be is not the same diagnosis as BAD today. In Olden Times, when I was young, a manic person was the maddest patient you would ever see. Usually brought in by the police, they ran around, tore their clothes off, sang, yelled, grabbed the anatomy of passing staff and laughed outrageously. They told jokes, had plans to save the world or make millions and angrily demanded permission to ring the prime minister to tell him what he was doing wrong. They talked and talked, their minds spinning faster than their tongues could keep up, ideas and plans tumbling over each other but they lost interest almost as soon as they appeared. They felt no need to sleep and usually didn't have time to eat. As the attack intensified, they became more and more disorganized, unable to complete a sentence, unable to lie down, panting, with sweat pouring down them, often becoming angry and suspicious, then bursting into wild (manic) laughter as another idea briefly took control. In a hot climate, they could develop serious dehydration in six hours so they were sedated as a matter of urgency. Acute mania was rare but it was seen as a medical emergency.

A few degrees below this florid clinical picture and more common was hypomania, meaning "just below mania." These people were usually aware that something wasn't right but, unless they knew where it might end, they mostly enjoyed it. They were very active, full of energy and needed only a few hours sleep each night. They would eat if reminded but mostly weren't much concerned about food as they were having such a good time. They buzzed around, talking to everybody, making friends, helping strangers with their problems, devising improvements in hospital procedures or making plans for a brilliant future. If they had money, they spent it or lent it to anybody who asked but they weren't concerned, money was neither here nor there. They were socially gregarious and sexually disinhibited, so the young women (and a lot of them were young women) had to be watched closely otherwise they would disappear into the garden with one male patient after another. A striking feature of these people was that they told lies, mostly silly, pointless lies that were certain to be discovered, then they brushed them off with a dismissive laugh.

Their depressive states were the same, only at the other end of the spectrum. Over a relatively short period, perhaps a couple of weeks, they would slip from managing their lives to sitting weeping in a corner, unable to eat or sleep, mostly apathetic and despairing but often agitated and restless with thoughts of searing, cosmic guilt churning their minds day and night. They lost weight at frightening speeds, up to 10kg in three weeks was not uncommon. Occasionally, they developed bizarre ideas of guilt, that they had caused an earthquake or some other catastrophe and deserved to die, or their intestines had rotted and the gas was poisoning their brains. The mental torture they suffered was palpable and there was no doubt that, left untreated, some would either die of inanition or make serious attempts on their lives. Mostly, they were brought to hospital by relatives or friends who feared such an attempt. Once admitted, they had to be watched closely as sudden, lethal suicide bids were common enough to keep staff nervous for their safety.

In the main, they came into hospital very disturbed, settled and went home in the order of weeks rather than months. Sometimes, in the course of a few days or a week, they would swing from a manic state to depression or vice versa, then their stay was longer but the expectation that they would always recover was rarely disappointed. Very few of them became long-term in-patients; very few of them moved into the psychiatric hostels and there were certainly not very many on pensions for chronic mental disorder. I remember saying to one new social worker: "Don't worry about trying to find work for the manic-depressives, they'll talk their way into any job." That's a generalization but that was how it was.

The modern picture could not be more different. What was once rare is now common, and rapidly becoming more so, and what was once a more or less normal, even productive life punctuated by bouts of disability has become a devastating condition that is now a major cause of permanent disability. The question then arises: why are there so many more of these patients now than there were four or even three decades ago? And of those who are given the diagnosis, why is the course of their condition so much more severe and disabling than it used to be?

In a detailed historical review, the investigative journalist, Robert Whitaker has argued that a very large part of the reason this condition has become so serious is just because of the effects of psychotropic drugs. In *Anatomy of an Epidemic* [4], he uses the psychiatric literature itself to chart the explosive increase in the rates of diagnosis of BAD and the equally disturbing deterioration in the functional output of individual cases. A person receiving this diagnosis in 2012 is not going to have the same life as a person diagnosed manic-depressive in 1974, on that point there is no debate whatsoever. Look at some of the famous people in history who were diagnosed or regarded as manic-depressives: Ludwig Boltzman, nuclear physicist; Edward Elgar, composer; Spike Milligan, comedian and actor; Edgar Allen Poe, Jack London, Virginia Woolf and Ernest Hemingway, authors; Edvard Munch and Jackson Pollock, artists; Friedrich Nietzche, philosopher and professional maniac; Ted Turner, billionaire; and any number of difficult, obstreperous, unpredictable, drunk or disreputable but brilliant musicians, actors, artists, politicians, sports men and women. Having seen many, many people who have been drugged to a near-vegetative state by the modern approach to medicating BAD, there is not the slightest doubt that those justly famous people would not have achieved at such high levels if they had received the same medication.

Whitaker's case is that the drugs themselves are very likely to be producing the epidemic: while it is not wholly an iatrogenic or doctor-caused condition, modern psychotropic drugs are greatly exacerbating it. Once a person starts the drugs, his condition is likely to deteriorate and he may eventually become disabled, just by virtue of taking the drugs. But as his mental state declines, so the numbers of drugs and the dosage levels are increased, in an ever-spiraling vicious circle of mental symptoms, drugs and disability. That is, a condition that, essentially untreated, had a relatively good prognosis has since mutated into a major, lifelong disability requiring constant specialist attention, numerous social and other supports that very often means a completely invalid life.

It is true that this conclusion has provoked intense negative reactions from the psychiatric establishment [5] and the drug industry. Predictably, psychiatrists have challenged his data or his interpretation of study results. What they haven't done is just what they would do if the tables were turned: propose a full, independent study of the charges, including an independent literature review and long-term field studies of the drugs *as they are used* (remember that the vast majority of drug trials are conducted in less than eight weeks, and patients take only the one medication). To illustrate, consider the case of another modern epidemic. In 1981, a previously rare pulmonary condition, *Pneumocystis carinii* pneumonia, was identified in a cluster of gay men in Los Angeles. At about the same time, a rare skin tumor, Kaposi's sarcoma, suddenly started to appear, but only in well-defined groups of younger people in certain parts of the world. Immediately, massive studies were launched and, in 1983, after a prodigious research effort, HIV, the causative organism, was isolated.

In historical terms, the discovery of HIV as the cause of AIDS was probably without precedent in medicine. As soon as the first alarming signs of disease were detected in the community, the enormous and enormously sophisticated investigative machinery of modern medicine swung into action, liberally funded and, despite Phillipics from naysayers in the deeper dens of fundamentalism (the people who put the mental in fundamental), with widespread public support. Public figures and celebrities of the very highest profiles threw their prodigious talents in public relations into the fight to find the cause and cure of this frightening new epidemic. And it worked. New infections and deaths from HIV/AIDS are now declining in most parts of the world except war-torn areas in Sub-Saharan Africa. Similarly, advances in the basic science of immunology have powered ahead. All of this serves only to prove what can be done if the political will is there.

In the case of the possibility that psychotropic drugs may be contributing to the unprecedented increases in the rates of diagnosis and morbidity of some major psychiatric conditions, the response of the psychiatric establishment has been notable only for their silence, leaving the field wide open to partisan observers such as Edwin Fuller Torrey. Torrey, who has had a long and varied career, adheres firmly to the strictest of biological interpretations of mental disorder. For example, he has long been involved in projects to find an infective cause for schizophrenia, focusing his efforts on the plasmodium, *Toxoplasma gondii*. Searches of this kind, previously derided as "the search for the elusive *schizococcus*," are definitely regarded as marginal by mainstream psychiatric circles but Dr. Torrey is nothing if not independent of mainstream opinion. However marginal, he has been able to convince funding agencies that the search for the schizococcus must go on. Given that track record, he could, if he wished, readily cobble together the wherewithal for a long-term, naturalistic study of treated vs. untreated mental disorders. He has not done so, the presumption being that he does not wish to do so.

There is only one method of disproving the hypothesis that psychotropic drugs are significantly adding to the total illness burden in the community. Mainstream psychiatric institutions all know precisely what that method is. They have vast experience in conducting those types of studies, they have access to essentially unlimited funds, they need research projects to justify their salaries, and they have done nothing. Moreover, my prediction is that they will continue to do nothing constructive but will denigrate any and every point raised by any person, anywhere, any time for any reason that calls into question their entire *raison d'être*: the belief that mental disorder is biological in nature and drugs prescribed by psychiatrists are the centerpiece of treatment. And there, for the time being, the matter rests.

14.3. Creating the New Plague

Meantime, back on the streets, or in the schools or factories or suburbs, rapidly growing numbers of people are becoming disabled by serious mental symptoms which appear to be increasingly unresponsive to the very latest of high-tech pharmacology. One theory to account for this has been described above: the drugs are doing it. Whitaker advances the suggestion that the main smoking guns are stimulants, both legal and illegal, and antidepressants. There is no doubt from the psychiatric literature that these drugs cause bouts of intense agitation as a predictable side effect, and that the standard psychiatric response of "take twice the dosage" serves only to make things worse. People can become psychotic on these drugs and on these drugs alone. Even more frightening are the reports that certain antidepressants actually cause episodes of suicidal and/or aggressive behavior, including homicide [2].

Mood stabilizers and antipsychotics are also prime suspects but these tend to come after the first event, i.e. after the first manic breakdown. People are not prescribed antipsychotics and mood stabilizers without a reason, and the reason is that they show a manic episode. The problem is that the first manic episode is, in fact, very often the predictable side effect of antidepressants. After the second group of drugs, antipsychotics and mood stabilizers, are started, their condition fails to improve as hoped and very often starts to get worse. We can't blame the antipsychotics and mood stabilizers for initiating the person's new career as a mental patient, although they may be responsible le for cementing it in place. The drugs were commenced for what seemed valid reasons. However, people definitely are put on stimulants and antidepressants without *good* reason, and this is where the psychiatric literature comes into its own.

In an earlier chapter, I showed figures for the evolving patterns of medication usage in the US. As usual, the rest of the world is following the American suit, with explosive increases in antidepressant consumption rates. There has not, however, been a commensurate explosive improvement in mental health, or even a dribble of an improvement. Every figure available, and they are readily available, shouts out: Look out, depression is the word and it's coming to your house soon. In the UK, the number of days of disability due to depression and neurotic disorders rose from 38 million in 1984 to 117 million in 1995, i.e. far from causing an improvement, the rapidly growing use of antidepressants was associated with a 300% increase in disability [4].

Like all English-speaking countries, Australia now has a psychiatric public relations industry that exists solely to pump alarming figures and news items into the homes of the general public. A hugely expensive program called 'beyondblue' (*sic*), run by a body called The National Depression Initiative, has a most professional website offering advice such as this: "Depression is currently the highest medical cause of disability worldwide and predicted to be the second highest medical cause of death and disability worldwide by 2020" [6]. Headlines shout that our (rather small) country loses half a million working days *each month* to depressive disorders, mixed with advice about telling your friends they look depressed and where to take them for help. Television advertisements run by this agency or posters in public toilets (yes, you can read them while standing at the urinal; perhaps the plan is that the poster will come to be associated with a sense of relief) posters in toilets urge anybody who feels they may be suffering this or related afflictions (anxiety and, essentially, all of what were once called neurotic disorders) to "see your doctor." Doctors, of course, prescribe drugs.

Antidepressants are now routinely prescribed for all cases of depression, including minor reactive unhappiness that many argue [7] should not even be called depression; for any and all cases of anxiety (DSM-IV-TR has eleven separate codes for anxiety disorders), including all post-traumatic conditions of any sort or anything that could be blamed on something unpleasant, like work or having a baby; all cases of unexplained physical disorders on the basis they may be a "depressive equivalent"; anything that could conceivably attract a label of "stress" (I say label because this is not a medical term); any and all cases of irritability, annoyance or bad temper; for any and all problems sleeping, including insomnia, nightmares and hypersomnia; for any condition involving pain, on the basis of augmenting the body's pain suppressant mechanisms or preventing depression; for grief (of course); for the large and growing group of obsessive-compulsive disorders; anything to do with the group known as autism spectrum disorders; anything to do with drug or alcohol abuse; and for anybody whose life isn't just A1 hunky dory, on the basis that, if they aren't overtly depressed then, if they were in their right mind, they must be covertly depressed but if they're not in their right mind, they need antidepressants anyway.

It goes beyond just recruiting ever-larger numbers of people to start drugs: they must continue them, too. The site WebMD says: "In general, doctors recommend that people stay on an antidepressant at least one year to experience the full benefits. Beyond that, when—and whether—you should to go off depression medication (sic) is a personal choice that requires serious thought" [8]. The implication is clear. Mainstream psychiatric opinion these days is that any person who has experienced two bouts of depression, or one serious bout, or one as a child or teenager, should take the drugs for life.

Now we start to see where all the alleged "bipolars" are coming from: they are recruited via a widespread and officially sanctioned policy of prescribing antidepressants unless there is a strong reason not to. Moreover, the prescribers are, in the main, busy general practitioners with, also in the main, absolutely minimal training in anything to do with psychiatry, who don't know how to conduct a psychiatric assessment and, if they did, wouldn't do it anyway because they don't get paid for it. That has recently changed in this country, and GPs are now paid extra to conduct psychiatric assessments in order to write a "mental health care plan," copies of which are signed and exchanged by GP and patient, as though they had some contractual nature beyond providing the GP with a modicum of legalistic protection. Having seen hundreds of these plans myself, you can be assured that, in terms of providing an accurate assessment of the patient's mental state, they are absolutely useless. It would be a brave GP who did the assessment and then decided to offer no treatment. The position now is: Patient complains of any of the above problems; GP completes a mental health care plan because he is paid extra to do so; patient is told of the outcome; patient expects drugs; most GPs will not say No. Once the patient opens his mouth to complain about his state, the chances of any outcome other than drugs plummet. Is that all? No, there's more.

Firstly, the criteria for making a diagnosis of a treatable depressive condition have been widened considerably over the years [7]. Second, and more important, a huge group of psychiatric conditions has simply been lifted from where they belong, and moved across to the category of depression. I am referring to personality disorders. This has been a two or three step process, depending on how you look at it. Regardless of the mechanism, for psychiatry, the particular value is this: many more people, who previously would have been discharged (perchance to feed the local crows), can now be prescribed drugs and kept in the psychiatric service. This did not happen overnight. It started in 1980, with the arrival of DSM-III. The sections on personality in this manual showed two features which, just for interest, were immediately and widely regarded as all-but fatal weaknesses of a very dodgy system of diagnosis.

The first problem was the fact that DSM-III opted for a categorical system of diagnosis for personality disorders. This means that each personality disorder is regarded as profoundly different from all others; essentially, there is no overlap. In Chap. 8 of *Humanizing Madness*, I have shown the folly of this system and how it was cobbled together by, in one word, *cheating*. The second was that psychiatry had no theory of personality disorder (because it has no theory of personality) and therefore regarded a diagnosis of personality disorder as of minor importance. Essentially, a personality disorder belongs to the afterthought class, something added to the stats sheet after the real work (of finding and treating a mental disorder) has been completed. All of this is true, but it doesn't explain why mainstream psychiatry has so little interest in personality disorder. The answer is that it has, in fact, no treatment for personality disorder. It used to be that some cases would be offered psychotherapy but, in these straitened days of managed care, insurers decide what they will pay for and what they won't, and personality disorder is one they won't. Since modern psychiatrists receive negligible training in psychotherapy, their choices are very limited.

Thus, psychiatry suddenly found that personality disorder could be relegated to Axis II of its schema, and there it has languished ever since, except that a remarkable thing has happened. Remember that psychiatry is based upon fee for service. In private practice, if you don't see patients, you go hungry and, despite claims, public services are no different. They exist only insofar as there is a demonstrated demand for their product, as governments now say. If nobody qualifies for public psychiatric treatment, then the services will be closed and all the nurses and psychologists, the social workers and therapists, the cooks, cleaners, drivers and gardeners and, above all, administrators, will have to find other jobs. As a career prospect, that idea does not go down well with all the nurses and etc. Medical staff tend not to mind, they can always go back and be real doctors but, for an overweight 58yo psychiatric nurse with arthritis, hypertension and a mortgage and an elderly mother to support, that option is not available. The thought of a service contracting, or even closing, is very, very frightening, and nursing unions and others the world over don't like it.

In Australia and other welfare states, hospitals can be "downsized" only so far; they cannot be closed, otherwise local communities, unions and other pressure groups become enraged and, when enraged, are apt to apply pressure to the tender parts of their local politician's anatomy. Despite any misguided beliefs to the contrary, the role of hospitals in welfare states is to provide jobs. Since hospitals are major employers of female labor, only a very resolute politician would risk closing one. In the US, hospitals are businesses, and businesses must make a profit, be they private for-profit businesses, government businesses (state and veterans' hospitals), not-for-profit hospitals (such as religious charities) or universities (very big business). In a capitalist state, hospitals exist to pull in money, as well as soaking up excess unskilled labor. However, as Mr. Hacker found [9], once opened, a hospital can never be closed. At the same time, they are not the sorts of businesses that can close in one town and reopen in another. Almost invariably, they have huge, ugly clusters of mismatched and absolutely useless buildings in bad parts of town that are hopelessly overcapitalized (the results of lobbying by the same pressure groups when times were better or elections impended) and conceal a tiny core of decrepit historical buildings that can't be bulldozed, so the site can't even be cleared for something decent, like a sports arena or a brewery.

The net effect is that, wherever one goes in the world, hospitals are full and are kept full. Deliberately. So the problem for psychiatry post-DSM-III was that, by decree, something like half the patients who had previously helped keep the show afloat were suddenly told they weren't wanted. Immediately, psychiatric administrators found themselves in a difficult position. On the one hand, they were selling themselves to the world as having a series of magic bullets [4] that could cure anything mental but, on the other, they were faced with a sudden shrinkage of their patient base as personality disorders, who are anyway immune to magic bullets, were excluded and yet, on the third hand, they had to stay in business. The solution took a little time in coming but desperate needs breed desperate measures: the swarms of rejected patients milling around the doors of the mental hospitals, angrily demanding to be allowed in, were given tickets and allowed in, but only if they pretended to be something they were not, like sick.

You can, I am sure, see the supreme artistry in this bureaucratic hand-spring. It's a bit like finding gold in the sewage: yesterday's turds become today's godsend. It didn't happen overnight, of course, it took the psychiatric establishment a little time to realize that they had been mistaken all these years, in that what they previously thought were signs of a true turd, such as outbursts of rage, or intense regret after being arrested, were really signs of an unrecognized sickness. Ironically enough, the sickness was, in this case, BAD. In the space of a few short years, naughty people were being relabeled as mad people, hospitals once more filled to bursting point, jobs were going begging, politicians had new buildings to open, there were commissions of enquiry into everything, laws drafted by lawyers legislating jobs for lawyers on the new mental health tribunals and, *mirabile dictu*, all the brand new mental patients were found to need drugs—for life. The reason they needed drugs for life was because they weren't getting better. Indeed, a lot were getting worse and needed extra services. The reason they weren't getting better was because they weren't sick in the first place, just difficult, so the only effect the drugs were having was slowly poisoning them.

The clearest example of this is seen in the reclassification of the most defenseless group in the community, children, especially difficult children who, coincidentally, are over-represented in abandoned or neglected children in care who, also coincidentally, are over-represented in the offspring of poor, ugly, stupid, drunk, violent or otherwise hopeless parents, including those of ethnic minorities who have lesser access to social services. Based largely on the work of the group around the proselytizing Harvard psychiatrist, Joseph Biederman, irritability in children was reclassified as a mental illness called PBAD. In one swoop, a huge new market opened for the manufacturers of a large number of drugs as children in care who played up were immediately put on the sorts of drugs that vets wouldn't dare use on thoroughbreds, in doses that would render a small thoroughbred insensible (can you seriously imagine a race horse running on olanzapine?).

It was, as Prof. Biederman later made absolutely clear in his friendly chat with Sen. Grassley's committee of inquiry, pure coincidence that he and his esteemed colleagues from his august institution were on the payroll of the same drug manufacturers to the tune of several millions of dollars which, by some oversight, had not been declared to the university authorities or, more to the point, to the psychiatrists who read the literature on PBAD and started prescribing drugs for the masses on the say-so of Prof. Biederman. Adult prisons weren't far behind and now, it seems, even the US Army has fallen into line, with soldiers going into battle zones stoned on psychotropics (the Australian Army is a little tardy: a soldier who needs psychotropic drugs is very likely to be discharged as unfit, so we don't have quite the same problem with mentally disordered troops as our noble allies).

It is now not uncommon for children in care to be placed on as many as seven or eight psychotropic drugs, including antidepressants, mood stabilizers, antipsychotic drugs, stimulants and tranquillizers—all at once. Does this matter? The drug companies and their supporters in academic psychiatry argue that it doesn't matter, that the drugs are safe when used for the purposes of treating mental disorders with a biological basis and, as we all know, that includes all mental disorders, even mental disorders that were previously wrongly classified as personality disorders. Any long term side effects of medication have to be balanced against the serious risks of an untreated mental disorder; it is, the psychiatrist will say, a case of balancing a very slight risk a long time in the future vs. the real danger of failing to treat what is known to be a rapidly advancing mental illness with suicidal and possibly homicidal tendencies. Very few parents can resist that. It is, in fact, a good example of the well-known cognitive defect in humans called "discounting the future."

There is now evidence to suggest that at least a part of the risk of deterioration from being diagnosed BAD (pediatric or adult) lies in the cocktail of quite dangerous drugs used to treat the disorder. Also, there is convincing evidence that some of the drugs actually cause homicidal and/or suicidal impulses, so the "disease" cannot be blamed for that (to my recollection, manic-depressives were pests but they were not a danger). But, as everybody knows, it's all in how you say it. As Sir Humphrey Appleby enlightened his minister, the browbeaten Mr. Hacker:

> "On the contrary, Minister, there's all the difference in the world. Almost anything can be attacked as a loss of amenity and almost anything can be defended as not a significant loss of amenity. One must appreciate the significance of *significant.*" (p133, *The Complete Yes Minister*).

Shall we pause here for an example? Let us begin with an item from CNN, dated July 6th 2011 [10]: "Children whose mothers take Zoloft, Prozac, or similar antidepressants during pregnancy are twice as likely as other children to have a diagnosis of autism or a related disorder, according to a small new study, the first to examine the relationship between antidepressants and autism risk. This class of antidepressants, known as selective serotonin reuptake inhibitors (SSRIs), may be especially risky early on in a pregnancy, the study suggests. Children who were exposed to the drugs during the first trimester were nearly four times as likely to develop an autism spectrum disorder (ASD) compared with unexposed children, according to the study, which appears in the *Archives of General Psychiatry.*" I should point out that the study involved 298 children with the diagnosis, and 1507 children to act as controls. Why CNN decided this was a "small" study is not clear, unless they had an eye on drug company advertizing on their service. Commenting on the same study, the *Wall Street Journal* noted:

> "In the antidepressant study, researchers tried teasing apart whether the mother's mental state or the antidepressants were linked with autism. The results indicated an association with the treatment, not with the mother's mental state" [11].

The message does seem to be fairly clear. It is a good example of the class of news items that would normally result in an immediate outbreak of mass hysteria among parents, teachers, nurses, psychologists and other experts, who would besiege the nearest politician's office and demand the offending drugs be removed, while squadrons of ambulance-chasing lawyers pulled up their sleeves and got ready for the fun. In fact, nothing much happened. As Sir Humphrey knew, it all depends on the meaning of the word 'significant,' and also whoever decides whether the results are 'significant.' In this case, the researchers themselves took an emollient line:

"A lot of people might get a little worried about these findings and change something they're doing—which they shouldn't. It indicates to us that there's more to look at," said the lead author [11].

A website maintained by a group called Autism Support Network™ reported on this study [12] for its readers:

"(The study) found that the 'use of antidepressant medications during pregnancy also shows a secular increase in recent decades, prompting concerns that prenatal exposure may contribute to increased risk of ASD (autism spectrum disorder).' It's a risk that Dr. Mathew Biel, who specializes in autism treatment at Georgetown University Hospital, says has to be weighed against the dangerous alternative. 'Trying to balance this risk ... what looks like a very small, but real risk of increased rate of autism, again very small, against the risk of leaving depression untreated and all of the negative consequences for the mother and her offspring,' is the challenge facing doctors and patients, he said. Biel says leaving depression or bipolar disorder untreated in pregnant women can be deadly for mom and baby. Biel says the study is intriguing and deserves the attention of a follow up."

Quite clearly, their expert is minimizing any risk associated with these drugs. The risk of autism from taking the drugs is "very small" (a 300% increase in risk is not normally regarded as very small, even if the absolute risk remains small) whereas the alternative, failing to dose the mother "can be deadly for mom and baby." However, any implied punches were pulled in the last line of their article: "Not taking medication may not be an option for some mothers." (It's not clear whether Dr. Biel said that or it was the reporter's own idea but it reads like Dr. Biel). That is, if keeping mother happy during her nine months of pregnancy costs the child's sanity forever, then so be it.

At this stage, not a year later, the report appears to have slid below the event horizon of the news services, indicating a well-orchestrated campaign has succeeded in heading off what could have been a highly embarrassing, not to mention hugely expensive, public relations glitch. Research that finds possible links between psychotropic drugs and highly visible mental disorders is not welcome. We should compare this doubly-muted response with the panic-stricken reaction to a paper published in *The Lancet* in 1998 which presented evidence that MMR immunization could cause autistic disorders. Very quickly, the rate of immunization dropped, leading to epidemics of measles and mumps which resulted in a number of deaths and numerous cases of severe, permanent brain damage. Over the next few years, the Wakefield matter (named after its author) swung back and forth until, after nearly twelve years of bitter vituperation, it was shown to be fraudulent. Wakefield has since been struck off the Medical Register in the UK but has moved to the US where he is apparently still able to pursue his bizarre crusade.

What began the process of exposing the fraud? A report published in the *Sunday Times* by an investigative journalist named Brian Deer. That is totally irrelevant, of course.

The facts of these two cases are worth scrutinizing. Firstly, autism is right at the front of public concerns for pediatric health. Whereas it was once considered very rare (less than 0.1% of population), it now affects 0.625% of the population in the US and in Australia [13], an increase of 525% in about two decades. The advent of "autism spectrum disorder" allows the diagnosis to be spread far and wide. Second, there are substantial financial and other rewards for a family with a child diagnosed with this condition. Third, the increased risk caused by mothers taking antidepressants is a risk imposed by the mother, whereas the supposed risk (there actually wasn't one) of MMR immunization was imposed by the (male-dominated) government and the (male-dominated) medical profession. Four, families fought ferociously against the risk imposed by outsiders but acquiesced in the risk imposed by the mother.

Thus, to return to the urbane Sir Humphrey, the totally spurious risk of autism from MMR was attacked as a significant loss of amenity for the child while the proven risk of ASD from pregnant women taking drugs was defended as not a significant loss of amenity for the child because banning the drugs during pregnancy was a significant loss of amenity for mother *and* child ("deadly," to quote Dr. Biel). "One must," purrs the well-oiled publicity machine, "appreciate the significance of *significant.*"

So to return to the maladventures of the group of people with personality disorders, who now have a new diagnosis of BAD: Is their loss of amenity from taking toxic drugs in the long term in order to gain a short-term benefit outweighed by the total gain in amenity for the hospitals, and nursing unions; and the psychiatrists who can claim treatment on private insurance; and the drug companies whose sales have reached unprecedented levels and show no signs of slowing; and the patients themselves who gain pensions and supported accommodation and counselors who deal with the social security department on their behalf and arrange legal aid lawyers for their infractions; and the probation officers who want compliant clients; and the prison officers who much prefer their guests to be stoned legitimately; and the defense lawyers who want a plea in mitigation after the plea bargain; and the judges who don't want to convict people if they can blame an illness; and the politicians who want to be seen as liberal and enlightened... And we must not forget the families, who desperately want an excuse for why their son or daughter turned prodigal and dropped out or couldn't hold a job or turned to drugs or alcohol, or was arrested for bashing a policeman; a ready-made excuse that pardons bad parenting and dumps responsibility for the whole problem on that Great Roulette Wheel in the Sky called genes.

When the ledger is balanced this way, slowly poisoning a small but pestilential bunch in the community is probably not too much to ask of them.

Two questions immediately arise. Firstly, the word 'poisoning' is very strong. Is there any evidence for it or is it just hyperbole? Second, is there any factual evidence for people being labeled BAD when, in fact, they have a personality disorder?

The first question can be answered in the affirmative: Yes, there is now a great deal of evidence to suggest that psychotropic drugs have major, long-term, deleterious effects on brain metabolism. Directly or indirectly, these drugs affect the genome. They can either work directly, say by inducing the cell to produce more of its transmitter or less of another enzyme, or they can have an indirect effect by destabilizing neurotransmission. In the latter case, they secondarily induce gene expression to counteract the effects of the blockade etc. However, they are now known to exert epigenetic effects, which are, by definition, extremely long-lasting or permanent and may even be transmissible across generations [14]. Thus, since the drugs crosses the placenta, it is perfectly feasible that pregnant women taking psychotropics could induce very long-lasting changes in the development of the fetal brain, changes manifest as, perhaps, the withdrawal of autism. This leaves aside such questions as whether psychotropic drugs can have a measurable effect on gametogenesis (it would almost certainly be a very small effect but, in view of the numbers of people now involved, and the dosages and the duration of their exposure, plus the early age at which they commence medication, even a minimal effect on an individual basis can summate across a population). In view of these very recent developments in the pharmacology of psychotropics, I do not see 'slow poisoning' as excessively strong language.

14.4. What New Plague?

The second question, of whether people with personality disorders are labeled as BAD, would normally be answered by a large, long-term, multicenter survey and even then, arguments would persist. I can't fund one of those studies, and nobody else shows any interest, so we will just have to rely on that rather dubious source, my clinical experience. Fortunately, a lot of the figures from my practice have been published or are otherwise in the public arena, so this is not the problem it may have been.

For six years from 1987 to 1993, I was the Regional Psychiatrist in the Kimberley Health Region of Western Australia. Initially, this appointment was an experiment, intended to run just three years, to see if having a psychiatrist on site could reduce the large numbers of patients who were being flown to the mental hospitals in Perth, at least 2,500km away. For Aboriginal patients in particular, travelling so far from their traditional homes, to a totally different climate where they knew nobody and nobody spoke their language was dislocating in the extreme. The Kimberley is very isolated, roughly equivalent to Canada's North West Territories. A youthful population of some 28,000 people was scattered over an area of 420,000 square km, about three times the size of New York State or more than three times the size of England. There was just one road into the Kimberley, and one road out. As the general practitioners were all busy, they were generally keen to refer psychiatric cases. In addition, the job involved constant travel to all but the smallest and most remote Aboriginal communities, so the psychiatrist knew very well what was happening at all times. The position also included full responsibility for mental health problems in nursing homes, prisons and schools.

In six years, no children were commenced on antidepressants or mood stabilizers. Three boys under age 16 were prescribed antipsychotic drugs for acute psychotic states; two ceased within six months with no long-term effects while the last, a boy with fetal alcohol syndrome, was still taking them after five years. It emerged that one boy of 14yrs was taking dexamphetamine prescribed by a pediatrician in Perth which was improper but not actually illegal at the time. Following considerable pressure from his parents, one boy of eleven was prescribed stimulants but they left soon after and the circumstances were rather suspicious.

In the whole region over the six year period, there were several hundred episodes of psychotic disorders among adults, the great majority of them associated with massive alcohol abuse. These were absolutely classic examples of what was formerly known as Alcoholic Hallucinosis. They did not show features of a manic or hypomanic condition. Following withdrawal from alcohol and a course of antipsychotic drugs and vitamins, the symptoms almost always resolved and the drugs were discontinued. However, the patients often had very little memory of their illness and would resume drinking after six to twelve months, so they were likely to suffer another bout. They were not given the diagnosis of schizophrenia and there were no plans for them to take drugs in the long term, partly because they didn't need them and also because they wouldn't have taken them, anyway.

No adult was prescribed any of the class of drugs known as mood stabilizers. Due to the risks of toxicity, lithium could not be prescribed in that climate, a semi-monsoonal region only a few hundred kilometers from the edges of the Great Sandy Desert, as daytime temperatures often reached 45C (113F).

No person received ECT during my six year period of office. Antidepressants were not widely prescribed, partly due to my own prescribing habits and partly because of a double-suicide a few days after I arrived in the region. In May 1987, two travelers went from one hospital to the next, requesting amitriptylline until they had about 300 tablets each, then drove to a secluded area 50km from town and took them. They were not discovered for several days, by which time their bodies had nearly liquefied in the heat. Subsequently, every GP became very wary of requests for these drugs. From recollection, I doubt I would have written 200 prescriptions a year for antidepressants, meaning 6000 tablets for 28,000 people each year. That's about one tablet for five people per year, so we hope they knew how to share.

At the same time, the numbers of aerial transfers to the city dropped precipitously, from over 50 per year (at about $5000 each time) to three or four per year, at a huge reduction in cost. Each year, a few carefully prepared patients were transferred by commercial jet rather than the Royal Flying Doctor Service. Quite apart from the massive savings to the region's health budget, this was of huge benefit as it meant RFDS aircraft were not being taken out of the region where they were needed. One benefit that does not appear on the balance sheet accrued to the local people who no longer felt they could not ask for help for fear of being dragged off, sedated, trussed in a strait jacket and flown the distance from New York to Hudson Bay. They rated the new service very highly.

What's the point of this? We can draw certain conclusions from this experiment (which has not continued in that style). I believe one major point is that, if one psychiatrist working in a remote area with people of diverse races and cultural levels (many of the Aboriginal people spoke little English and lived a semi-traditional lifestyle), in an area with the world's highest alcohol consumption, with no dedicated hospital beds, no psychologists, no psychiatric nurses and no administrators, if one psychiatrist can do it, then so can all the clever psychiatrists in the world's great academic centers. If I didn't need an ECT machine in the Kimberley, nobody in the world needs one (I haven't used ECT since I graduated, in 1977). The differences between my practice there and in Darwin, and any of the large academic centers I have visited in Australia and overseas, was simple: low-key psychiatry, carefully tailored to the patient's needs as he verbalized them, free of doctrinaire or dogmatic preconceptions, with a minimal intervention and a heavy expectation that the patient was going to recover and return to normal life, and therefore he ought to get started straight away produced excellent results at low cost.

No person was ever told: "You have a biochemical imbalance of the brain." No person was told his disorder was genetic, that he would need drugs for life or that he must lower his personal expectations. To the contrary, great pressure was (and still is) applied to people to the effect that they will return to normal life or very close to it even if they need long-term support to do it, but having a psychiatric diagnosis is not a reason to give up.

Point No. 2: True manic-depressive psychosis was extremely rare. This is not to say that I didn't see people who showed intermittent bouts of agitation or overactivity, with or without impulsive behavior, separated by bouts of misery, because I did. They were not, however, treated as BAD. It happened that, after assessment, each one of them was seen as a primary personality disorder with secondary or reactive bouts of agitation and/or misery. That is, their disruptive behavior caused the agitation or the unhappiness; dealing with the disruptive behavior without using psychotropic drugs resulted in a satisfactory resolution of the acute stage. Some continued treatment thereafter, others disappeared until the next bout of trouble but the important point was, and still is, that they were not afraid to come back and resume where they had stopped a year or two before. And so they could be managed after the fashion of what we used to call "jollying them along." That is, when they wanted help, it was available, but when they didn't, it paused until they changed their minds. That is how I practice to this day.

My figures for my solo private, office-based practice in Darwin were similar. I was seeing up to 550 people per year, of whom about 250 were new cases. Of these, about 100 were seen for pension or other medicolegal purposes, so treatment was not usually offered. I averaged about 3,500 individual consultations with patients ("occasions of service") per year, defined as a face-to-face contact with a person for the purpose of treatment of a recognized psychiatric disorder (phone calls etc. are not occasions of service and cannot be charged). Patients had to be referred by a medical practitioner, so there was a minimum standard of disorder before I saw them, after which my own standard of what is or is not psychiatry acted as a further filter.

Because of the national health insurance system in this country, unemployed people or pensioners can be seen in private practice if the psychiatrist is prepared to accept a reduced rate of payment. The Health Insurance Commission sets all medical fees on a national basis. The basic rate for a psychiatrist is about $170 per hour, but Medicare pays only 85% of this rate for services to people holding a government health care card. In addition, practitioners can choose to "bulk bill" all patients to Medicare if they wish, so nobody has to pay anything. In return, the practitioner is guaranteed prompt payment, so there is no problem with people leaving town with unpaid bills or arguing over what they should pay. It isn't perfect, but it works.

My practice in Darwin was one of very few bulk-billing psychiatric practices in the country, so I was able to see the same sorts of patients as would be referred to public mental health services in other parts of the country. This suits me, as I am by nature a "bin doctor" and don't own an Armani suit or a Porsche. In addition, I have worked for years in public services, so I know exactly what patients they see. Except on one point, my patients are, and always have been, absolutely stock standard mental hospital fare. The only exception is that I no longer see patients who have been arrested by police because of violence, nor do I see patients detained against their will. If anybody asks, I advise them that I am required by law to refer them to a specialist psychiatric unit under a detention order if they are a direct danger to themselves or others, and that danger arises from a recognized mental disorder. Otherwise, they are on their own. I can't recall the last time I detained anybody, probably about eight years ago. I do not admit people to hospital as I have no admitting rights, but hardly any of my patients ever go to hospital. Sometimes, a new patient will take an overdose and go to hospital, but they rarely try that twice. A small number of patients with long psychiatric histories were in the habit of coming for a while, then disappearing. Next I heard, they were back in hospital, happily telling the staff they were seeing me and I was keen to have them back. Needless to say, the hospital staff were keen to send them back, although I was usually not keen on seeing them again. Needless to say, this did not help my reputation with the local hospital but one lives with these things.

In the past fifteen years, only two patients currently in treatment have committed suicide. Both were very secretive men with numerous long-standing problems they did not reveal. However, I would say that over fifty percent of my patients express suicidal ideas during their initial assessment. They are still managed as outpatients and are almost never given antidepressants at the first appointment. Last time I checked, my prescription rate for antidepressants was on the 8th percentile for private psychiatrists in this country, but my rate was dropping whereas the national average was climbing.

I never prescribe mood stabilizers and never use antipsychotic drugs in any but actively psychotic patients, and then for the shortest possible time. In fifteen years, I inherited one patient who had an iatrogenic addiction to dexamphetamine and was able to reduce his dosage by about 70% over a number of years but, that man apart, I do not prescribe stimulants. At least one patient a month arrived with a history of taking stimulants, usually started interstate. I continued these in only one patient, a quiet and very pleasant youth, only because he told me he spat most of them out and his mother, a singularly unstable woman, shouted that if he didn't get the prescription, she would send him back to his alcoholic father: "Can't you get it through your head?" she demanded, trembling with outrage. "He's unmanageable without his damned dexies." As he didn't want this, I broke my own rule and wrote the scripts although I had no doubt who the real patient was.

It will be agreed, I am sure, that this is not your usual psychiatric practice profile. Three possibilities suggest themselves:

1. I am a grossly incompetent psychiatrist, unable to see standard syndromes that medical students must recognize before they can pass their courses, and my thousands of patients have survived by luck alone or there was nothing much wrong with them in the first place.

2. I am a uniquely eccentric, if not frankly delusional, psychiatrist who, purely by chance, has stumbled over a weird formula that works for the people of northern Australia who are clearly as silly as their psychiatrist, but which couldn't possibly be generalized to a more typical setting.

3. It is possible to practice a low-impact type of psychiatry with good cost-benefit ratios, without exposing people to expensive, potentially dangerous and life-changing drugs, if and only if the psychiatrist is prepared to diagnose people with, and treat them for, personality disorders. In essence, not all that has ups and downs is BAD.

Options 1 and 2 rest with the Medical Board; be assured that a complaint in December 2003, by the then president of the Royal Australian and New Zealand College of Psychiatrists (RANZCP), an eminent professor of psychiatry, to the effect of option 2, was extensively investigated by the NT Medical Board who, in August 2004, advised that the president's complaint had no basis in fact. Remarkably, he declined to apologize for his astounding clinical error.

Moving to option 3, this is the point at which the question should be rephrased so that it can be answered by a carefully constructed research project. I would expect that the minimum would be a long-term, multi-center project, carefully coordinated by a transparently independent management team, with absolutely no affiliations between any of the research staff or project management and the drug industry. The project would take considerable time to organize, as it would necessitate training psychiatrists to assess personality disorder as part of their routine assessment, and then how to manage people as long-term out-patients using very low doses of medication and minimal paramedical involvement. I would expect a preliminary report after the project had been running three years, a more detailed report after five years, and the full project to run for as much as eight years. Anything less would leave the results open to manipulation by vested interests. Vested interests include the drug industry and an entire generation of psychiatrists who have irrevocably committed themselves to the model of biological reductionism.

Needless to say, I don't have the resources to implement such a project, or the influence to convince somebody who does have them to implement it. The people who have either the resources (in their departments) or the influence (over funding bodies) are also the people who stand to lose most if this project had any degree of success, so we can't expect much interest from them.

14.5. Conclusion

It's rather strange, you know, you would think that any eager young psychiatrist keen to make his or her name would be only too pleased to have the chance of finding the cause of an epidemic but it seems they're not. It seems they are quite happy to let it rumble along, treating the patients but showing no concern about why more and more of them just keep coming back.

No, on second thoughts, it's not rather strange, it's really strange, inexplicable. I wonder if it's really one of them sociological questions, you know, not so much a question of science as a question of the sociology of science. Looks as though we'll never know. Pity.

15

Testing the Biocognitive Model: Clinical Syndromes (2) Not all Ups and Downs are B.A.D.

"Many orthodox people speak as though it were the business of skeptics to disprove received dogmas rather than of dogmatists to prove them. This is, of course, a mistake." ."

—Bertrand Russell

15.1 Introduction

Where do all the bipolars come from? I believe This is a critically important question for modern psychiatry because if the "bipolar epidemic" is allowed to run on its present course, it has the potential to devastate the profession, if not destroy it. That doesn't take into account the lives destroyed by wrong use of long-term antipsychotic drugs. In this chapter, we will look more closely at the complex relationship between personality disorder, anxiety and winning a diagnosis of bipolar disorder.

15.2 Case 1: Mr. KA.

A 42yo man was referred for assessment of "mood swings and mania." He had recently been commenced on venlafaxine, an antidepressant, quetiapine, an antipsychotic drug, and valproate, an anticonvulsant used as a mood stabilizer. He had been married twice and was now living with his fourth partner and his eldest two sons (the first aged 25yrs) who both worked in the family businesses. Mr. A owned two businesses, a transport company with depots in several towns, four trucks and various other machines, and a garage and service station which his elder son managed. He was referred after he assaulted his partner while drunk; she offered him the choice of psychiatric treatment or separation. He freely stated he chose treatment over the thought of yet another property settlement.

His history showed some depressive symptoms, mainly a general sense of hostility and resentment against the world, but probably not enough to justify the medication. He was not suicidal although when he saw his GP two weeks before, angry suicidal ideas were noted. He was suspicious, distant and dismissive of psychiatry in general. His history showed a life-long pattern of erratic and impulsive behavior, with fairly regular bouts of intense agitation during which he did not need sleep and was physically and mentally highly active. With the bouts of agitation, he experienced a range of physical symptoms, including shaking, sweating, churning stomach and pounding heart. He was dizzy and light-headed, short of breath and he stumbled over his speech. To control them, he tried to work harder. Alcohol controlled the agitation. Although he knew that these periods were abnormal and people were suffering because of his behavior, he didn't mind them as he got so much done. He would take on a new project that people said was impossible and complete it before they knew he had started. However, he didn't like the bouts of misery that overwhelmed him from time to time.

At first, he said they came "out of the blue" but closer questioning revealed they always followed some sort of reverse, e.g. his first wife leaving him, losing custody of his sons, having to sell his businesses as part of divorce settlements etc. He drank most days but, when feeling miserable, he drank himself to sleep every night until the mood passed. He had a police record of mostly minor offences that could have been avoided. In his twenties, he often got into fights when drunk and had been imprisoned briefly for resisting arrest and assaulting police. His relationships usually broke down because of his quick temper, his threatening and sometimes violent behavior, his drinking, his jealousy and his affairs.

His own family background was poor. His father was a violent alcoholic military veteran and Mr. A ran away from home at age 14yrs, to work on cattle stations (ranches) in the outback. From the age of fifteen, he was driving big trucks and other machinery (trucks in the north of Australia tow three trailers each holding a forty foot container [1]). By twenty-one, he owned two trucks and was employing men twice his age. In his mid-twenties, when his second relationship broke down, he began drinking heavily and took several overdoses but refused treatment. He was contemptuous of formal education and loathed police and "other parasites," especially anybody connected in any way with Aboriginal welfare, etc. He despised anybody who didn't work, all other races except Philippinos ("real good workers"), governments, homosexuals, religion of any form, lawyers, anybody from the south of the country, psychologists and social workers (he had had extensive dealings with them through his divorces), the mentally ill... Anybody who didn't meet his exacting standards of hard work and independence. He believed he could do anything he turned his hand to and had ideas (revealed later) of declaring the north of Australia independent and importing low-paid Asian labor to develop the region's vast mineral wealth for the benefit of the white inhabitants who were not receiving welfare. From time to time, these ideas seemed to grip him and he would make appointments to see politicians to get their support.

He described a recent bout of feeling very low and hopeless with a strong sense of guilt and worthlessness. He had been suicidal, feeling that nobody needed him and his sons could take over the businesses and run them better. That followed a period of overactivity when he had been working very hard to set up another depot for their transport business. This involved long hours of travelling to remote communities and tortuous negotiations with two government departments and an Aboriginal community (all of whom he loathed). He made no secret of the fact that he bribed the Aboriginal elders and "bought off" the officials with fishing trips on his large and powerful boat, well-supplied with alcohol and marihuana. During this period, he started an affair with a nurse who worked on the community; his partner found out, he began drinking then developed the idea she was having an affair which led to the assault.

The mental state showed a stocky, muscular man of a little below average height with deeply tanned skin who was wearing clean but faded work clothes and dusty industrial boots (he had come from work for the appointment). He had a number of old tattoos and a heavy gold chain around his neck. He had two days' growth, his hair was dusty and tousled and he smelled of dust, sweat and fuel oil. His manner was wary, tending to defensive, alert, quite abrupt and impatient. He tended to sit jiggling his leg and fiddling with his mobile phone, repeatedly checking messages as they came through but was still able to answer questions without interruption. He was still angry and unhappy, very resentful of his partner's threats, but he was fairly sure he could ride the storm until life got back to normal. Further questioning showed the repeated bouts of over-activity were driven by an intense need to succeed and a deep-seated fear of failure. If he thought things were going badly, he redoubled his efforts and forced himself to stay awake for very long periods. From time to time, he still used amphetamines for this reason. He was fearful of social interactions and much preferred to get any social life through work (on the boat trips, he piloted the boat and left the socializing to his sons). He had a number of life-long fears, including spiders and snakes, confined spaces, darkness and murky water. He was easily agitated by arguments or confrontation of any sort and had a compelling need to be on good terms with people, even those he loathed. He described an overwhelming fear of making mistakes or letting people down and often got into difficulties by promising to help people he knew he should abandon. He was frightened of physical and mental illness, blood, hospitals, dentists, police and all aggressive people, but forced himself to deal with his fears even though this often made things worse. He described strong paranoid ideas and was a rigidly fussy and punctual person. If things were going badly, he experienced repeated intrusive thoughts that he was no good or people disliked him. There were no psychotic features and nothing to indicate an organic impairment of brain function. He was of superior intellectual ability but educated well below his capacity. His self-esteem was generally very poor although, during his over-active periods, he often felt he could do anything.

At the end of the interview, he revealed that people had been telling him for years he was "bipolar." This was the diagnosis his GP had provided and it frightened him. He had not been taking the drugs regularly as they caused drowsiness, difficulty thinking, loss of energy and poor sexual function. His partner had found some websites devoted to Bipolar Disorder and he completed their questionnaires, scoring very highly on all of them. However, he had also done some on ADHD and on a site for autistic disorders, and boasted he was "off the top" on all of them. He greatly feared admission to hospital and said he would not, under any circumstances, agree to admission. Any attempt to take him by force would be resisted "force with force" (he had numerous firearms in different places). Death was far preferable to going to a mental hospital.

Management:

He was told that, while he actually met the criteria for Bipolar Affective Disorder, the diagnosis was misleading as his main problem was anxiety caused by abnormal personality factors resulting from his early life experiences. He did not need major psychiatric drugs but would benefit from specific treatment of his anxiety and panic attacks. If they could be controlled, his life would run smoother but he would never be what people call normal. At this, he grinned broadly for the first time in the interview, saying he didn't believe he was mentally ill. He agreed he was a difficult person and his father was probably to blame but he didn't hold any grudges: "He was normal when he joined the Army and it wrecked his head. He couldn't help himself." If the panic could be controlled, he expected his life would run better but he had no intention of any sort of major change: "I couldn't see myself as a nice bloke. Nice blokes don't survive in my industry, it's a tough life."

The last of the psychiatric drugs were withdrawn over a period of a week and he was commenced on beta blockers to control the somatic agitation. He responded dramatically and was enormously gratified by his improvement. Because of his constant travelling for work, he could not attend regularly but always kept contact, even if it was only through his partner coming for further scripts (she revealed he was not much interested in talking of his life as he felt it was 'girly'). .

Discussion:

The bipolar disorder is a syndrome, that is, a relatively stable collection of signs and symptoms of unknown cause. It is not a disease or illness *per se*. Normally, when we talk of a syndrome, we expect to find a single cause, so that it will be converted into a formal disease, i.e. all the signs and symptoms will eventually be shown to be the result of a single defect state. Consider an example we learned at medical school, Kartagener's Syndrome. This is a rare recessive autosomal condition characterized by chronic sinusitis, situs invertus and bronchiectasis. Forty-five years ago, nobody could say what the cause might be, the features were too diverse for a single cause so we just learned it as a cluster of symptoms and that was that. Needless to say, I never saw a case. Now we know that the disease is caused by a variety of genetic defects that affect cilia, so embryonic development is thwarted and the sinuses and bronchi cannot clear mucus secretions. It is a heterogeneous disorder, the causes being defects in genes that code for proteins in the outer dynein arm of the cilia. From such a tiny defect grows a life-threatening disease state. Amazing.

The bipolar syndrome is most emphatically not the same. Yes, I am fully aware that the vast majority of academic psychiatrists in the world are resolutely determined to prove that it has a single genetic cause, or perhaps they will settle for a group of genetic causes, but what they will not accept is that the clinical picture can have a multitude of causes, many or most of which are not genetic at all. The whole point of the DSM project has been to isolate pure examples of the various clinical conditions so that these can then be mapped directly to the genome, the final goal being a single drug for each disease condition (if a genetic defect is found, then the syndrome, now called a disorder, would become a disease state). As noted in Chapter 11, on the NIMH RDoC (and as predicted long ago), this project has failed. There is absolutely no reason to believe that the (vague and unstable) clinical picture now known as BAD will have anything like a single cause, and definitely not a genetic cause. That's not how brains work. In fact, orthodox psychiatry knows the syndrome has many causes, that's why they give it a different name when it occurs after massive psychological stressors (PTSD): same symptoms, different cause.

In the main, researchers will acknowledge that non-genetic factors make a variable contribution to the clinical syndrome. One eminent researcher told me that heritability accounts for 80% of the total causation of BAD. However, this assumes the subjects in the studies were accurately selected. I will argue that they are not accurately selected, that the researchers' net is set too coarse and is sweeping up cases that are not, in fact, bipolar. What does it mean to say "not in fact bipolar"? A person making a career out of proving that BAD exists and should be treated in a particular way will reply: "A patient who meets the criteria for BAD as defined in DSM-IV-TR is a person with BAD." My response is: "Yes, but the criteria are so badly defined that a person you diagnose as bipolar I would not so diagnose. Where does that leave your objective science?" After a bit of sparring, it would be agreed that we have to disagree. There is no formal, objective criterion, no authority, no test, no gene study, no post-mortem study, nothing, that can resolve the question. It becomes a matter of one person saying: "I am an expert, and if I say he is bipolar, then he is and that is the end of the matter."

That, of course, is not science. That is how witches were exposed, how blacks were deemed genetically inferior, how communists and fellow-travelers were exposed by McCarthy and so on. As a result, all the genetic studies of this disorder are worthless. The claim that 80% of the variability in BAD is due to genetic factors is false science.

Mr. KA showed a very typical finding in people who arrive with a diagnosis of BAD made elsewhere, the cluster of intensely discomforting and intrusive anxiety symptoms that he always tried to conceal. When he felt normal (admittedly, not very often), he was inclined to take short cuts in his business as he didn't like waiting for other people or officials. If he started to feel miserable for any reason (such as business worries, constant anxiety, various social upsets), he usually spent money on himself and others to try to feel better, mostly on things he didn't need. If he was feeling insecure or that people thought he was incompetent, he would usually engage in inappropriate sexual encounters to reassure himself he could still "pull them in." By controlling the anxiety with medication, he was able to manage his daily affairs without the inner sense of losing control. His sense of his own self-worth improved quite dramatically, so he became less intrusive and less impulsive leading to improved behavior at work and in his social and private lives.

Essentially, the cause of his bipolar syndrome was a decidedly abnormal personality with strong anxious and paranoid elements. This led to bouts of agitation with poor sleep, racing thoughts, distractibility, irritability and so on. If we check the diagnostic criteria for BAD, it is immediately clear that they do not sort anxiety states from the more serious psychotic disorders. The criteria have been loosened to the extent that they conflate two separate conditions with totally different etiologies, treatment and natural histories.

The DSM-IV-TR criteria for a manic episode are as follows:

A. A distinct period of abnormally and persistently elevated, expansive or irritable mood, lasting at least one week (or any duration if hospitalization is necessary).

B. During the period of mood disturbance, three (or more) of the following symptoms have persisted (four if the mood is only irritable) and have been present to a significant degree:

- inflated self-esteem or grandiosity
- decreased need for sleep (e.g. feels rested after only three hours of sleep)
- more talkative then usual or pressure to keep talking
- flight of ideas or subjective experience that thoughts are racing
- distractibility (i.e. attention too easily drawn to unimportant or irrelevant external stimuli
- increase in goal-directed activity (either socially, at work or school, or sexually) or psychomotor agitation
- excessive involvement in pleasurable activities that have a high potential for painful consequences (e.g. engaging in unrestrained buying sprees, sexual indiscretions, or foolish business investments).

The condition has to interfere with normal life in some way and is not due to intoxication or any medical illness. It can, of course, be seen after a brain injury but that is not considered the pure syndrome. Hypomania is essentially the same symptoms persisting for four days but the diagnosis implies they are not quite so severe.

By these criteria, a person who is irritable for a week, who can't sleep well, who paces around, talking rapidly but who is distractible, disorganized and complains of his mind spinning too fast or too many thoughts tumbling around, who impulsively spends money or makes an unwise decision, is suffering a psychotic disorder. It is necessary to remember this point at all times: BAD just is a psychotic illness, an SMI (Serious Mental Illness). On this basis alone, it is not a diagnosis to be bandied around. The problem is, those features are also a perfect description of an acute anxiety state: that is just what anxiety is, but anxiety is *not* a psychotic condition. Faced with two conflicting diagnoses, psychiatrists never opt for the lesser of the two. If the choice is anxiety or BAD, then BAD wins, every time. Part of the reason is that making a false negative diagnosis (saying it's not there when it is) is regarded as a worse mistake than the false positive diagnosis (saying it's there when it is not). This is due to academic conceit: the really clever doctor is the one who finds the diagnosis that everybody else missed. This is one path by which patients are wrongly recruited into the ranks of BAD sufferers, why there is now a rapidly growing epidemic of the disorder, and why they don't get better with the drugs. The problem is, there are far more anxious people than genuinely manic-depressive. The supply won't dry up.

From a distance, Mr. KA appeared to match the bipolar syndrome very well but, as soon as a proper history was obtained and he felt able to speak openly of himself, the reasons for his behavior became obvious. This is the critical point: in a cognitive model, people have reasons for acting as they do, even if they are not entirely sure what the reasons are. In a biological model, there are no reasons. When talking about brain enzymes, the very idea of reasons is irrelevant: making a diagnosis becomes a matter of genes and transmitters vs. reasons and motives. Manifestly, these are ontologically different concepts, occupying different realms of discourse with no overlap, no points of intersection. The biological psychiatrist is of the view that reasons amount to nothing in the face of the determinism of the genetic state. Of course, this claim has no rational basis. It is simply accepted as an established fact and is therefore an ideological commitment, not scientific. The psychiatry starts at that point and continues merrily on its way, unhampered by any rational constraints.

15.3 Case 2: Ms ML.

This 46yo woman was referred by her lawyer for a medical report to be used in a claim of wrongful dismissal against her former employer. She had been employed as a divisional head in a major public institution, on a salary of about $140,000 plus substantial benefits (subsidized rent, a car, regular airline travel, conference leave, etc.) but had been terminated after all the staff in her office jointly signed a letter of complaint, alleging constant bullying, sexual harassment, lack of leadership and other shortcomings. During the preliminary investigations, it was learned that she had been misusing the departmental credit card and had made several unauthorized purchases of up to $5000 each. She was told to resign or face further investigations which may lead to criminal prosecution. She refused, claiming that she had been mentally ill throughout, so she was dismissed forthwith (in fact, the employer had not followed due procedure and she had a minor claim under some workplace legislation). Her post had subsequently been abolished and she could not be re-employed so, effectively, her claim amounted to a demand for a cash settlement from the employer for not recognizing her medical condition.

When she arrived, she was quite intensely agitated. Gabbling loudly, she said she had "proven" bipolar as her sister and her mother had both been diagnosed with this condition at a prestigious hospital in Melbourne. They had been taking large doses of medication for years and each had been in hospital a number of times. She said they had always insisted she had the same illness and should get treatment. Now, she realized it was correct and, as soon as the case settled, she would come back for proper treatment.

She gave a clear account of frequent periods of disturbance from early teenage years, to the extent that she said she didn't really know what normal meant. At times, she would feel fantastic, on top of the world, full of energy with her head stuffed full of brilliant ideas but this never lasted. For no reason, just when it seemed she had everything she needed, her mood would "crash" and she fell into a state of misery, apathy and resentful despair. In these moods, she developed a black hatred of the world and often acted very cruelly toward people, especially her juniors. She admitted that one of the complaints against her was true, that she did sexually harass her staff, "but only men," she added helpfully. During the low moods, she targeted young, married men in the office and maneuvered them into sexual liaisons by promising advancement if they complied or "a hell of a life" if they didn't. As soon as she had achieved her goal, she pushed them aside: "It's like I've got to have them, an obsession, but I don't actually care about them, they're just things for me to play around with. I prefer my cats to people." She was emphatic that there was neither rhyme nor reason to these moods, they came upon her with no warning and no pattern that she could see.

Everything in the memorandum of complaint from the employer was quickly explained away in terms of her unstable moods. She insisted she had spent the money in a state of such black despair that she didn't know what she was doing and was appalled when she realized. When she felt good, she would decide to reorganize her department but her mood usually changed before it was complete so she lost interest. She agreed she was very jealous of any attractive young women in the department and "gave them hell," but this was again in the bad moods. When she felt good, she would try to make up for her previous misbehavior by being friendly, inviting them out to dinner for their birthdays, and even giving some of them quite expensive gifts. She had always been like this.

Socially, she came from a middle-class family in Melbourne but attended an expensive girls' school, mainly because of pressure from her father's family. She hated the school and never made friends. The disturbed moods began there. On leaving school, she trained as a primary school teacher but never worked as a teacher because the children "drove her mad." She had no trouble getting work and quickly gained senior administrative posts. Along the way, she was married several times and profited handsomely from the divorce separations but never had children: "I've got cats instead. Children just aren't me." She said she had no previous psychiatric history as she had refused to accept there was anything wrong with her, and no prior criminal record. She drank every day but didn't drink to excess and used no illegal drugs. She did not gamble and her general health was good.

She presented as an attractive woman who looked ten years younger than her age. She was dressed in expensive clothing with high quality, tasteful jewelry and elaborate make-up, nails and hair. At first, she was agitated and disorganized and close to tears but, as the interview progressed, she settled and soon became expansive and confiding. After about fifteen minutes, she sat back and smiled pleasantly: "This is a lot better than I'd expected," she purred. "I was quite terrified about coming here. I've never seen a psychiatrist so I didn't know what to expect. I'm surprised, but you're actually quite human. You've got a lovely office, not overdone, it's very tasteful. That's a lovely wedding ring you're wearing, do you mind if I have a closer look... later?"

About five minutes later, she leaned across the desk: "You know," she said breathily, "I've done my homework about you. People said you've got the most dreadful temper but I don't find that at all. I find you... professional. Yes, that's it. You've got an amazing calmness about you, I feel so much better for coming here. I'd like to come back, if I may." After another five minutes, she moved her chair closer and brushed her hair back. In the process, her blouse was loosened and dropped revealingly. "You obviously take very good care of yourself, Doctor," she said, with a heave of her chest. "A healthy body means a healthy mind. I totally agree with that, we could talk about that later. I think how you present yourself physically is terribly important."

After one hour, the interview ended. "Oh," she said with a radiant smile. "That was quicker than I expected. I was sure learning about me would take you several hours at least. There's so many things I need to tell you. Perhaps we could go somewhere for coffee and discuss them?" She was advised the next patients were already waiting and ethical rules forbade any social contact with patients. "Oh, but you don't really see me as a patient, do you? I mean, we're both professionals, we're both mature people. I'm sure nobody would mind if we continue this meeting... Would it help you to go somewhere private? Perhaps even... my apartment? That's very private."

She was told the report would be ready in two days and would go to her lawyers, meantime, she should settle the account on her way out. "So when will we meet again, Neil?" (That's not my name and I do not use first names at work). "Probably in court, I should imagine. Good afternoon, Ms L. Mr. Smith? Come this way please."

Routine enquiries with her employer showed a pattern of disruptive and dishonest conduct from the beginning of her employment. Unfortunately, the employer was unable to find the reports from her referees, so I rang her previous employer interstate. As expected, the human resources officer described exactly the same behavior throughout her period with them. She was disruptive, seductive, dishonest, manipulative, disorganized, demanding and was constantly surrounded by chaos of her own making. He had actually known her twenty years before and said she was no different then. She had been imprisoned once for embezzlement but he was sure most of her crimes were concealed by the men she had seduced. She was a notorious gambler and most of her juniors were convinced she used stimulants illegally. She was always "borrowing" money from junior staff in her office and had left town owing tens of thousands. Every time she got into trouble, she pleaded mental illness but he had heard that her family were very nice people and he was sure they had no record of mental disorder. "She's just a lying bitch," he added. "You'll never know the damage she did here. She's a home-breaker, a liar, a thief and then she smiles that lovely smile and everybody falls over. Did she invite you to her apartment for further meetings?"

Discussion

It is absolutely characteristic of these people that their references are not checked in the recruitment process. It always happens. There is always a reason, the letters are on the way, or still packed, or the referees were busy, but the real reason is they know that their lies and flirtatious behavior will pull them through. If it doesn't, well, move on.

The report to her lawyers said that she had a severe personality disorder of the type previously known as the creative psychopath. She did not fit any of the modern categories of personality disorder but narcissistic personality with antisocial traits came closest. She was most assuredly not mentally ill and had no psychiatric defense. The lawyers were happy with the report and, thus armed, convinced her to accept a small settlement and leave town. With her cats.

These days, everybody is bipolar when the police are closing in.

15.4 Case 3: Dr. VM

This 29yo clinical psychologist was referred for treatment by his employer. He had been in his position for about two years but there had been concerns about his behavior almost since the beginning. His job was half clinical and half administrative. The letter of referral said that when he did his work, it was brilliant but he was terribly disorganized and constantly had to be pushed to complete routine work, especially administrative tasks. However, if there was anything out of the ordinary, especially if it involved meeting people or appearing in public, he threw himself into it and achieved at the highest level, even while his routine work was in complete disarray. He took a lot of time off work and was suspected to have forged a medical certificate. On the occasions his superiors had tried to speak to him about it, he burst into tears and said it was all due to being bipolar, could they just bear with him while his medication was tweaked and he was sure all would be well.

On questioning, he described "mood swings," meaning some days he woke feeling brilliant and the day went fantastically well but others were a disaster and he would often not get out of bed. Closeted in a darkened room, he would speak to his friends interstate and overseas for hours, complaining how nobody cared and he might as well be dead. A bad day could be transformed if one of his dear friends rang, or a good day ruined if somebody ignored him: "My entire life is a roller-coaster, up and down, no stability whatsoever." When asked about medication, he giggled: "I wouldn't take drugs, I made that up to get them off my back. Drugs ruin everything, your mind, your figure, your sex life. Not me, no way." Questioning did not reveal any significant mental symptoms at the time, apart from worrying about the interview and the report: "You won't bag me, will you, Dr? I mean, I'm telling you the truth. I need that job, I owe so much money, you wouldn't believe." He had made a series of unwise investments on the stock market even though he clearly knew nothing about it: "I read somewhere it was all stats, I'm brilliant at stats so I thought I'd have a go. At first, I made a mint, then it all went bad so I borrowed more. So silly of me, I know, please don't roll your eyes like that."

He spent money all the time, paying for extravagant dinner parties for his friends but they never seemed to invite him back. He always had to have the latest fashionable clothing and rarely wore a shirt more than half a dozen times: "I don't want anybody to see me looking drab. I have to be the best-dressed at the party, I want everybody to look at me when I walk in the room.

My hair costs a fortune, my teeth, my skin, everything has to be absolutely perfect. If I wake in the morning with a spot on my face, I won't go to work."

His family background in the UK had not been happy. His father was an Indian doctor who married a nurse at his first chance so he could stay in Britain. He was a mournful, distant man who didn't drink or smoke but spent his free time raising cacti in a shed in the garden. His mother was "the most pretentious creature you ever met, full of airs and dramas, had to have the latest fashion, be seen at the best parties, everything. We're so alike it's scary. God but we fight." Two sisters had followed their father into medicine and were both junior consultants at major teaching hospitals before they turned thirty ("You wouldn't believe how dull and boring they are, clones of Dr. Cactus"). His schooling was reasonably happy but he never had a sense of belonging. He felt the white boys looked down on him and he, in turn, despised the Indians who kept to themselves and whispered in Hindi to each other. Whatever he did, he did brilliantly, but he never kept anything going: "I could have been an international star at half a dozen sports, every teacher pleaded with me to enter their field and win a Nobel Prize. I wrote plays at twelve, novels at thirteen, prizes, awards, you name it. God it was boring." At high school, he found he was too shy to approach girls although if a woman wanted to put the effort into seducing him, he was happy to join in but soon lost interest.

At university, he didn't know what to study but it had to be glamorous so he enrolled in psychology. Everybody lusted after him and, in his second year, he allowed a male teacher to take him overseas on holidays but they argued as he was often impotent: "I'm a terrible flirt. It's all a game with me but people take it seriously and I can't tell them to nick off because I'll hurt their feelings. Everybody thinks I'm gay but I'm not, I'm really not that committed to anything. Can you see me marching up and down the street with a sign for gay rights? God, what a hoot." He tried modeling but the other young men learned they could reduce him to tears by criticizing his appearance so that didn't last. He loved drama and music and joined the drama society but lost interest after the first few productions: "All my life is an act. Why would I bother acting about acting?" On graduating, he completed his PhD with no interest in the field, then was horrified to find he had to get a job: "Teaching? At a university? Oh, no, I couldn't do that. They work them too hard. Research is fun and I'd love the conferences but can you imagine me staying up at night to mark papers? Never happen."

He agreed he was much more anxious socially than he wanted anybody to know, so he tended to have a few drinks before he went out. At parties, he was constantly worried that people were talking behind his back, so he flitted around talking to everybody. He needed company as, when alone, he started to worry about his appearance or his intelligence or his accent or his charm... However, he had trouble keeping flat mates and often ended up living alone, which he hated. He had tried "every drug known to man and a few more" but wasn't much interested and mainly took them because people expected it of him. From time to time, he was caught telling lies: "Silly lies, lies I don't need, I know when I'm saying it I'm going to be found out but I just keep going. Then I have to tell some more lies to cover them up. It's all too much, gets me down." He had never been in trouble with the police: "Absolutely no way, never happen. They terrify me." Socially, he had a large number of fears that dominated his life. He was fussy, pedantic, ritualistic and totally disorganized, all at once: "I lose a phone a week and I never know where my car keys are. But I never forget a name or a face, I have an absolutely photographic memory for anything I read."

He was tall and strikingly handsome with faultless light olive skin, flashing dark eyes, thick, wavy black hair and perfect, gleaming teeth. He was very well built from attending gym but it was not overdone. He was dressed like a model from Vogue and sported an expensive watch and the latest smartphone. He spoke quickly with a rich upper middle class London accent, using a remarkably extensive vocabulary and could do the same in Hindi and in French. His talk was often punctuated with bright laughter. His movements were fluid and a little exaggerated, with slightly effeminate mannerisms but he was never theatrical. Initially, he was edgy and rather wary but he soon settled and began to enjoy himself. He showed no signs of anxiety, depression, hostility or suspicion but his mood was obviously very reactive as, when talking of his troubles, his eyes moistened and he would then change the subject with a laugh. He was clearly of very superior intellect.

The end of the interview startled him: "I'm so sorry, is it time to go? I was having such a good time that I forgot what this was about. I mean, my job's on the line and I can't afford to lose it. My father will shoot me if he hears of any more trouble. So what's the verdict? And the sentence? Bipolar with a life of drugs?" Again, his eyes gleamed wetly but this time, he was not laughing: "I don't think I could do that, I swear, it would kill me..."

Management.

He was told he did not have a formal mental illness, that his problems were entirely personality-based and drugs were not just unnecessary but were highly likely to have an adverse effect on his life. He could consider psychotherapy if he wished but it would be strictly controlled with no Freudian nonsense. At that, he sat up, one hand creeping up to his throat: "Is that true?" he asked breathlessly. "You mean I'm not bipolar? Oh my god, Dr, you don't know what you've just done for me. Just a PD, is that it? Thank you, thank you so much, I can't tell you how happy I am to hear that. Well, do I get the jackpot? A sociopath? Malignant narcissism with self-indulgent traits? Give me your worst. I can take it... I think."

"It's pure hysterical personality, as we used to say, or Histrionic Personality Disorder in modern terms. You're really just Joan Crawford in trousers."

He covered his face and began to cry. "That is absolutely the best thing you could possibly have said to me," he said tearfully. "I could never tell you the fear I've endured since they told me to come here. I told you I'd never seen a psychiatrist before but that wasn't quite true. I was pushed to see one at university and he wanted to give me twenty diagnoses and a drug for each of them. I ran out and vomited in fright and refused to go back." Leaning back, he wiped his face delicately and began to laugh. "Mommie Dearest. That's me, except I'm not a bitch. I would never hurt a fly. Well, I see you're getting ready to put me out, may I come back? There's so much to talk about, we've hardly scratched the surface. Oh my god, I'm a PD, a PD. Oh how frightful, how delightful. Rex Harrison, but you know that, I'm sure."

Discussion.

DSM-IV-TR defines personality disorder as:

"A. An enduring pattern of psychological experience and behavior that differs markedly from cultural expectations, as shown in two or more of: cognition (i.e. ways of perceiving and interpreting self, other people and events); affectivity (i.e. the range, intensity, lability, and appropriateness of emotional response); interpersonal functioning; or impulse control.

B. The enduring pattern is inflexible and pervasive across a broad range of personal and social situations.

C. The enduring pattern leads to clinically significant distress or impairment in social, occupational or other important areas of functioning.

D. The enduring pattern must be stable and of long duration, and its onset can be traced back at least to adolescence or early adulthood.

E. The enduring pattern is not better accounted for as a manifestation or consequence of another mental disorder.

F. The enduring pattern is not due to the direct physiological effects of a substance (e.g. drug of abuse or a medication) or a general medical condition (e.g. head trauma)."

Let's see whether this fascinating and rather pathetic young man (who responded very well to standard psychotherapy) met the criteria.

"Enduring pattern..." Yes, it hadn't varied at all since he was about ten.

"Psychological experience and behavior that differs markedly from cultural expectations." Absolutely. He was a glittering, brilliant failure in a family of stodgy successes.

"Defective cognition." I don't know how defective an IQ of 165 is, but he had no control over it. The Social Conscience of Minnesota, Garrison Keillor, says: "Intelligence is like a four wheel drive: it lets you get stuck in much more interesting and isolated places." A science fiction writer once said: "Intelligence serves insanity quite as well as it serves sanity, which is to say, very well indeed." Undirected intelligence is like an unguided missile, it may just head back where it came from. Dr. M's prodigious intellect was at the mercy of his emotions, rather than the other way around.

"Defective affectivity." Exactly. His emotions were like a cloud of rainbow-colored mirrors falling from a great height, sparkling in the sunshine then shattering into a million brilliant razor-sharp shards.

"Defective interpersonal functioning." There was no question about this point. He needed people's approval as he had no self-esteem at all, but he could not get close to them for fear they would find him shallow and tiresome and would lose interest in him. He was sexually immature and used his body to attract people but then became anxious when he had to perform as a man as he didn't believe he was a man. He was quite convinced that whatever men feel like inside, it was nothing like the mess of emotions that ran his life.

"Defective impulse control." This presupposes the individual feels any need to control his impulses. He did only after the event, and then not for long. Everything he did was for the purpose of impressing people and gaining their approval. When it didn't work, he immediately tried something else but once he had started something, he couldn't stop or back down for fear of looking weak.

Behavior is "inflexible and pervasive across a broad range of personal and social situations." Beyond doubt. As soon as he came into contact with another human, he had to start his act.

"...clinically significant distress or impairment in social, occupational or other important areas of functioning." True. All of the above.

"The enduring pattern must be stable and of long duration, and its onset can be traced back at least to adolescence or early adulthood." Unquestionably. At the age of ten, he learned he could conceal his shyness and sense of inferiority by acting the brightest boy in his class or on the sports field, even when he wasn't interested (I don't know who wrote this, surely 'enduring' means 'of long duration'? It is just another example of fluffing the criteria so they seem different when they are not, the DSM intuition pump again).

"Not due to a medical illness or brain disease, not due to drug abuse." All true.

"The enduing pattern is not better accounted for as a manifestation or consequence of another mental disorder." Aha, now we come to the crunch. With a bit of pushing and shoving, he could be made to fit the criteria for BAD, so which one takes priority? According to DSM-IV, Axis I disorders take priority. How do we know? Because, as anybody who can read knows, Axis I comes before Axis II. One always comes before two, so anything on Axis I must take priority over something on Axis II.

That does seem to be begging the question, so we can look at it from another point of view. Psychiatrists do not have a theory of personality disorder. They have no convincing forms of treatment for personality disorder and they don't get paid much for seeing personality-disordered patients. To cap it off, they don't actually like seeing these people because they are not passive, compliant and respectful patients. They are most definitely not like schizophrenics. They are rude and ungrateful; they object if they are kept waiting; they complain about the mess in the waiting room and no paper in the toilets; they ring after hours but won't talk to the duty nurse; they search the Internet and often know more about psychology and pharmacology than the psychiatrist; they ask impossible questions; they want to be treated as an equal and not as an inferior; and they are not delusional so their complaints can't be dismissed in court as the rantings of the deranged. So why would a mild-mannered, somewhat insecure psychiatrist want to see the average personality disorder (it's different if the PD is the lubricious Miss Holly Woodstar, the must-have fashion accessory of the year for the socially aware; a young Alan Turing or a Franz Kafka would be turfed out).

On the other hand, psychiatrists all agree they have a wonderful theory of mental disorder (reductionism); they have lots of drugs they can give to people with mental disorders that keep them quiet, usually for life, and they get paid for seeing people with traditional mental disorders, again for life as they don't get better. And the good thing about psychotic people who complain about their drugs is that they can be given more drugs. I recently interviewed a man who had been confined to a security ward because he "complained too much." Who had he complained about? The doctor who locked him up.

You are still mystified. "So why," you ask, "do mental disorders come on Axis I and personality disorders on Axis II?"

Are you serious?

You are persistent if nothing else: "But," you object, "where's the science?"

To answer that, go back and read the papers on the NIMH Research Domain Criteria project, seen in Chapter 11. There, brimming with confidence, is an exposition by the world's leading experts of "the science of mental disorder as the science of the brain." You want science, son, we'll give you science.

The simple truth is that the whole of DSM is written to bias psychiatrists into diagnosing conditions that they think they understand, they think they can do something about and they are sure they will get paid for, without running the risk of having a clever, vengeful "PD" launching a series of tort claims. This is done by artfully rewriting the various criteria so that it looks as though they are different when any medical student can see they are not. Medical students, however, can be bullied into keeping quiet whereas personality disorders can't. And personality-disordered medical students? Well, there's always academia.

15.5 Case 4: Mr. SP.

This 32yo man was referred for a routine review of his disability pension, which was granted when he was about eighteen. He had been diagnosed as BAD at the age of 16yrs, and had been taking medication most of the time since then. When seen, he was taking quetiapine, olanzapine, valproate, benztropine, clonazepam and a variety of somatic medications for asthma, peptic ulceration, skin trouble and arthritis. Questioned about the last, he reluctantly admitted he was getting morphine from his GP.

He was a small, thin man with narrow features and bad teeth. His receding, straw-colored hair was straggly and untidy, he was unshaven and there were numerous old tattoos, many self-inflicted, on his arms, legs and chest. He was wearing dirty, stained old clothes including a shirt missing most of its buttons, scruffy football shorts and dirty rubber sandals. He smelled strongly of dirt, sweat, tobacco and alcohol. When warned that people who have been drinking will not be seen, he began to wail and blubber that his pension would be cut off as he had already missed two appointments. He lived in a small government flat but he was constantly in trouble for noise for allowing drinkers to camp on his floor. On pension day, he would start drinking and continue until the money ran out three or four days later. Groups of drinkers came to his flat to join in and fights were common. He said he had a girlfriend, an alcoholic part-Aboriginal prostitute who drank even more than he did but she was in prison so life had been a bit quieter. If he lost his pension, he would automatically lose his home.

He said he was always "up and d-down, never normal, always m-manic or d-depressed." At the time of the interview, he felt miserable and hopeless. He often thought about death, mostly when he was sober but he was too scared to try suicide. He had trouble sleeping, his appetite was poor, he had no energy or interests, no sexual interest and was unable to perform, drunk or sober, as he was too nervous. He had trouble thinking, his memory and concentration were poor and his thoughts were either "dead in the water" or he had too many thoughts tumbling through his head. Sometimes when he was very agitated and was unable to sleep for days, he had the impression of hearing voices but he wasn't sure if they were real or not.

He described frequent bouts of intense agitation, with shaking in his limbs, sweating, pounding heart and churning stomach. During them, he felt short of breath from a choking sensation, and he could barely speak due to stammering. He was clumsy and unsteady on his feet ("It might be the g-grog, doc, I g-gotta admit I h-hammer it"), and he felt frightened to the point of vomiting. Each bout lasted up to half an hour, with perhaps a dozen episodes a day when sober so he tried to stay drunk. The agitation was caused by having to deal with people, such as going to shops or offices, any sort of friction or confrontation with people, and the thought of people getting angry at him or people not liking him. He could not speak in public or ask anybody for help of any sort due to feeling panicky. He feared crowds, queues, big dogs, officials, especially the police, hospitals, dentists, blood and needles. He was frightened of any aggressive-looking people and always tried to keep on their good side, usually by giving them alcohol or letting them stay on his floor.

He always had the feeling people were looking at him and talking behind his back, judging him and disapproving of him. He often felt people were likely to attack him so he never carried money or any credit cards. He had the feeling his neighbors were plotting to have him evicted but agreed they would be pretty crazy if they weren't. Physically, he was in poor health. He had Hepatitis C from using dirty needles as a teenager, his chest was poor from smoking and he seemed to have physical symptoms affecting every part of his body.

The only times he felt reasonable was when he had his first few drinks when his pension money arrived: "It calms me, all that t-tension goes and I feel I can t-talk to people. Sometimes I try to talk to m-my neighbors and be f-friendly but they tell me to fuck off, they know what happens when I get on the t-turps. That upsets me so I d-drink more and then it's on."

Questioned as to the reason he was given the diagnosis of bipolar disorder, he looked perplexed. "It's like I tolja, doc, I get manic. You know, shakin an' sweatin, heart goin mad, can't siddown an' all that." When it was pointed out that they are actually symptoms of anxiety, he shrugged: "Everybody tells me it's manic. Chemical imbalance of the brain, that's what I got. Not much f-fuckin b-brain left, I reckon."

He was then asked in detail of the true symptoms of elevated mood. He said he had never felt good or on top of the world in his life. He had no self-esteem at all: "Me? Like m-meself? You gotta be f-f-fuckin jokin." He never spoke quickly as he stammered when nervous, and he was always nervous around people ("Like now, d-doc, no offence but I'm sh-shittin meself"). He never had any energy but, when really nervous, he couldn't settle so he would often walk long distances to try to get relief. Sometimes he had the idea that if he went to another town, life would be different. He might even tell people he was leaving and fix a date but, the closer it came, the more nervous he became so he would make up an excuse not to go and then start drinking again. That was the limit of his big ideas. He had no plans beyond making sure his pension was secure, no goals, no ambitions in life. He didn't expect to live long but it didn't worry him: "Who wants an old stiff hangin round? Get to f-f-forty, that's it, jump in with the f-fuckin crocs. They won't get f-fat on me, though."

There were no true psychotic symptoms. Cognitively, he was aware of poor concentration ("That's m-me, doc, ADD as a kid, bipolar since I g-grew up"), poor memory, inability to organize his thoughts, either too many thoughts tumbling through his head or none at all, a blank head. He had trouble finding words so he tended to just keep swearing and mumbling. The thought content was either miserable and hopeless or terrifying thoughts of what might go wrong. In between, he worried about getting his next drink.

For the record, his family history was quite appalling. He was born in a small country town in a poor part of the state. He never knew his father. His mother worked at roadhouses or in bars and was constantly on the move. He thinks he went to about twenty schools before he left at fourteen. "She was on the g-game, mate, she was the truckies' m-moll, the biggest, ugliest, fattest, drunkest whooer b-between 'ere and Adelaide" (3200km). She had a long succession of men in her life, mostly violent alcoholics, but she could trade curse for curse and blow for blow. She had half a dozen children who were all taken into care at different times. This one was fostered several times but always ran away as he was terrified. Always terrified. He was extremely small for his age and had a very late puberty so he had trouble getting work. He was placed in institutions several times and lived in fear of sexual assault but it never happened. At eighteen, he was imprisoned for stealing petrol but, because of his small stature, he was placed in a juvenile detention center where he saw a psychologist. The psychologist diagnosed BAD and the visiting general practitioner commenced medication but he felt it was never much help. He took the drugs when he was sober as they helped calm him a bit but forgot when he was drinking. Since then, he had been seen by a couple of psychiatrists, once in prison and once after he took an overdose. They agreed with the diagnosis. Did they take a full history? "Nah, nuffin like what you j-jus' done. They jus' talk to m-me a coupla minutes an' write a b-bit an' then it's outa there, You 'eard the d-doc, take yer fuckin d-drugs an' shut the fuck up, prisoner P."

As an adult, he had drifted around from town to town, drinking, getting into trouble and moving on when the police told him to. Sometimes he found a bit of work but he never lasted as he became too nervous of the other men and left. He had had one or two girlfriends but they were all drunken "whooers" who mainly used him for his money. He was emphatic that he never pimped as he was absolutely terrified of their clients. He didn't know about children but doubted it as he had severe premature ejaculation: "That's 'ow f-fuckin useless I am, doc, I can' even m-make it up the spout wivout c-comin to the boil."

His pension was confirmed on the basis of about ten separate diagnoses, but the primary diagnosis was his severely anxious personality. BAD was not one of the diagnoses. He was advised that his medication should be reviewed and he could probably manage on a lower dose of medication with fewer side effects (meaning beta blockers). He said he would think about it and maybe come back but he was not seen again.

Discussion:

This man had the two most common diagnoses that lead to a false diagnosis of BAD, a severe anxiety state with phobic features and panic attacks, and a severely disturbed personality. He was not a bad person; his police record was for a series of minor offences spread over half a dozen towns and a dozen years, mostly drunk and disorderly, giving a false name to police, failing to pay fines, failing to heed a police officer, the usual nonsense. We will start with his personality.

15.6 Three Psychopaths.

A strange thing happened with DSM-III, a lot of people who previously were neatly labeled and filed under personality disorders suddenly found themselves without a diagnosis. This was particularly the case with the group with the rather chilling name of psychopath. In one day, the disparate group of creative, aggressive and inadequate psychopaths disappeared, to be replaced by the slimmed down Antisocial Personality Disorder. The latter is much more homogenous but, in terms of the idea behind categorical clusters, something important has been lost. The antisocial personality selects a group of persistent, highly aggressive, impulsive, dishonest and irresponsible people. Essentially, it gives a label to recidivists, the unstable men who can't keep out of prison, especially men of ethnic minority background. They were more than adequately covered by the term aggressive psychopathic personality, but what about the other two?

The term 'inadequate psychopath' picked out a group of men like Mr. LP in the example above. They led lives of constant, low level chaos, drinking and fighting, breaking the law, in and out of custody, unable to form stable relationships, always letting people down, disinterested in social conformity but not necessarily wanting to bring society down. They were deceitful in a petty, mean-spirited way, manipulative, dependent but hostile about it, mistrustful, querulous, resentful, miserable and lonely, demanding and blackmailing. They couldn't keep out of trouble but when they were arrested, which they usually were because they didn't plan their crimes, they would try to inveigle themselves into favor by informing on other people. They were called psychopaths mainly because of their failure to learn from experience, as seen in their long police records for the same sorts of silly offences, and their inability to relate on any emotional level except hostile dependency. They had children but neglected them then, when the children were placed in care, they ran weeping to somebody, anybody to get them back again but, if they recovered them, then the same thing would happen again in six months. In big hospitals, they were pests, always hanging around trying to get a bed, wanting a pension or some extra benefit, wheedling, probably stealing, borrowing from other patients, threatening trouble then wailing like a child when pulled into line. When their (highly descriptive) label was abolished, the behavior pattern wasn't abolished, so where did they go? A significant proportion of them popped up as BAD.

The third leg of the unholy triad of psychopathic personalities was a variant considered rare by most authorities. The term creative psychopath was reserved for truly outstanding, even inspirational depredations, far beyond the workaday brawls and quotidian homicides of the suburbs. It appears to have originated in Germany, in the writings of Kurt Schneider, who also defined the cluster of symptoms known as the First Rank symptoms of schizophrenia. In 1923, Schneider published a book called *The Psychopathic Personality*, which attempted to put the notion of personality disorder on a value-neutral basis (I have never seen a copy). It was actually an old word; *pathos* comes from the Greek, meaning to suffer (as in the patient), so psychopathic meant a person who suffered mentally, meaning any mental disorder. However, Schneider restricted it to what we would now call the personality disorders. This probably reflects his experience as a medical officer in the Imperial Army during the Great War, when the first attempts were made to sort recruits according to their temperament and, hence, their reliability as soldiers. Three groups were recognized, reliable, weaklings and destructive. The constitutionally hopeless were set to peeling potatoes but I don't know what happened to the menaces. Post-war, Schneider studied psychiatry and became an influential author. During World War II, he refused to have anything to do with the Nazi policies on the mentally ill (mass murder through the T4 program) and served in the Wehrmacht as a medical officer.

Schneider apparently recognized ten abnormal personality types and his influence appears to live on in DSM, except he did not see personality disorders as being distinct categories. One type was the amoral or affectless psychopath, which was quite distinct from the explosive type and the weak-willed or feckless type. Interestingly, he also saw fanatics as personality disorders, which would not have endeared him to the Nazis. He had no problem with the idea that there were no clear boundaries to these types. The amoral psychopath was a very clear-thinking, determined person who could calmly plan crimes, or wait years for revenge, then strike out of the blue and show no regret if he was caught, although he probably wasn't. So the concept grew of a person who had no feeling for the human race, who used them as objects or pawns to achieve his own goals.

In 1948, the British analyst, John Bowlby, wrote an influential book called *Attachment and Loss*, which formalized the notion of affectionate bonding between infants and mothers (fathers came much later). Bowlby said the affectless (emotionless) psychopath was the product of repeated rupturing of the primary affectionate bonds, resulting in a person who was totally self-sufficient in his emotional needs and therefore independent of others. From all of this came the idea of the creative psychopath but, for some reason, the old textbooks always gave the example of Col. T.E. Lawrence, of Arabia fame, as the archetype. I always thought that was completely wrong, Lawrence was a clear example of a personality disorder, but not that one. Be that as it may, we now have the records of the twentieth century, which may go down in history as the Century of the Psychopath.

15.7 The Creative Psychopath

The creative psychopath was not a ranting Hitler or a quivering, neurotic Himmler, he was much more like Stalin, calmly ordering the destruction of his entire group of old revolutionary comrades and his officer class in the Great Purges (when Himmler visited the Ukraine in 1942, he ran from the hall and vomited when his SS officers put on a demonstration of how they shot their prisoners in the head). German creative psychopaths such as Goering and Heydrich translated Hitler's insensate ramblings into precisely detailed death machines. The same thing happened in the Soviet Union in their purges. Mao Zedong was almost certainly a creative psychopath, as was Pol Pot; Idi Amin and Muammar Gaddafi were just psychopaths, nothing much creative about them. Closer to home, we have the astounding example of Bernard Madoff, who calmly embezzled the life savings of thousands of the New York-Long Island-Palm Beach multimillionaire Jewish country club set. He did this, not aggressively, not violently, but carefully and seductively, dispassionately creating an entirely new class of crime, the tribal plunderer. He took advantage of the strength of a race under siege, the fact that they can rely on their own. With great care, over three decades, using his prodigious brainpower allied with endless charm, wit and *savoir faire*, he looted them as though he were a Nazi general sauntering through the Jewish quarter of Vienna, choosing the old masters for his study and the modern masters for his wife's country house. Indeed, just to show that he truly was beyond the pale (*sic*), Madoff helped himself to the funds of the saintly Elie Wiesel's Foundation for Humanity. He did this while bestriding the arcane world of high finance in New York as, perhaps not a Titan, but not far off. When he was exposed, he did not hang himself (as his son did soon after), he went to court and then to prison where, by all reports, he is having quite a good time giving financial advice to the other inmates. Madoff I can label as he is convicted; Ken Lay wasn't far off in his machinations at Enron but he died; Raj Rajaratnam has been convicted; others who led huge banks into disaster have all the hallmarks of the creative psychopath but they are still on the loose so discretion dictates that I should say no more.

Now the important point about Bernard Madoff is that, for all his breathtaking crimes, his monstrous inhumanity, he was not exceptional. There are so many of these people in business, calmly getting on with the serious business of separating the innocent from their money. The newspapers are full of those who are caught; it's those who are beyond the law, the few thousand who set up the conditions for the global financial crisis who are the real villains but they don't see it that way. Then again, nor did Adolf Eichmann. They will plead that they are not murderers, they're not violent, they don't bash their wives or fellate their children; they are often pillars of the society, renowned for their generosity, supporting charities, founding schools, donating to medical research and so on.

It is their very ordinariness that, after they are arrested, stuns people and makes them say: "He'd have to be sick to do that." No, they are not sick. They are just... naughty. They don't care what people think because people don't actually count in their worlds—apart from as raw material, an ore body to be mined and then discarded when the resource is exhausted. They see a loophole, they put their finger in and pull out a plum, so they do it again, and again, then they set up a conveyor belt and really get serious in the plum business. But if it doesn't work, they move on to try again somewhere else, very often the same story or a small variation on a proven formula. Once they are arrested, they usually cooperate with the police and carefully trade information for a reduction in sentence. In prison, they quickly sniff out the power structure and insinuate themselves straight into it. They get the cushy jobs in the prison hospital or the library, the quietest cell or the cell with a view. Soon, they have the prison officers running errands for them, conveying messages, bringing in aftershave, getting shoes that fit better and so on. They are always the same: they waste no time on regret or recriminations but they hit the ground running every time.

Every suburb has one or two, every big corporation, every political party (especially); they flit through expensive clubs, sniffing out the power and their next victims. When their cases come to trial, their lawyers rush around to all the usual psychiatrists to get a report saying their client wasn't himself, he was sick, a victim—anything, in fact, that he wasn't. Now it was not good form for the expensive psychiatrist to stand up in court and say, "Yes, Your Honor, I have examined the defendant and I find he is a psychopath. Creative, mind you, but still a psychopath." This was especially true when the defendant was a younger man and his parents, who truly were pillars of the society, renowned for their generosity, supporting charities, founding schools, donating to medical research and so on, were still very much around. It doesn't look good if they have to hear this in court, then see it on TV that night and read about it as they are chauffeured to work or while sitting under the dryer in the exclusive beauty parlor. Imagine the whispering: "My dear, did you hear about that Winston van Vielgeld? Yes, the very one. A psychopath, the psychiatrist said so in court." But later, the doubts start: "My dear, it couldn't be true, I know what a psychopath is and he isn't one. Psychopaths are killers or gangsters, drug dealers, like blacks and foreigners. They're dreadful people but Winston's so charming and considerate, one of us. A lovely boy, I've known him since he was a child. And his parents, such upstanding parishioners, how devastating. It can't be right, he must have been sick, you know, not himself.... They should get another psychiatrist, go to the top, get the very best. What's money when your entire family reputation is at stake?" Indeed, and what about when your own son and Dear Winston were good friends and you used to boast how very alike they were? Cuts close to the bone, doesn't it.

Creative psychopaths are a reality. They are not sick and, mostly, they are not killers. They are clever, meticulous, charming, seductive in the most insidious ways (and nothing so elementary as inviting psychiatrists back to their apartments to get a better report, that's *Psychopathia vulgaris*); they are courteous, considerate, cultured, tasteful, amusing, discreet and, above all, fascinating. Charisma lightly seasoned with panache and understated flair is their style. Alan Stanford was a loud-mouthed vulgarian compared with the true creative psychopath. So if you meet a person who is clever, meticulous, charming, courteous, considerate, cultured, tasteful, amusing, discreet, fascinating and, above all, interested in you, run. Hold tightly to your pants and your wallet and run, because he or she is just about to strike. The reason is this: if it were not for your money or your connections, why would anybody who is all of those things be interested in a boring little grub like you? By the way, there's no shortage of female creative psychopaths although they can usually find a ticket to Hollywood or the catwalk, per expense of some silly old man who has more money and ambition than testosterone and brains. Fortunately, most wealthy men can usually out-psychopath the ambitious young hopefuls who flock around, drawn by the scent of a Bentley Continental in heat. Did you hear the one about the senile billionaire Italian prime minister and the 17yo Moroccan dancer called Ruby Heart-Stealer? (it's on Youtube, along with him pretending to bugger a female police officer and picking his nose and eating it; I love the thuggish bodyguards [2]. You can tell a man by the company he keeps. Those bodyguards should worry about their reputation)

That's by the by; what matters is that the very real personality disorder called creative psychopathy was abolished by a group of people who, as the record shows, aren't above a bit of monkey business themselves. As a result, charming naughty people had no category of their own in the Bible of Psychiatry; hence, no faulty genes to keep them out of the slammer so they had to come up with something else, and "bipolar" filled the gap. These days, it's all the rage among the cognoscenti. Lawyers ring me to announce the diagnosis: "He's bipolar, you know. He'd have to be sick to do that. Imagine stealing from a charity, a normal person wouldn't do that." Nor would a sick person, just on the basis that sick people are most emphatically not "clever, meticulous, charming, courteous, considerate, cultured, tasteful, amusing, discreet and fascinating" for as long as it takes to organize and run a truly original scam. Selling Sydney Harbor Bridge or the Golden Gate Bridge to elderly Japanese tourists is old hat and takes only an hour or two of fast talking but setting up an Enron or a Bank of Credit and Commerce International, now that takes time, planning and connections, smooth talking and panache plus [3]. Madoff ran his racket for thirty years. Did you hear about Nugan Hand Bank, late of Australia [4]? They over-reached themselves. They were the bankers to the CIA in the 1970s who handled all the money from the CIA's drug-running to finance the Hmong insurgency and various other shady deals but they went a bit too far and tried to scam the CIA which is not the brightest thing to do. No, not very bright, the CIA are not renowned for their forgiving nature, as the late Mr. Nugan soon discovered. Talking of psychopaths...

Fascinating. We could talk about this for hours but I'm running out of space. Suffice it to say that, just as Schneider knew from his vast clinical experience, these people are not a category. The really clever ones merge imperceptibly with the not-so-clever-but-think-they-are ones, who stand next to the rather stupid ones in the line-up who, in turn, rub shoulders with the really dumb ones. Another branch veers out to religious fanaticism, such as the fundamentalist Mormon, Warren Jeffs, across a very small speed hump to David Koresh and his Branch Davidians, and then to Jimmy Jones, who slipped unnoticed into a paranoid psychosis in his last years. Religious dictators fit somewhere in here, one foot in the religious crank camp but mostly in the political psychopathic stream, along with so many other meticulous, charismatic, homicidal people who believe they can do no wrong, so everybody who opposes them must be wrong and therefore should be eliminated. And they, in turn, are only a few rules of life away from the rest of us. As Thoreau didn't quite say, they march to the sound of a different drum. That is all there is to it. Creative psychopaths are *not* sick. Almost invariably, they have very fine brains, they just put them to a different purpose from you and me.

You could be forgiven for thinking that creative psychopaths saw to it that they were removed from the DSM section on personality disorder and relabeled as mentally ill. That would be right up their alley—supremely creative and diabolically psychopathic.

15.8 DSM and Personality Disorder

DSM wants to give everyone a label and there are even labels for those who fall between the cracks. However, the computers in medical records didn't like too many people being classified as Personality Disorder NOS (Not Otherwise Stated, meaning abnormal in so many ways we can't make a choice). So the files were sent back for reprocessing, and the busy staff in the emergency centers just chose the most obvious label: substance abuse, somatoform disorder, borderline personality disorder (especially if the patients were young people from rich families) but the *crème de la crème* was, of course, BAD. Why this? Because people with personality disorders were constantly up and down, all over the place, in fact. With only the slightest effort, it was possible to manipulate their complaints so they matched the very elastic diagnostic criteria of BAD. With just a few questions, the diagnosis was established and last week's pests emerged from the hospital as genuine, authorized mental patients, with a diagnosis, drugs, social workers who had to listen to them and help them find somewhere to live, a permanent excuse for court, and a pension. There are no pensions for personality disorders; pensions are reserved for people who are sick and not just naughty, so having a diagnosis as a person with a genuine *psychotic* disorder based in genes was a vast improvement over feeling like (and being told you are) a failure.

The next question is: why were they up and down all the time? On this, you will have to trust me because nobody, to my knowledge, has bothered to do the study but Mr. LP shows the problem with great clarity. He was a most severely anxious personality, doubtless due to his appalling early life, and being anxious is a total pain. Anxious people have ups, kindly donated by the nice people in the DSM office, except we all know they are not the real McCoy, they are pseudo-ups, impressions of ups, just bouts of anxiety masquerading as ups. They also have downs, some of them brought on directly as the effect of being up all the time, where up = anxious, and being anxious is a total pain and gets you down; and some because of the totally messed up lives they lead, some of it due to being anxious and the rest due to being generally scrambled by their parents, schools, detention centers, police, work mates, drinking mates and so on.

If any reader doesn't believe that being anxious wears you down (and such people do exist, they still believe that being anxious is a sign of moral weakness and can be cured by a bit of willpower), then we can easily arrange a little experiment that will cure you of that false belief. Take it as read: being anxious is a singularly powerful "depressogenic" factor. I tell my patients that the commonest cause of recurrent depression is an unsuspected chronic anxiety state, just as this particular patient had. Very commonly, they say something like: "Well, that makes more sense than being told I have a chemical imbalance of the brain."

Orthodox psychiatry, of course, doesn't believe that being anxious causes depression, partly because their world view says that depression is a categorically separate disease with its own, distinctive genetic fingerprint, and partly because they don't accept that psychological factors have anything to do with mental disorder—ask that pre-eminent authority, Dr. Thomas Insel at NIMH (Dr. Insel's CV on the NIMH website reads as though he has practically no clinical experience. I'm sure that can't be right). To the real experts in mental disorder, the academics, anxiety is *comorbid* with depression, meaning the two disorders coexist in the same person but are not causally related (there is some dispute over this point but we won't quibble). However, to me, chronic anxiety *causes* depression just as chronic pain and disability *cause* depression, and for essentially the same reasons: life eventually becomes unbearable due to constant distress and loss of amenity with no end in sight. Thus, the biocognitive approach can explain the appearance of "ups and downs" in anxious people. The ups aren't in fact true bouts of elevated mood, they are simply the normal symptoms of anxiety (agitation, irritability, inability to concentrate, etc) conflated with the superficially similar but phenomenologically distinct features of a true hypomanic state.

Here is a sound bite: Orthodox psychiatry conflates the diagnoses of anxiety and hypomania by eliding their differentiating features.

If a psychiatrist can't tell the difference between a genuine elevated mood (and yes, hypomanics can be irritable) and anxiety, then that psychiatrist is not fit to practice. In fact, I have no hesitation saying that any such psychiatrist is a danger to the general public because s/he is likely to give the 15% of the population who are significantly anxious the dangerous and debilitating drugs that should be restricted to genuine manic-depressive psychosis. This error is a major contributant to the explosive increase in the incidence of BAD over the past three decades. Genetic diseases don't explode. If an allegedly genetic disease rises by several thousand percent in less than half our allotted three score years and ten, then there is something seriously wrong with the model. In my less than humble opinion, what is seriously wrong is orthodox psychiatry itself, and the rot starts with their failure to develop an articulated, scientific model of mental disorder. To rephrase that, if they had a valid model of mental disorder, they wouldn't make such breathtaking mistakes as conflating anxiety and hypomania, or thinking that anxiety and depression are unrelated when they coexist in the same person. Try asking the patients themselves: they all know that anxiety causes depression but they hate admitting it. To most people, anxiety is a moral failing but genetic diseases are not.

In this context, a paper studying over-diagnosis of BAD is highly relevant. In a detailed study of 700 consecutive outpatients, Zimmerman's group found that bipolar disorder is "...frequently over-diagnozed" [5]. By carefully reappraising the patients using standardized interview techniques, they found that only 44% of people who had previously been given the diagnosis actually met the criteria. The most common mistake was for a depressed person to be labeled bipolar when he wasn't but, consistent with my views, both personality disorders and anxiety disorders were also heavily over-represented in the group of misdiagnosed patients. Of the 82 patients who were misdiagnosed as bipolar, 35 had primary anxiety states. There were also 41 diagnoses of personality disorder, mainly antisocial and borderline personalities, spread among 35 individual patients. That is, a depressed person who also shows an abnormal personality or anxiety features (which would account for a large proportion of depressed people) is very likely to be misdiagnosed as bipolar—and then, totally inappropriately, be treated as such.

Why is this happening when the whole purpose of the DSM project was to standardize the process of diagnosis, reducing positive and negative errors? The authors were cautious in their opinions, so I should quote them at length:

"We believe that the increased availability of medications to treat bipolar disorder and the accompanying marketing efforts are chiefly responsible. Many continuing medical education programs on bipolar disorder begin with a summary of research suggesting bipolar disorder is underdiagnosed, and this is followed by a discussion of methods clinicians can use to improve the detection of the disorder. These discussions of diagnostic practice are usually not balanced by a summary of studies demonstrating overdiagnosis and the risks associated with overdiagnosis. Because clinicians are probably inclined to diagnose disorders that they feel more comfortable treating, we hypothesize that, in patients with mood instability who do not meet criteria for a hypomanic episode, physicians are nonetheless inclined to diagnose a potentially medication- responsive disorder such as bipolar disorder rather than a disorder such as borderline personality disorder that is less medication-responsive (p 30)."

It is, they concluded, difficult to differentiate BAD and personality disorder, especially borderline disorder, because "...many of the correlates of each disorder are the same. Both bipolar disorder and borderline personality disorder are characterized by young age at onset. Both disorders are also characterized by high rates of diagnostic comorbidity, particularly with anxiety disorders, impulse control disorders, and substance use disorders."

As part of the study, they assessed the remainder of the 700 patients and found a total of 560 diagnoses of a depressive nature, and 801 diagnoses of anxiety states. On that basis alone, there is a prima facie case that anxiety is more likely to be causative of other conditions than the other conditions are of anxiety.

I should add that this study comes from Providence, Rhode Is., in a privately insured, essentially white, upper middle class population. I have not the slightest doubt that if the study were repeated in a poor black neighborhood, where poor education, unemployment, high rates of imprisonment, drug and alcohol abuse, family breakdown et cetera, are ten times more common, or in a prison, then the results would show this finding in much stronger form. Bearing in mind that the diagnostic criteria for the various categories of mental disorder in DSM-III-IV are subtly misleading and deceptive just because they are artificial, that they are very often mere distinctions without a difference, then the act of diagnosis is debased to the point where it becomes an artful exercise of personal prejudice masquerading as science.

There is one other personality disorder of note in this respect, but it is no longer deemed a personality disorder, it is now a fully-franked illness in its own right. The cyclothymic personality was just as you would expect: somebody whose life consisted of ups and downs but normally not so bad as to end in hospital. They were usually discovered when one or other of the swings brought them to attention, often after trouble with the police or via a lawyer's office when they had been found embezzling money or some other fraudulent activity, such as overspending on credit or failing to return hired goods. Overdoses after bust-ups with boyfriends were another source, as well as people who were abusing drugs or alcohol.

The cyclothymic personality met the criteria for a personality disorder, that is, an enduring pattern of disturbed behavior and inner experience, affecting all aspects of life including cognition, affectivity, interpersonal functioning and impulse control. Like all abnormal personalities, they were not regarded as suitable for drug treatment, not the least because of their propensity for overdoses. Their problems were too diffuse for behavior therapy and they were utterly unresponsive to any form of moral suasion (which is, of course, what personality disorder means). If treatment were offered, it would be a form of introspective psychotherapy only, with occasional prescriptions of mild, non-toxic drugs if they could not be avoided.

Today, the picture is different. Cyclothymic Disorder is an Axis I diagnosis, meaning an illness in its own right. Anybody diagnosed with an illness is highly likely to receive drugs. The helpful people at WebMD [6] suggest the incidence is 0.5-1.0% of the population (i.e. about five times the incidence of the old manic-depressive psychosis). At first, they take a rather cautious view, suggesting that treatment of this condition is not very helpful, but then the scary warnings start: "Cyclothymia may wreak havoc on the personal lives of people with the disorder. Unstable moods frequently disrupt personal and work relationships. People may have difficulty developing stable work or personal relationships, instead moving through short-lived romances or erratic job performance. Impulsive behavior can be self-destructive and lead to legal problems. People with cyclothymic disorder are also more likely to abuse drugs and alcohol. Up to 50% of people with cyclothymia may also have a problem with substance abuse. Over time, people with cyclothymia are at increased risk of developing full-blown bipolar disorder. Limited data suggests they are at higher risk of suicide. Treatment with mood stabilizers may help to reduce this risk."

Clearly, anybody who has self-diagnosed cyclothymia will immediately be thrown into a panic by this as it reads unmistakably: "Things are going to get worse. OK, so you haven't committed suicide. Yet." Most will rush off for treatment, meaning drugs. And this is exactly what happens. Once they start the drugs, they will develop side effects. A proportion (perhaps 7%) of people taking antidepressants can expect a period of agitation which will be diagnosed as "Mania" or "Hypomania," because the drugs will have "exposed" the genetic disorder (intense agitation is not regarded as a predictable side effect of the drugs), and they will then be put on the full cocktail of drugs for BAD for life.

15.9 Acute Psychoses

In the old days, meaning pre-DSM-III, orthodox psychiatry accepted the idea of an acute psychotic state with a similar clinical picture to schizophrenia but with a completely different onset and prognosis. This group was well-known in public mental health services. In the main, they were taken to hospital by relatives and friends or by police after being taken into custody. Despite a number of different names over the years, the history and appearance was much the same. After a period of a few days' or weeks' fairly intense psychological pressure, the person became confused, agitated and paranoid, couldn't sleep, eat or work and his speech became a disjointed rambling with a strong religious content. Mostly, he showed fleeting delusional ideas and often seemed hallucinated but this was more often deduced by observers than admitted. Sometimes the pressures were external, sometimes they were internal; sometimes the personality was normal while others seemed a bit odd. The important point was that, after a fairly sudden onset, they tended to recover fully in one or a few weeks, rarely months, with very little risk of a recurrence. These features are important: they were going to recover regardless, and they had a good to very good prognosis.

Over the years, this picture was described by a number of authors, mostly European, who named them as they saw fit, also mostly with little regard for what others had said. Christian Langfeldt named them schizophreniform psychoses, meaning having the clinical form of schizophrenia but a completely different clinical course. Karl Leonhard named them the cycloid psychoses, distinguishing them from manic-depressive psychosis and from schizophrenia. Faegermann named his group the psychogenic psychoses, meaning the psychotic state was a reaction to inner pressures, while another cluster was labeled reactive psychosis as they seemed to have been pushed into a psychotic state by external stressors. Finally, the original descriptions of the borderline personality disorder noted that the patients quite often developed acute but transient paranoid psychotic states in response to real or imagined stressors (in keeping with DSM's penchant for diagnostic creativity, these have been reworded as "transient, stress-related paranoid ideation or severe dissociative symptoms" which is a euphemism for psychotic). In each diagnosis, the prognosis for the individual psychotic episode was very good but they were at heightened risk of developing further bouts.

Having seen several cases in rapid succession, and as a fully-paid-up lumper, I decided in my first year of psychiatry that these were all the same condition. Any differences were either the product of wishful thinking by the psychiatrist or they meant nothing as they were neither causative nor reflected on the etiology: they were differences without a distinction. This un-nuanced opinion was reinforced by the fact that all these people got the same treatment (because there was nothing else) and they all recovered at the same rate, regardless of who or where they were treated.

There were other acute psychotic states as well, especially those associated with drug and alcohol abuse. Alcoholic hallucinosis was an uncommon condition in whites but, in Aboriginals, it was extremely common. When they stopped drinking and were treated with antipsychotics and massive doses of vitamins, they recovered. If there were no antipsychotics available, then morphine did the job about as well. Very often, after they recovered, they had little or no memory of what had happened to them.

In the main, people with acute psychoses were very easy to treat, it was just a matter of keeping them safe while we gave nature a bit of a nudge in the right direction, then they went home and were rarely seen again. There weren't many of them, perhaps two or three per ten thousand of the population each year, so they were curiosities in the rush of chronic madness that was public psychiatry at the time. Today, these diagnoses are all but forgotten. Almost nobody would use these terms and they have no currency in the psychiatric literature. They get very little mention in DSM (Brief Psychotic Disorder 298.8) so, in another small example of cultural hegemonism, that is essentially the end of the matter. So what has happened to them? Where are the acute psychoses of yesteryear?

Psychiatric syndromes have fads, just like every other human activity, but going mad isn't quite in the same class as wearing your cap backwards or see-through earlobes. Madness does change from one culture to the next or one era to the next, but only its content. The form doesn't change. For example, a hundred years ago, paranoid states were all about religious persecution (who remembers Masons?), then persecution became political (our friends the commies) and finally it took up where science fiction ran out of credibility (unless your name was Hubbard, in which case it did a full circle). X-rays shining down from geostationary satellites nudged the Archangel Gabriel out of orbit, while microchips implanted by mad scientists have replaced the devil's whispering. The form of madness hasn't changed at all, and one classical form is the acute agitated confused psychotic state as a reaction to psychological stressors. Today, almost all people presenting with this form of disorder are given the diagnosis of bipolar disorder and treated with the usual drug cocktails.

Now this is a problem because we have taken a small group with a good prognosis who, in the past, were carefully not labeled with anything long-lasting, and have relabeled them as having a permanent disorder with a genetic basis. Therefore, in tune with the modern concept of defensive psychiatry, they have to be treated for their condition. It avails them not to plead that they no longer have a condition, because modern psychiatry doesn't recognize the idea that psychotic disorders can be just a passing whim. Psychosis is genetic and, as the oft-repeated parables of diabetes and hypertension show, genetic disorders have to be treated to prevent complications. Why is a psychotic state presumed to be genetic? If you ask a conventional psychiatrist that question, you will not get an answer. He will either look at you strangely and move on, or start talking about neuro-transmitters until you move on. The short answer is because that is what they believe. Since they believe it, certain other imperatives come into play, as in: "This is a case of psychosis. Psychosis is a genetic disorder. Other untreated genetic disorders deteriorate, e.g. diabetes and hypertension. As a physician, my job is to cure or to prevent deterioration. Since we cannot cure a genetic disease, I have to act quickly to prevent deterioration. In psychiatry, as in all medicine, deterioration is prevented by life-long prescription of large doses of medicaments. Here, Patient, take these and be grateful."

There is a corollary: "If the patient objects, then he is more deteriorated than we suspected so he must be given even more medication." How does this arise? It arises because one of the cardinal features of psychosis is lack of insight. If anybody refuses medication after being told he has a genetic disease which must be treated to prevented deterioration, then he must be suffering a lack of insight, which is a cardinal feature of psychosis, so he is clearly worse than superficial appearances indicate and must therefore be treated against his will to prevent deterioration. How do we know he will deteriorate? As proof, the psychiatrist points to the thousands of deteriorated patients in his care: "That is how we know," he says. "Huge numbers of patients all over the world confirm this to be a general truth." What he doesn't do is point to the very large numbers of ex-patients around the world whose acute psychotic states resolved with little or no specific treatment, and who now show no signs of mental disorder.

The idea that the patient may have developed a psychotic state as a pure psychological reaction to life stressors, or to an interaction between his social environment and abnormal personality factors, is not entertained. It is not entertained because psychosis is a chemical imbalance of the brain and everybody knows that chemical imbalances are genetic, not psychological. The notion that psychological stressors could cause a genetic disorder, be it diabetes or psychosis, is too silly for words. The logical errors are perfectly apparent.

This is another path to the burgeoning lists of deteriorated BAD patients in Western countries. Acute psychotic states are now almost entirely diagnosed as BAD and treated as such. Most of the remainder will be diagnosed with schizophrenia and will be given standard treatment, i.e. more or less the same long-term drug cocktails as those with BAD. This point should not be overlooked: drug treatment of any serious mental disorder is now essentially standard, regardless of the diagnosis. Anybody under treatment for schizophrenia who seems depressed will be given an antidepressant; if he doesn't respond or the antidepressant causes a state of acute agitation (always known as mania but it is actually akathisia), he will be given "mood stabilizers" as well, if not ECT. Effectively, there is now a generic dosage regime for any psychotic state (and BAD is a psychotic condition, don't forget), consisting of quetiapine by day, olanzapine by night, an antidepressant, and an anticonvulsant such as valproate as a "mood stabilizer," with or without benzodiazepines for agitation and anticholinergics for motor side effects.

The fantastically successful remarketing of anticonvulsants as psychiatric drugs has an interesting history. In the early 1970s, there was only one drug used as a mood stabilizer, lithium. While it seemed effective, it was toxic and required regular blood tests to monitor the blood levels. In addition, patients didn't like it as it was very sedating, caused slowing of the thought processes, motor discoordination and loss of enjoyment. As a result, and despite intense pressure from mental health staff, they often stopped it. Unfortunately, when they did so, many of them had further breakdowns which was always seen as proof of the fact that they needed it, not of the possibility that they may be suffering withdrawal effects.

In 1966, a man in Texas was given a prescription for phenytoin, an anticonvulsant [7]. I don't know why he was given that particular drug because he did not suffer epilepsy but he was an extremely wealthy man who was also decidedly unstable. This combination tends to result in people getting all sorts of treatments they don't warrant. Jack Dreyfus (a distant relative of Capt. Alfred) was hugely impressed by this drug and began a campaign to have it accepted as a standard treatment for nervousness and depression. In the early 1970s, he sold his companies which gave him the time and money to indulge his passion, including writing a book and sending a copy to every medical practitioner in the US. By that stage, he was well and truly a billionaire so he probably didn't notice. Nor did anybody else. His zeal was not contagious, not the least because phenytoin, a folate antagonist, is a very unpleasant drug with many toxic side-effects, plus (tellingly) it was out of patent. There was no money to be made from conducting the expensive studies to have it approved for use in psychiatry, so nothing happened. Certainly, Mr. Dreyfus didn't undertake them, which was probably the business man talking, not the zealot. Eventually, in his nineties and still fabulously wealthy, he passed from this vale of tears, unremembered by most psychiatrists despite his prodigious efforts.

Soon after phenytoin hit the ground (face-first, not running), there was a push to prescribe carbamazepine, another heavily sedating anticonvulsant with a huge list of dangerous side effects, but this also didn't go far. In those days, it wasn't thought to be specific for mood disturbances but as a sort of all-purpose personality restorer for the obstreperous neurotic. It also didn't take off, not the least because it is highly unpleasant with a worryingly low ratio of toxicity to therapeutic effect. Not so sodium valproate, which arrived in the mid 1970s and soon gained a reputation as the drug for all reasons. In no time, anticonvulsants were marketed as effective in preventing elevated moods, although they were mostly ineffective in preventing depression. And so a new industry, the "mood stabilizers," was born, the end result of which is that any psychiatric patient who shows more than brief unhappiness with his mournful lot in life (i.e. about 90% of them) is very likely to be placed on an antidepressant and an anticonvulsant "to rectify the imbalances." The problem is, there is now very worrying evidence that indicates the imbalances are caused by the drugs themselves, and the drugs are given to patients who don't need them, either because their primary conditions (anxiety, personality disorder) don't respond to them or they didn't actually need any drugs at all because they were going to get better quicker than any medication can work.

This last point is part of a general trend. The psychologist Irving Kirsch has studied placebo effects in antidepressants, and concluded that these drugs are no use in mild or even moderately severe depression, and have a significant risk of making people worse [8]. Needless to say, this news has not been well-received by all the psychiatrists who have made their reputation by putting more and more people on bigger and bigger doses of antidepressants for longer and longer. A recent review and meta-analysis [9] disagreed with Kirsch, concluding that antidepressants are in fact equally effective across the spectrum of severity but, in cases of mild depression, it is necessary to wait eight weeks to detect the improvement because it isn't evident at six weeks, the normal cut-off point for this type of study.

This study was of interest, partly because I don't recognize a condition called Mild Depression, or mild Major Depressive Disorder, or Minor Depressive Disorder, or anything that puts the words 'mild' and 'depression' in the same sentence. To me, with my comorbid afflictions of pedantry and gross insensitivity to the human condition, that is like saying "mildly dead," "mildly pregnant" or a "mild case of ventricular tachycardia." Just as you can't order a steak tartar well done or a non-alcoholic scotch, so you cannot be mildly depressed. It is an oxymoron. Anybody who thinks he is mildly depressed has been watching too much daytime television and should take up a vigorous and preferably painful outdoor hobby.

Be that as it may, I admit there are some foolish psychiatrists in the world who don't share my views, who actually see patients, diagnose "mild depression" and, horror of horrors, put them on antidepressants. They must then wait eight weeks for the "patients" to show an improvement. Why anybody who was not on death's door would persist with antidepressants for eight weeks, we do not know, especially when we do know that 95% of them will have got over their attacks of the vapors in six weeks, anyway.

The idea that any deviation from psychological normality, no matter how trivial, represents a "disease state" and must therefore be treated with drugs, either to rectify the present symptoms or to prevent future deterioration, drags psychiatry into disrepute. It constitutes a serious lack of clinical maturity and a gross underestimation of the commonsense and resilience of ordinary human beings. If the famously unstable and irresponsible people of the Kimberley region of Western Australia can get by sharing one antidepressant tablet a year among five, then so too can the civilized world.

15.10 Conclusion

This chapter provides some basic clinical evidence to suggest that BAD is overdiagnosed at the expense of "less important" diagnoses. Daily clinical practice will yield a steady stream of people who have been incorrectly diagnosed as BAD, meaning specific treatment of their other conditions is then neglected in favor of chronic polypharmacy of a diagnosis they don't have. Needless to say, they don't get better. The fact that they don't get better should start alarm bells ringing but it doesn't. Why not? Zimmerman's group concluded much as I did, that psychiatrists are keen to diagnose the conditions that interest them, conditions they can treat and the conditions they have been seduced (my term, not theirs) into seeing which are not, in fact, present. The reason this goes on with no apparent concern in the community or from the responsible government authorities is because the Supreme Authority, DSM-IV and soon to be -5, is so badly worded that, to paraphrase Justice Sol Wachtler, "If it's what you wanted, I could bring in a diagnosis of Bipolar Affective Disorder on a ham sandwich." (Now his was an interesting career...)

I have shown that the criteria for BAD in DSM-IV-TR do not distinguish adequately between true affective disorders and the very much more common classes of anxiety disorders and personality disorders. There is epidemiological evidence to support this conclusion, but a definitive answer could only come from a very extensive literature review in association with a very large scale, long-term, precisely organized field study. Anything less will leave the field of psychiatry wide open to allegations of mass misdiagnosis and mistreatment. In my view, those claims would be so widespread, so expensive, and so irresistible as to bring about the end of psychiatry as an independent specialty. "Good," you may say, but the evidence is that whatever replaces it would be no improvement, and probably worse.

My warning is not directed at the senior members of the profession who have made their mark over the past two or three decades by instituting and institutionalizing a grossly defective parody of a scientific system of classification. Quite frankly, they've made their names and their packets, so, with one or two brave exceptions (Spitzer and Frances come to mind), we cannot expect any of them to recant. I suppose this is why Shaw snarled: "Every man over forty is a scoundrel." As a group, the psychiatric "authorities" will take the fight to whatever low level they feel they need to win: witness the disgraceful behavior of the Center for Addiction Mental Health at Toronto University Dept. of Psychiatry, in 2000-01 toward Dr. David Healy. As soon as the institute had the idea that Healy's (highly regarded) work might cut into their cash flow, they ditched him. Talking to such people is manifestly a waste of time: their minds are made up, money trumps academic freedom and the devil take anybody who tries to question them. In the higher echelons of orthodox psychiatry, this type of behavior is not regarded as out of place.

Instead, my warning is directed at the younger members of the profession, the residents, trainees and medical students who regularly contact me to say they detect some fell influence lurking at the intellectual heart of the profession. They are right. Where we ought to be creating and nurturing a compassionate theory of mental disorder, there is only a cash register next to a pile of degrees for sale.

If this keeps up, soon we'll all be BAD.

Testing the Biocognitive Model: Clinical Syndromes (3) ADHD

"Fallacies do not cease to be fallacies because they become fashions."

—G.K. Chesterton

16.1 Introduction

In this chapter, I want to establish a case to show why so many people are being put on drugs they do not need, drugs which may well be causing serious, adverse mental problems in the long term. I need to show in what way orthodox psychiatry is making a serious mistake in diagnosis, and why their biological model leads them inexorably to this mistake. I will also have to give an alternative formulation of the problem their model is trying to explain, then show that the alternative explanation meets standard criteria of what constitutes a superior scientific explanation, and that it will not lead to the same mistake itself.

This is quite a lot to ask of a single chapter, so I will have to tread my usual tightrope. If I explain things at a level I think is sufficient, people complain that it is incomprehensible so they decline to read further on that basis. If, instead, I spell out each and every step in the explanatory sequence so there can be no misunderstanding, they complain that I am being patronizing and pedantic so they decline to read further on that basis. This chapter will veer toward being pedantic because, for orthodox psychiatry, the concepts involved are sometimes counter-intuitive.

16.2 Case 1. Mr. JMcK

A 25yo man moved 4000km across the continent after being recruited to a most lucrative and responsible position in the technical division of an international energy giant. With a salary of some $130,000 plus substantial benefits, and the chance of rapid promotion in the most technical section of one of the world's fastest growing industries, he was naturally pleased and excited with his opportunity. A few weeks after he arrived, he obtained a referral to see a psychiatrist. The purpose, as he put it, was to "get some more of my dexies" as he had run out a week before. He explained that he had been commenced on dexamphetamine 30mg per day by a pediatrician and had been advised to continue it for life. He was surprised and a little irked to hear that the laws regarding these drugs varied from state to state, and I was required by my state law to take a full history and assessment, then base my decision on that and that alone.

"That's, ah, a bit of a waste of time, isn't it?" he asked with a slight blush. "I mean, I was assessed by Prof. X at the University of Y institute of neurosciences, it has an international reputation. I had all the tests, scans, blood tests, I saw psychologists, the lot. You could see the diagnosis on a PET scan, do you know what that is?"

I did, and advised him that it was purely a research tool of no indicative value.

Again, a slight frown creased his smooth brow: "Are you sure? I was told quite the opposite by some leading authorities."

I assured him that, in the context of local law, it carried no weight so we would proceed if he wished?

He had two degrees, in petrochemical engineering and IT, and his contract was to develop three dimensional depth analyses of the earth's crust using geodetic data from a number of incompatible sources (or something, it was far beyond me). He came from a well-to-do family in an old money suburb and attended the top school in his home town where he took several prizes, then went straight to university. At school and at university, he played both cricket and rowing at the level of the state schoolboys' team, a superhuman effort. While studying, he remained on the best of terms with his family and felt his parents had played a big part in his success as they were 110% behind him at all times: "I know it sounds bad," he said with a laugh, "but I never made a bed or even picked up my clothes until I moved here." He had a good social life with a bit of sporty drinking but nothing excessive. He did not use drugs. After being snapped up by a local oil company, he was soon head-hunted by another, and now this one: "I've gone from fifty to a hundred and thirty in barely two years. Seems remarkable, doesn't it." Through gritted teeth, I agreed that it was indeed remarkable and we pressed on (I had already checked his car, he was driving a company car, a locally-made Ford with private plates, not a Porsche).

The mental state showed a fit, lean and healthy young man of a little above average height, well-dressed in neat city clothing with no visible tattoos, studs, scars or jewelry. He was well-groomed with neat hair and clean nails. He had a pleasant, open look, a mild but self-assured manner and a measured way of speaking in his courteous private school accent. He was not anxious, depressed, hostile or suspicious. There were no signs of a psychotic disorder and nothing to indicate an organic impairment of brain function. It is difficult to assess the intellect of an engineer without tests as they usually see no point in verbal pyrotechnics but there was no doubt that he was of very superior intellectual ability. In particular, there was nothing to suggest a primary defect of attention or concentration, or of his arousal level. In short, he presented as a fairly enviable package from anybody's point of view.

After completing my notes, I advised him that there was no evidence to suggest that he was suffering a diagnosable mental illness or that he had ever done so. He was, I assured him, a picture of mental health. So what was the purpose of the drugs? Why were they prescribed.

He was the youngest of the family. At the age of three, his elder brother's first born son had been diagnosed by the pediatrician as suffering a severe case of ADHD "and some other diagnoses, I'm not sure, Asterisk...?"

"Asperger's."

"Yes, that's it, Aspergers. And a touch of ODD and OCD."

"That's quite a collection for a three year old but what does this have to do with you?"

"Oh," he said with a warm smile as he recrossed his legs and straightened the crease in his trousers, "the doctor wanted to see all Josh's male relatives because it's a genetic disease. He wanted to check everybody to see if they needed treatment because the condition is quite serious if it's left untreated."

"He said that?"

"Indeed. Anyway, the long and the short of it was that I saw him and was given a huge battery of tests, I mean I was really taken with the PET, I'd never heard of them, fantastic, I was actually thinking we might be able to use it in detecting hydrocarbons at depth by seeing if the drill cores supported lipophagic bacteria. But I digress. The professor took one look at me and muttered "classic case" and so, after a quick check and completing a questionnaire, I walked out with a handful of orders for all the tests and a prescription, and I started them at lunchtime that day."

"You started the tablets before he had the test results?"

"Of course, it's quite serious."

"Do you think the tablets may have biased the PET results? No, don't worry. How long were you in there?"

"Hmm, he asked some questions, then he gave me a 12 item questionnaire to complete. I did it at his desk, then he quickly checked my heart and blood pressure and my knee jerks and that was it. Fifteen minutes at the most, no, more like twelve minutes. Including taking my shirt and tie off."

"I see. And if you don't mind my asking, how much did this cost?"

"His fee? Five hundred, about that. The scans were extra, of course. Twelve hundred all up."

"I see. Five hundred for twelve minutes."

"Oh, the waiting room was full. Queues of people. He's so busy, I don't know how he does it. He had to see ten members of my extended family alone, all our cousins."

"All at five hundred for twelve minutes?"

"Now don't be like that, doctor," he chuckled. "He's a renowned researcher. I suppose if one wants the best, one has to pay for it. I'm not unhappy with the outcome. I think it's important to know what the future holds. I was given a brochure that suggested that, when the time comes, I should have my own offspring assessed at the earliest possible time, even before they've left hospital. The disease can be arrested and held at bay but only by intensive management."

"I see."

He laughed and brushed his hand over his eyes: "Don't keep saying 'I see.' You unnerve me. You asked me whether I was shy and I said no, but I really am a bit. I'm fine on a cricket field or presenting a PowerPoint to an audience of executives who don't even know how to spell geodesy, but one-to-one is not my strongest point."

"I worked that out. Anyway, enough of this pleasant chat. Back to business, and the business is that the law in this state says you cannot have that medication."

He shrugged politely. "In that case, I'm sure I could get Prof. X to courier them here."

"He could, but he would be breaking the law. Transporting S8 drugs across state borders is a very serious offence."

"Really? I had no idea... He told me they were very widely prescribed and there was a vast literature relating to them."

"Indeed, they are and there is, but that's not the point. The point is you don't qualify as you are not mentally ill and that is the end of the matter in this city."

A look of mild exasperation crossed his brow, so I decided to pull out a bigger gun. "Have you told your employer you are taking these drugs?"

"No. Should I?"

"I think not. At least until you know whether you can go on board an oil rig with amphetamines in your bloodstream."

The color drained from his face. "Are you serious?"

"Do I look like a comic? Don't answer. I can check, but oil rigs come under Federal law as well as state law and it tends to get murky."

Drawing a deep breath, he licked his lips slowly. "I'd rather you... perhaps I could make some discrete enquiries?"

"Absolutely not. Don't say a word. I can do it and nobody will know a thing. I'm used to this, I have the same problem with the military and the medical board. It's very widespread, especially where you come from. I was hoping for a quiet day but still... Sorry, how long have you been on them?"

"Three months."

"I beg your pardon. At 25, you saw a pediatrician...?"

"I was still 24."

"At 24, you saw a pediatrician, a physician, who examined your chest and said you had a mental disorder. In twelve minutes? How long have we been going this morning?"

He glanced at the elaborate chronometer on his wrist. "Good heavens, nearly an hour. Time flies when you're having fun, except I'm no longer having fun."

"Do you need them? What do you take them for?"

"ADHD."

"Mr. McK, please don't do that to me, it's unbecoming for a psychiatrist to shriek and bite the table. What are your symptoms? Don't worry about the label, what's the trouble in your... sanctified life?"

Beads of sweat were forming on his upper lip. "Dr, I don't quite follow...?"

"Are you suffering? Are you crazy?"

"No... Oh, I see. No," he laughed, rocking back with obvious relief, "no, I'm not mentally ill. I can go on the rigs without wanting to blow them up. Truth is, I take them because they enhance my lifestyle."

This caught me unawares. "They what?"

"They enhance my lifestyle. I feel I... expand to fill my role."

"You already function at a level just below beatification, what more do you want?"

"I don't follow..."

"Forget it. Alright, time's up. At five hundred for twelve minutes, one hour makes.... Don't panic, young man, it's my little joke. Today costs you nothing but a tax burden. OK, don't tell your employer and don't attempt to courier S8 drugs into the state, the police have a very effective surveillance system in place in this town. And don't, whatever you do, attempt to buy them on the street, regardless of who offers them or for what reason, even free. That is the first step on a very short, slippery slope into a criminal lifestyle. I will sort something out. Come back next week."

By now, he was pale and slightly tremulous. I could see his pulse pounding in his throat. Slowly, he cleared his throat and swallowed hard, then rose to his feet without a word. In the waiting room, he collected his appointment and swiped his card while checking his iPhone, then bade the receptionist and me a pleasant good morning and strode briskly out to his car.

Driving home that evening, I berated myself: "Why were you such a puritanical arsehole? Why didn't you give him the bloody stuff? You can see he's anxious and he uses it to suppress performance and social anxiety, and now he's addicted so just go with the flow." On the other hand, if I simply lie down and wave him through, am I not being complicit in a crime of some sort? Maybe not in terms of the criminal code but in terms of that principle somewhere that says we are all responsible for each and every action we take, so if it was wrong for a pediatrician to start him on the drugs, then it would be wrong for me to continue them. There is an important point buried in this case, the difference between getting it wrong and doing it wrong. Getting It Wrong is where you follow the correct procedure, you take the history and do the tests and then prescribe a form of treatment. But because medicine is very imprecise and we are only scratching the surface in terms of our knowledge of the complexity of the body, and not even in the right mental space in terms of the mind-brain axis, then the treatment can fail. The surgeons have a pithy epithet for this conundrum: The operation was a success but the patient died. Getting It Wrong is not a crime.

At the far end of the spectrum lies Doing It Wrong, which is a crime of some sort. The pediatrician who saw my adult patient as he whirled past on the production line was Doing It Wrong. Just as I don't see children for their asthma, or 24yo women for placenta previa, or 24yo men for mid-shaft fractured femurs (all of which I have done in the past but that was the past), so pediatricians do not see 24yo men for psychiatric reasons. End of discussion. We stick to our area of expertise and that's that; anything else is adventurism and deserves whatever punishment the Medical Board throws at it. The idea of some amateur assessing a psychiatric problem in anything under an hour, without following a formal protocol, and in the absence of anything approximating an articulated model of mental disorder, is a crime. Gouging the general population for over $2000 an hour just to put them on dangerous and highly addictive drugs they don't need, with long-term effects we can hardly predict, is a crime. Giving people amphetamines for the wrong reasons is as much a crime as selling them on the street. The police in this country are presently just about at war with bikie groups who control the illegal manufacture and distribution of stimulants. But this fast-talking professor (professor!) can buzz around his office, spouting the most arrant pseudo-scientific claptrap about putting newborn babes on stimulants for life, and he doesn't go to prison? I can't stand it, I thought as I drove through the bush to my very isolated home. As I went for my run at sunset that night, with the enormity of the monsoon season nearly upon us, I was close to despair but the sight of a vast flock of magpie geese whirling excitedly in the face of an advancing thunderstorm cheered me and it didn't feel so hopeless. And so we move to the next part of this story.

As it turned out, I never saw him again.

16.3 Setting the Doctors Right

Western Australia is physically a long way from the geographic center of the universe, and even further intellectually, if you ask anybody from the eastern part of the country. West Aussies are not much fussed by this, their attitude is that not having the vast burden of thinking you are better than everybody else lightens the processes of thinking. So it comes as no surprise to find that one of the world's foremost critics of the ADHD industry is from WA, and he isn't even a doctor. Martin Whitely belongs to that most despised of Australian sects, a member of parliament. To be precise, he is a Member of the WA Legislative Assembly, the junior in a bicameral house in a very isolated part of the globe. He started his professional life as an accountant but found he didn't have the attention to detail to be a bean counter, so he decided to try teaching. Oddly enough, in a wealthy independent boys grammar school (private college), he found his niche; he loved the work. I say oddly enough, because he is a member of the Labor Party which, traditionally, has opposed the alleged privileged elitism of the private school system. However, he found that boys are the same regardless of the uniform; they weren't strange at all.

What he did find strange was the number of students who were taking drugs for mental disorders. Further, he found that the drugged boys lacked the verve and vitality of their undrugged peers, so he presumed it was an unwanted side effect of whatever treatment was being offered for their unseen "disease." However, in the course of the year, he found that if a boy stopped his medication for any reason, the drugged effect went away and he recovered his verve and vitality. Even more peculiar, in his newly undrugged state, his disease didn't reappear so it was all a bit mysterious. After a long, roundabout route, it finally dawned on him that their verve and vitality just was their disease, that they were being sedated to suppress what, based on his own childhood and his experience as a teacher, he thought was normal behavior for boys. This led him to find the name of the disease, then to read about the subject. Eventually, it became a sort of crusade to stop the endless drugging of the coming generation for doing exactly what boys have done since Adam was one himself.

In 2001, Whitely entered parliament and, following protocol, rose to give his maiden speech. By hallowed tradition, which not even young Labor radicals would snub, the maiden speech can address any topic as long as it doesn't reflect on the government's agenda, or lack thereof. I don't know what its purpose is, to string out the day and keep the Honorable Members out of the Members' Bar, or maybe to give them a good reason to stampede there when the final bell rings, who knows, but for his topic, the newly-minted Hon. Member chose the vexed matter of stimulant use in schoolchildren. He used his free airtime to raise his "grave concerns that ADHD misdiagnosis and the resultant over-prescription of amphetamines (is) a threat to the health and happiness of many West Australian children" [1]. He could have said children all over the world but, by the same tradition, the maiden speech should reflect something about WA's population of barely two million spread over their (largely empty) one million square miles of territory.

Well, you can imagine the squeals of vested interests who could see their games being brought to a sudden halt. The production-line stamping and labeling of mental disease by doctors, the planes flying in drugs, the pharmacists unpacking the boxes and ringing them through, the line-'em-up-an'-dose-'em nursing posts at the schools, and the endless black market in the school playgrounds as the drugs percolated back up another channel to surface in dark corners at all-night rave dance sessions in nightclubs and hotspots. Millions upon millions of dollars, going round and round, people being pushed in at one end and spat out, zombified, at the other. Children getting to eighteen, totally habituated and dependent on stimulants, only to find their disease had abruptly run its course. It only affects children, you see, if you look in DSM-IV-TR, you won't find it listed among the mental illnesses of adults. So, as Whitely soon discovered, the 18yo drug addicts, because that is what they had become, simply stopped buying their tablets at the chemist and started buying them on the streets. But illegal drugs cost money, a great deal more than when your parents are buying them at hugely subsidized rates at the local pharmacy, so some of the boys turned to crime to finance their habits and some of the girls turned to prostitution. In no time, WA had one of the world's highest rates of prescription of these incredibly helpful drugs and, commensurately, one of the world's highest rates of addiction to these incredibly dangerous drugs. Because, you see, you can't have one without the other.

Eventually, somebody put two and two together and realized that, if a boy could be mentally ill the day before his eighteenth birthday party, he probably still had the same condition the day after the party. So adult ADHD was born, a new industry was unleashed and the party went on. This time, it wasn't quite so easy. When it comes to anything to do with child health, however esoteric or removed from reality, governments turn to jelly. With adults, especially crazy adults, it's not so much a problem so they had long clamped rules and regulations on amphetamines, all the while knowing perfectly well that the schoolchild legal drug industry bred an adult illegal drug industry.

They also knew that stimulants had become the point of entry of the increasingly well organized and ruthless bikie gangs, white Australia's answer to the tribal crime families of the Sicilians, the Calabrians and the Vietnamese triads. Under Whitely's increasingly effective scrutiny, it became clear that the pediatric drug industry had slipped out of control and was now largely unregulated. An anomalous situation had arisen where doctors prescribing Schedule 8 drugs (S8; narcotics and other drugs of addiction) for adults had to ring the Federal Dept of Health for each prescription, and answer questions as to why they were prescribing them. For a busy practitioner, this is a nuisance so they avoid S8 drugs where possible. It was also true for S8 drugs for children but, because there were so many children taking the drugs, and relatively so few specialists to prescribe them, the Health Dept. had waived the regulations, allowing specified practitioners to prescribe them without restriction. And so they did. One enterprising pediatrician commenced 2000 new patients on S8 stimulants in 20 months.

Between 1989 and 2000, the number of people taking stimulants in the isolated state of WA rose some 2,300%. Of 20,650 people taking the drugs in 2000, nearly 90% were children, meaning some 4.5% of all children aged between 4-17 in the state were taking this particular class of drugs [2]. Zero to 4.5% in eleven years: it is unprecedented in medical history in this country, if not in the world. Yet no alarms were ringing. So readily were people convinced by a small group of medical practitioners that it has to be seen in a single context: that of the phenomenon of mass hysteria. Witchcraft. Tulip mania. The Yellow Peril.* UFOs. Reds under the bed. Royal Free Disease. Repetitive Strain Injury. Not even the Second Coming could sell so many tickets to the laconic and suspicious citizens of West Oz. The mass hysteria is not in the children, it is in the adults. The children are only responding to psychosocial pressures for the full range of private and social reasons. But why were allegedly scientifically trained medical practitioners such an integral part of it? Was it money, or hubris, or fearing to appear ignorant by not recognizing the condition, or a case of a little bit of knowledge being a bad thing? Yes.

In any event, this rampant medical growth industry was reined in, but not by the usual method of more regulations, more inspections, more intrusion. No, this was far more subtle. Under the influence of the energetic Mr. Whitely, the anomalous position of stimulants for children was brought back into line with the rest of the pharmacopeia. Any new scripts for stimulants had to go through the normal authorization procedures, meaning the enterprising Prof. X who had seen Mr. McK in twelve minutes would have spent an extra five minutes or more on the phone, waiting for a clerk in the bowels of the Health Dept. to give him an authorization number. Oh dear.

In remarkably short order, the bubble-epidemic collapsed. In just a few years, the number of children taking these drugs (because, we presume, of having the genetic affliction) dropped by 60-70%. Perth became the only ADHD "hotspot" in the world to apply the fire extinguisher and bring the conflagration under control. Does this matter? Well, one of the immediate results was a collapse in the black market for these drugs, partly because they were no longer freely available outside every school for dealers to buy, and partly because there were fewer takers. Police statistics had always shown a very clear correlation between adolescents and young adults who were abusing amphetamines, and their history of having been prescribed them as children. That is, far from preventing illicit drug use by mentally disordered people needing to self-medicate, the legal prescription of the drugs actually set up the conditions for an epidemic of illicit use three to five years later. In Sept. 2007, the Premier of Western Australia told Parliament: "The evidence shows that if amphetamine prescribing rates are decreased, abuse rates are decreased" [2, p410]. As a bonus, with something like 14,000 ex-patients at about $100 a month, that meant anything up to $20,000,000 a year saving for the community. This figure did not include the costs of treating drug addicts, police and legal costs, etc.

The picture is actually worse, much worse than this brief summary can show but my intention is not to repeat Whitely's diligent work (and I believe his book should be on the curriculum of every medical school in the world) but to relate this to my themes: Firstly, that while orthodox psychiatry does not have an agreed, articulated, publicly-available model of mental disorder, abuses will inevitably occur. The reason they occur is because nobody can (or will) stand up and say with full authority: "What you are doing is wrong." The appalling scandal of the lobotomy (leucotomy) era shows this with crystalline clarity [3]. Such was the state of theorizing in psychiatry that, regardless of what anybody thought, nobody could say to Freeman: "This procedure has no basis in a science of psychiatry and you must stop." It was only when the complaints grew too loud that the medical profession acted.

The second theme is that, in the absence of a working model of mental disorder, any nosology consists of simply arranging a very large set of unrelated observations (unrelated because there is no model to relate them to or to dictate their collection) in patterns that happen to suit whoever is arranging them. That is, they become little more than a projective test of the organizer's prejudices. In the case of the DSM, the prejudices are that mental disorder just is a special case of brain pathology which, in turn, has a primary biological cause in the genome. Thus, each clinical disorder has its own discreet pathology in the genome. *QED.* Moreover, since the causes are genetic, there can be no overlap so any relationships between the separate disorders is essentially random, not causative in any biologically conceivable sense. But, and here the DSM thesis runs into an insuperable problem, what is biologically inconceivable is perfectly conceivable in a non-biological framework. If mental disorder is not biological by nature, then another model may look at the relationships of, say, depression and anxiety, or personality disorder and anxiety and thence depression, and say: "Makes perfect sense. Where's the problem? Depression is the result of an accumulation of adverse life experiences. Sometimes the experiences are here and now, sometimes they are echoes from the past. Sometimes they are out in the real world, and sometimes they are internal and private. Sometimes they are known, and sometimes they are not, they are latent or unconscious events. There is nothing contradictory in any of this, but if you disagree, then show me the fault in my reasoning."

It is at this point that the highly polished public relations machine of biological psychiatry switches off. They have nothing to say, just because they have no rational objection to a cognitive science for psychiatry. As has been said in another context: They know the truth about biological psychiatry and could tell us this afternoon; they just haven't worked out how to still be in power tomorrow morning.

16.4 ADHD and Normal Behavior

Let's look again at the nature of ADHD. The first part of my case is that there is no such condition. It does not exist. It is wholly a social construct, practically unique to certain English-speaking Western countries, and its spread shows a very close relationship with a number of sociopolitical and secular trends in the past four decades. It is not a disease, there is no biological basis to it *apart from* the biological basis of any human behavior (e.g. we have a genetically-determined speech center; male behavior is heavily influenced by the effects of testosterone at different stages of development, etc.), so the search for a biological cause is like the search for a biological cause for preferring crosswords to Sudoku.

Second, the artificial construct called ADHD represents a unique concatenation of socioeconomic and mass psychological phenomena, which are closely related to... the way our education system has changed post-war; the rise of married female employment; the spread of television; the loss of physical exercise in adolescent boys due to urbanization; obesity; the feminization of schools; changing power structures in the nuclear family; lack of supervision due to working parents; the growing fear of the effects of failure of education, especially for boys, and so on.

Third, in decreeing that certain sectors of the normal range of young male behavior represent disease states, the institution of psychiatry has merely responded to secular expectations by "creating" a disease where none previously existed. As my six years in the Kimberley region of Western Australia proved, the genetic disease had not penetrated that admittedly backward part of the country, even as it was exploding out of control south of the Tropic of Capricorn. In a similar context, Eric Dean noted: "...the salient point is that the mental health professions have a track record of advancing diagnostic categories that lack clear underlying unity based on scientific evidence, but that, nonetheless, have the effect of responding to popular needs and aggrandizing the power and authority of mental health professionals" [4]. The drugs came first, a rare condition was found by the medical profession, parents came to believe in it, an industry involving psychiatrists, teachers, psychologists and under-employed pediatricians sprang to life and then, for a vast range of private and social reasons, the children started to behave in the way they thought everybody expected them to. If society expected unhappy, difficult, bored or dissatisfied children to become pale, anorexic, apathetic and withdrawn, then they would all take to their beds like phthisic poets. If it expected them to become possessed by a spirit that could only be exorcised by expensive gifts, then they would all show the features of Zar possession.

Fourth, the lack of scientific validity for the concept of ADHD has been sacrificed in favor of an entirely artificial diagnostic system that provides a spurious reliability if and only if the practitioner accepts without question the constructs from which it derives. The moment anybody questions any of the criteria, the whole concept falls apart. One either accepts it as beyond question, or there is no choice but to reject it out of hand. That is to say, it has one of the central definitions of a religion built into it: "Accept on faith this construct which we, the authorities have handed you or be cast out." I do not believe that anybody today could pass the examinations to be a psychiatrist in this or most English-speaking countries by denying the reality of ADHD. Psychiatry has become an ideology, not a science.

These are bold claims, so we should look at them a little more closely. I have repeatedly said that DSM established the separate categories of mental disorder by an entirely spurious process using two closely related ploys. First, the inclusion criteria for each disorder are not separate but are merely the same small number of features cleverly rewritten so that they seem different when they are not. Thus, I can put a person in the category of Avoidant Personality Disorder if I like or, using exactly the same item of behavior, slot him in the Schizoid Personality Disorder. Same phenomenon, he doesn't do anything different, but he gets a different label. I have already shown that anxiety and mania overlap at all significant points, even though their criteria seem different. It has been said that this was deliberate, that the purpose was to ensure that no disorders had criteria in common—but they do. Of course they do: the mere fact of setting out to change the very description of the features in question shows that they need changing, just because they can't otherwise be differentiated. Second, there were no exclusion criteria to distance the categories from each other (allowing that a category excludes a diagnosis is not an exclusion criterion as it presumes the existence of the categories that the criteria are supposed to establish).

Bearing this in mind, a proper analysis of the features of ADHD shows that it does not exist as a separate category. If we take the essential features of personality disorder, as per DSM-IV-TR, we find that ADHD matches them perfectly, i.e. they don't overlap, they actually overlay.

PARAMETER	ADHD	PERSONALITY DISORDER
Long term	+	+
Childhood onset	+	+
Family history	+	+
Friction with social surroundings	+	+
Failure to perform	+	+
Antisocial behavior	+	+
Drugs and alcohol	+	+
Inner distress	+	+

Fig. 16.1: ADHD vs. Personality Disorder (DSM-IV)

This says that the *career path* of ADHD is indistinguishable from the career path of personality disorder; it is then open to the psychiatrist to assign a person to either category as he sees fit. The allegedly objective process of assigning a diagnosis under the "decision tree" of DSM becomes a projective test of the psychiatrist's prejudices. When Mr. McK saw Prof. X, he wasn't handed a questionnaire on personality factors or on psychosomatic disorders, he was handed a questionnaire designed to elicit a particular condition. Unremarkably, that is the condition he showed. Entirely non-specific symptoms were converted into the (vague, value-laden) symptoms of ADHD by artful rewording and subtle realignments.

In the alternative, if we look more closely at the actual clinical features for ADHD, and not at the form or career path, we find that they are all found in personality disorders; not all of them occur in all personality disorders but they are all absolutely characteristic of personality disorder even if they are not specified in the diagnostic criteria for personality disorder (mainly because they are so common as to be entirely non-specific; no amount of rewording could have differentiated them).

The first group of diagnostic criteria, those relating to defects of attention, include failing to pay close attention to detail or making careless mistakes. That sounds like most personality disorders except the obsessional and the avoidant, who pays attention to detail in order to avoid leading a real life.

"Often has difficulty sustaining attention." That is just another way of saying the same thing, to give the impression that there is a large group of criteria when there is not, but it is still typical of most of the personality disorders. Watch a histrionic personality in action.

"Often doesn't seem to listen." For a start, I don't know any child who listens except when you don't want them to, but ask any army NCO if his charges listen and he will say they don't (I have always thought this criterion reflected more on the adult's need to control than a defect in the child, but we won't start that debate again). Ordinary children listen when what is being said interests them. If not, they don't. Perhaps teachers need to attend to their presentations.

"Doesn't follow through on instructions or finish jobs." Sounds like every disorganized, insecure or passive-obstructive personality disorder I've ever known.

"Difficulty organizing tasks." "Avoids tasks that require sustained mental activity." "Loses things." "Easily distracted." "Forgetful." These are absolutely classic features of personality disorder. Granted, they are not regarded as diagnostic criteria but they are part and parcel of the concept of a physically healthy person who isn't mentally ill, isn't intellectually handicapped, knows the social rules and culture and the language and still makes a mess of everything. That is, they describe a person who should be able to function but never quite seems to make it. That is what is meant by "personality disorder," that's what personality disorder *is*.

The rest of the criteria are so widespread that we can't even use them to nominate personality disorders:

"Often fidgets or squirms." This can indicate boredom, a wide range of anxiety conditions and some, but not all, personality disorders.

"Jumps up and down." This is completely non-specific. In Aboriginal children, it is so normal that if a child didn't jump up and down, we would take his or her temperature. I could point out that, back in the Dark Ages when I was at school in classes of 48 children in huge, draughty classrooms with hard wooden benches, no child jumped up and down. Teachers had canes.

"Runs around or feels restless." All males run around. It is part of the species. If they don't run around, they get fat and feel miserable. I once went to a deserted beach at Bali to watch the sun set. As it lowered toward the sea, small groups of teenage boys and young men began walking down to the beach, then a football appeared, then more young men, then more footballs until the entire beach was crowded with several thousand healthy, happy, handsome Balinese boys playing football, shouting and laughing, running around until the sweat poured down their bare chests. As the sun set and the light faded, the process reversed until, by darkness, I was once again alone on the beach. Those young men were not hyperactive, they were normal. Those who were not playing were abnormal. Actually, I forgot to watch the sunset but who cares, we have good sunsets here. Also, in my school days, we either walked a mile or two to school or rode our push-bikes. At breaks and lunchtime, we ran around and played games. In between bouts of exercise, we had no trouble sitting in our seats for 75 minutes at a time. After school, we walked or rode home, then we played outside until the evening meal was ready. We were not allowed inside until we were called but who would want to go inside, anyway?

"Difficulty playing quietly." Girls (some) may play quietly but boys don't. It is not natural for them.

"On the go, driven by a motor." Same as "Runs around or feels restless," it artificially inflates the score and allows a teacher who doesn't like a boy to give him a bad mark.

"Talks a lot." Who doesn't? Ever seen an academic or a politician who knew when to stop?

"Often blurts out answers before question is finished." This is precisely the sort of behavior that Skinnerian token reinforcement schedules were designed to eliminate, and they did, very effectively. However, token economies take a lot of effort from the teacher; far easier to have the children drugged instead.

"Doesn't wait his turn." When I was at school, if we pushed or shoved or didn't wait our turn, we went to the back of the queue. Teachers watched like hawks and enforced rules consistently. They did not wander around the back of the playground, drinking coffee and talking distractedly on their mobile phones to their divorce lawyers. Teaching is hard work, I don't know anybody who has tried it who disagrees. I like teaching but I also find it exhausting. Easier to hand out pills.

"Often butts in." Do we want our children to be active and involved and excited, or do we want them to be solitary little class potatoes, too frightened to say boo?

When we see the paintings and photographs of upper class children from the nineteenth century, we laugh at the way they are depicted as small adults. They don't seem like children at all. When we complain that children don't sit quietly at their desks and refrain from speaking to each other, don't listen closely to what is said, answering when told to and only the question asked, don't wait for each other to speak in turn, can't wait until the breaks to go to the toilet and are forever losing things and forgetting things, we are making exactly the same mistake, but on a behavioral level. We are criticizing children because they are not small adults. Children are not just "little adults." Anyway, has anybody ever watched parliament in action? It's like watching feeding time in the baboon cage.

We pride ourselves on no longer using corporal punishment to ensure compliance in our schools; instead, we drug our children to achieve the same end.

These diagnostic criteria are all seen in normal children and adolescents as well as in more extreme form in personality disorders. From the way the diagnosis of ADHD varies according to the child's address, we know that the labeling process is essentially random. We now know that the chances of getting a diagnosis of ADHD vary according to the child's date of birth. Children whose birthdays fall in the earliest part of the academic year (i.e. the older children in the class) are much less likely to acquire the diagnosis than children born late in the year (i.e. the younger group). That is, the symptoms of ADHD fade with the passage of time, otherwise known as the normal process of maturation [5]. A huge and long-term study from British Columbia looked at 937,943 children who were between six and twelve years of age at any time between December 1st 1997 and November 30th 2008. This compared the child's month of birth with the risks of acquiring the diagnosis of ADHD and of being treated with stimulants, for boys and for girls. Methodologically, the study appears very sound.

The researchers found that the risk of the diagnosis for boys born in December, the last month of the academic year, was 30% higher than for boys born in January, while for girls, the increase in risk was an astounding 70%. This means that children born in the month of December were at much greater risk of having a genetic illness than children who dragged their feet and arrived in January. Similarly, the risk of being prescribed stimulants was 41% higher for December boys while, for girls, the increase in risk was a completely improbable 77%. In boys, the rates of diagnosis and prescription were approximately three times those in girls. Boys, of course, are physically more active than girls and verbally less proficient until well into adulthood, differences which are never entirely obliterated in the community.

The calendar has a baleful influence on children's genes, as does geography: cross the border into another suburb, or county, or state or country and the figures gyrate wildly. It is considered an epidemic in the US, Canada, the UK and Australia but, with few exceptions, it is simply not recognized in France [6] (here's an interesting thought: what about French Canadian children?). To illustrate how geography affects health, when I worked in the Kimberley region in WA, deliveries by caesarian section were quite common. The young Aboriginal women often did not attend their antenatal visits and so they would present in labor with PET, anemia, untreated diabetes or renal disease, pelvic difficulties and fetal distress. As a group, and not for lack of devoted effort by the isolated nurses, they had the worst maternal health in the country. However, at the same time, the caesarian rates in the wealthy eastern suburbs of Sydney, a city larger than Chicago or Berlin, were almost twice what they were in the Kimberley. That is, very fit and healthy, wealthy and educated women in upper class suburbs, with the finest of antenatal care, needed twice as many surgical interventions as their poor, illiterate, sickly black sisters living in shanties in the bush. I don't believe it. Since Medicare paid for each operation, it represents at the very least a gross misallocation of resources, especially as the surgeons in Sydney were paid far more than the surgeon in the Kimberley.

When figures like that are seen, or the rate of prescription of toxic drugs for children rises 2300% in eleven years, we medical practitioners have failed in our professional duty. The reason psychiatrists have failed is because we have not articulated a formal model of mental disorder to guide our daily practice, our teaching and our research, thereby allowing ideologues and adventurers to set the pace and direction of medical practice.

16.5 Adult ADHD as a Personality Disorder

Perhaps I am making too much of this, maybe childhood syndromes are difficult to isolate and the various DSM committees have done the best they could under demanding circumstances. Yes, that may be the case, so perhaps we may even have to wait until adulthood before making the definitive diagnosis. But DSM-IV doesn't recognize adult ADHD, even though very large numbers of men are now prescribed stimulants for just this diagnosis. Indeed, after 2006, when Major League Baseball banned players from using stimulants prior to games, the incidence of diagnosis of Adult ADHD among league players soared to 8% by 2009, twice the average for children and far more than the incidence of childhood ADHD among the same players. Compliant doctors were responding to pressures to provide a medical cover for a social demand.

Since DSM does not allow a diagnosis of adult ADHD, we can only use the unofficial formulae as they are used in the community. A popular website maintained by WebMD [7] lists ten criteria after a warning that Adult ADHD is itself an "enduring pattern of deviance": "Unlike other psychiatric disorders, including anxiety and depression, ADHD doesn't begin in adulthood. So symptoms must have been present since childhood for a diagnosis of adult ADHD to be made."

Their criteria are as follows: Difficulty getting organized; reckless driving and traffic accidents; marital difficulties; extreme distractibility; poor listening skills; restless and difficulty relaxing; difficulty starting tasks; chronic lateness; angry outbursts; and difficulty prioritizing matters.

These do not distinguish between an alleged primary disorder of brain function and the large group of personality disorders. In fact, three of them (reckless driving and traffic accidents; marital difficulties; angry outbursts) practically amount to an operational definition of personality disorder. Others have no biological connection: chronic lateness has nothing to do with angry outbursts, nor does difficulty starting tasks relate to marital problems (Orwell's "sausage and a rose, their purposes hardly intersect"). They simply cluster together because they are results of the same prior cause, a personality disorder. The term "extreme distractibility" is absurd. The word "extreme" means "at the limits of human experience, the point beyond which there is no return." It does not mean rather, somewhat, a fair bit, quite often or such like; people who use this expression have clearly never seen a case of "extreme distractibility."

To confirm this gloomy opinion, we can look at the group of general diagnostic criteria in DSM-IV-TR for personality disorder. The "enduring pattern of deviance" is manifest in two of four areas:

- Cognition (ways of perceiving and interpreting self, others and events);
- Affectivity (range, intensity, lability and appropriateness);
- Interpersonal functioning;
- Impulse control.

Each of these is either stated or implied in the list of criteria for Adult ADHD given above. I say that if an adult shows the ten criteria for Adult ADHD listed above as "an enduring pattern of inner experience and behavior that deviates markedly from the expectations of the individual's culture..." then that is *ipso facto* personality disorder. It is *not* an illness in any sense of the word. The problem for the advocates of the new illness of Adult ADHD is that they cannot prove my claim wrong. They are not able to show that their syndrome is *not* just a case of personality disorder. They cannot prove, for example, that "angry outbursts" are not a clear example of affective disturbance when assessed against the criterion of "range, intensity, lability and appropriateness" for personality disorders. They can say "We think you are wrong" or "We feel you are looking at it the wrong way" or something similar but of proof, they have none. There is none.

However, any minor quibbles against the concept of Adult ADHD by naysayers such as my unworthy self are eliminated when we turn to a website called Helpguide, a site jointly produced by a non-profit organization with Harvard Medical School [8]. This wins hands down. To ease the passage of any unwilling adults to their new state of illness, this site helpfully explains:

> "ADD/ADHD looks very much like a willpower problem, but it isn't. It's essentially a chemical problem in the management systems of the brain... A person with ADD/ADHD is six times more likely to have another psychiatric or learning disorder than most other people. ADD/ADHD usually overlaps with other disorders... Many adults struggle all their lives with unrecognized ADD/ADHD impairments. They haven't received help because they assumed that their chronic difficulties, like depression or anxiety, were caused by other impairments that did not respond to usual treatment... In adults, attention deficit disorder often looks quite different than it does in children—and its symptoms are unique for each individual."

The unwarranted claims in these few lines are astounding: it is a matter of public knowledge that Harvard Medical School does not know enough about the brain to say anything about a "chemical problem in the management systems of the brain." Their claim is without scientific warrant, i.e. they were using their prestige to compel acceptance of an assertion for which they had no factual evidence. The fact that the symptoms of ADHD also occur in many other conditions confirms my assertion that they are unique only by virtue of sly rewording of the descriptions. If ADHD "usually overlaps with other disorders," then the most parsimonious explanation is that it is part of those other disorders, and not a separate disorder *sui generis*. But the most remarkable assertion is the last: that the symptoms of Adult ADHD are "unique for each individual." This means the symptoms are whatever you want them to be, so nobody who makes the diagnosis can be proven wrong. This is from a center which claims to be a "key opinion leader" in the development of a modern science of psychiatry.

My goal in this section is to show that the diagnosis of personality disorder is no longer being made, but the patients are being wrongly diagnosed as suffering mental illnesses. They are then prescribed drugs, either stimulants or antidepressants, which are known to lead to severe disturbances of mood. These unstable moods, the result of an unknown combination of the drug and the personality disorder, are then wrongly classified as BAD. As soon as they are given this diagnosis, patients are prescribed very large doses of major drugs which have serious side effects on brain function, so they become permanently mentally ill and require intensive social support in the long term. I have not proven that case, because the evidence that would constitute proof can only be obtained by a very large-scale research project. However, if this claim is correct, then the risks are so great that it has to be given credibility, just as the claims of impending financial destruction were not given credibility prior to the global financial crisis.

16.6 ADHD as a Manifestation of Anxious Personality Disorder

If, as I claim, ADHD does not exist but is simply a case of self-interested slicing and dicing of the limited number of mental symptoms, then what is generating those symptoms? As I have described above, a lot of them are not, in fact, symptoms, they are variants of normal—or normal behavior which society no longer chooses to countenance. That still leaves a significant bunch of behaviors requiring explanation. Calling them personality disorder tells us how to approach them but it doesn't say much about their causation. For example, temper outbursts can have any one of dozens of causes, or dozens in the same person at different times. I will state that most of the actual symptoms of so-called ADHD, child and adult variants, are caused by anxiety. I fully appreciate that, because of their prior commitments, many psychiatrists will not agree, so the issue will not be settled in what remains of this chapter.

The symptoms of ADHD are, almost without exception, also extremely common in anxiety. We can see this in a side-to-side comparison of the DSM criteria for ADHD:

PARAMETER	ADHD	ANXIETY
Poor attention to detail	+	+
Makes silly mistakes	+	+
Attention not sustained	+	+
Doesn't seem to listen	+	+
Fails to complete instructions	+	+
Can't get organized	+	+
Avoids prolonged tasks	+	+

Loses things	+	+
Easily distracted	+	+
Fidgets and squirms	+	+
Gets up and down	+	+
Over-active, restless	+	+
Excessive noise	+	+
Can't settle	+	+
May talk a lot	+	+
Talks impulsively	+	+
Can't wait turn to talk	+	+
Interrupts or intrudes	+	+

Fig. 16.2: ADHD vs. Anxiety (DSM-IV)

People may object on the basis that not all of the symptoms listed above appear in the section on anxiety in DSM-IV. This is true; as any clinician knows, there are very many symptoms of anxiety that do not appear in the section on anxiety in DSM-IV. Others may object, saying: "My son doesn't look anxious," or "My husband doesn't complain of anxiety." That is also true. Firstly, as DSM-IV acknowledges, children don't have to look anxious or complain of anxiety before we accept that they are anxious. Second, adults generally don't like acknowledging anxiety, as the case history above shows. It was clear Mr. McK had mild social anxiety; he wasn't good "one-to-one" but, put a cricket bat in his hand or give him a pointer in a lecture theater and his mild sense of somehow not quite measuring up ("I know it sounds bad, but I never made a bed or even picked up my clothes in my life") could be kept under control. I had picked him as a mummy's boy and I was right: he had very little sexual experience for a man of his age and station in life. He was too shy but, as is so common, he initially denied being shy. Men see anxiety as a moral failing and will do practically anything to avoid admitting it. So he used drugs that are renowned for relieving anxiety. Touting a genetic defect is a vast improvement over saying "I'm weak, women make me nervous."

Third, and most significantly, DSM does not recognize the concept of an anxious personality, so this requires a digression.

16.7 Can There Be a Biological Disease Called Anxiety?

For orthodox psychiatry, all anxiety is a medical illness; it is an Axis I diagnosis, along with depression and schizophrenia, and *ipso facto* is classed as another chemical imbalance of the brain with a genetic basis. In the broader context, this claim is unsustainable. Anxiety is a reaction to life events; it has the very clearest parallels in the animal world (no suggestion of using knock-out mice to get an animal model of anxiety, just let normal mice see the lab's pet cat) and it has the very clearest, most minutely-detailed and substantiated role to play in survival of the species. There is absolutely no precedent in western science for claiming that something which is both universal and has the same role in every other species known to man suddenly jumps to being a disease in humans. On this basis, we would have a much stronger case for saying that speech, laughter, self-decoration, art, tool-making and (especially) organized warfare are diseases. Anxiety is a normal part of all life on the planet. It becomes a problem for *H. sapiens* only if it is experienced too often or too intensely for the social setting. Crucially, social settings change, from place to place, context to context and from one generation to the next.

In the animal world, under normal circumstances, organisms are not anxious. Being anxious is biologically very expensive, so the anxiety (fight or flight) reaction is not switched on unless it is required. However, its switch is biased toward over-reacting rather than under-reacting: animals survive by their wits, by their alertness and responsivity to the environment. So how is this generic alarm system switched on? By a variety of direct stimuli. The sheep becomes anxious when she smells a dog. The cow does not become anxious while she can smell her calf, but if she cannot, she calls; if it doesn't respond, she panics. The hatchling freezes at the sight of a snake, and so on, but humans are different. We can switch on our fight or flight reaction without a direct stimulus. We can panic if we think we have left the gas on or about a coming job interview. We can fear stimuli that are ten times removed from the original feared object: we can panic over the very *thought* that we may panic. That is, activity in the cognitive system can feed directly into whatever circuits subserve anxiety.

This is where we fall into the trap Kuhn described so well: people do not see the same events, just because of their mental sets. Thus, a biological psychiatrist looking at a panicky patient does not see a naked ape who has accidentally switched on his fight or flight reaction, he sees a case of brain disease, same as if he were looking at a case of Parkinson's Disease or of Huntington's Chorea. The problem is, people who believe reductionist biologism is the correct model of mental disorder also don't believe in mental sets. I don't have a survey to prove this but, from long experience, they believe that mental sets are what other people have whereas they, being superior types of fellows, are inherently objective and therefore incapable of bias. It then follows that anybody who challenges them is *ipso facto* acting immaturely, mischievously or maliciously, the exact reason depending on which of their prejudices is on top that day. Oh, and they also don't have prejudices, which makes it difficult to argue with them because if you show they are acting in a prejudiced manner, they get angry and stamp off: the difference, you could say between Dr. Insel's "constructive criticism" (meaning, what he is prepared to accept, i.e. anything that matches his prejudices) and the rest.

Late in life, the great Lord Lister said: "I remember at an early period of my own life showing to a man of high reputation as a teacher some matters which I happened to have observed. And I was very much struck and grieved to find that, while all the facts lay equally clear before him, only those that squared with his previous theories seemed to affect his organs of vision" [9]. Or, as Gene Simmons said, "Life is far too short to hold anything but delusional notions about yourself."

The model being developed in these chapters is essentially cognitive. It says that the cognitive contents, meaning what we think and believe, including implicit beliefs, are causally effective in determining our behavior, often in ways we don't understand. This is not exactly a revelation; the idea of unconscious causation has been around forever. But unconscious does not mean 'biological.' It means 'of the cognitive realm but not able to be expressed verbally.' In cognitive speak, it means the clusters of rules that together form the basis of our habitual modes of interaction, i.e. the rules that generate what DSM-IV calls "the enduring pattern of inner experience and behavior." When this pattern of behavior "...deviates markedly from the expectations of the individual's culture," it does not mean that the causation has suddenly switched from quotidian ideas to disease states, it may only mean the cultural context has changed. My case is that the biological approach to human mental function explains nothing, that 2+2=4 is to be understood in its semantic context, not in the context of an analysis of the genome. The relationship of mind and brain is metaphysical in nature, meaning it is not the sort of question that can be answered by empirical evidence. As the following quote shows, reductionists keep claiming that biology will somehow explain the relationship between mind and brain:

> "The connections between physical and mental health have never been clearer theoretically... Moreover, we are just beginning to formulate integrated mind–brain models that incorporate both the genotype and its expression in hierarchical and complex phenotypes of the brain, and the bilaterally causal interactions between brain phenotypes and the physical and social environments... This is just one example of neuroscience driving progress in understanding of psychiatric disease, from erroneous dogmatism to a gradually consolidating empiricism... In short, we are lucky enough to be living at the start of a golden age for neuroscientific discovery in relation to psychiatry and there has never been a better time for psychiatrists to pursue physical models of the mind and mental disorders " [10].

These claims are false: "Against dogma disguised as science, objectivity fails" [11]. This group does not have anything approximating an "integrated mind-brain model" that can explain any kind of relationship between the genotype, phenotype and "the physical and social environments." The only "erroneous dogmatism" standing in the way of a theoretical understanding of the mind-brain interactions that produce mental disorder is the blind and baseless conviction that "a gradually consolidating empiricism" can answer questions of a metaphysical nature. Biological psychiatrists are now the major obstruction in the path to a "golden age of discovery in psychiatry." For example, their model cannot explain human anxiety. They can only look at the suffering patient and say "Chemical imbalance of the brain." Scans may say the man is frightened, they may eventually say (but I don't believe it) what frightens him, but the one thing they can't say is why he is frightened. There can be no treatment of a damaging idea apart from a better idea.

So can there be a biological disease called anxiety? No, there cannot. Do we need it, is there anything about anxiety that "erroneous dogmatism" (usually called psychology) cannot explain more succinctly and with greater heuristic power? No, there is not. Do we need to invoke an unprovable entity called "chemical imbalances of the brain" to explain a context-dependent variant of normality? No, we do not.

16.8 Can There Be a Cognitive Explanation of Anxiety?

The cognitive model looks at the same anxious person and sees, not a festering heap of neurotransmitters firing erratically, but a brain in the peak of condition. Agreed, its owner doesn't feel too flash, as they say, but the brain is fine, nothing wrong with it. There is no reason to try the hack and slash of Freeman's transorbital antemortem dissection, nor any reason to believe flooding his brain with chemicals that affect *every* synapse will influence just the ones we want and no others. There is, however, very good reason to believe that some mental factor is inadvertently activating his fight or flight reaction for *no good reason*, just as it does in you and me for good reasons. He has simply misclassified an event as threatening, and his mind-body continuum is reacting perfectly appropriately to the signals it is receiving.

Now, in terms of final causes, or goals, that is an explanation. It is not, of course, an explanation in terms of efficient causes, meaning the mechanism by which a goal is achieved. If a man kicks a ball between two upright posts, we can explain his action at two levels. The first is the physical machinery of brain, body, leg etc., of how he stays upright, how his eye detected the white ball against the green of grass, how instructions went from his motor cortex via the pyramidal tract and all the olivopontine influences thereon, out through his anterior horn cells to the motor end plate, why his muscles twitched and, because of his cholinesterase levels, did not go into spasm ("Footballer carried off with leg in air") and so on. I am in total agreement that the whole of this is vastly fascinating, a source of wonder and delight that I am alive now and not a hundred years ago when none of it was known, but there is more to a game of football than biology. There is another level of explanation that is not open to biological investigation.

There is nothing about his motor endplates or his inferior olive that can explain why he was running around a windswept field on an icy Saturday afternoon, and why he kicked the ball through that goal and not the other, or why he did not pick up the ball and run with it (different football code) and so on. This is the doctrine of final causes, the notion that mere mechanism is not enough, that an explanation of how a leg kicks a football is not also an explanation of why it bothered. There are always two levels of explanation, the physiological as well as the psychological notion of a game, so there are perforce two questions of "Why?" We cannot explain a game of football without invoking explanations at both levels; one or the other alone is inadequate. At the same time, a single answer cannot satisfy questions on two levels of causation. It is the same as language theory: we cannot nominate an entity and define it in a single illocutionary act.

If we go back to the anxious man, there are two levels of explanation. In the first place, we need to know what is the *mechanism* of anxiety (the same as we share with chimps and probably a lot of other animals), which we expect the neurosciences to tell us, but we also need to know what *ideas* this frightened man has that are activating his anxiety systems. "Why is he anxious?" is not the same question as "How is he anxious?" Consider Mr. McK again. He was not anxious at sport so, if he had a biochemical disease called anxiety, why did it switch off when he walked onto the sports field? There is no biological answer, but there is a psychological answer. He played calmly and confidently because he *knew* full well that he was perfectly capable, that he *understood* the rules and did not *doubt* that he had the physical prowess and experience to perform. He also *knew* it didn't matter if he failed to perform. He *had no doubt* his team mates would *know* he had tried his best but he just had a bad day, same as could happen to them. That is, as he *knew* failure was unlikely and there were no great consequences to failure, his mind generated no anxiety. Knowing is irreducibly a psychological event. However, his experience of work was quite different from sport. He knew he had the intellectual ability, he knew he had the technical training and experience to achieve his goals but the consequences of failure were now enormous. Therefore, he was always a little edgy at work, always a little apprehensive and concerned, watching his colleagues' faces for the first signs of disinterest or disapproval, and he found this sense of constant mild apprehension wearing. Not devastating, just tiring.

His social life, however, was a very different matter. He did *not* know if he could perform, he did *not* know if he could satisfy the demands of an autonomous person. Sure, he had always known that whatever he did in life was immensely satisfying to his parents and other relatives but that was no precedent for the greatest challenge still before him, to attract and retain a mate. And knowing of this gap in his knowledge base did cause anxiety. That is, he did not know what he could do, he did not know if he had the ability, and the consequences of failure were potentially catastrophic. This caused quite immense anxiety and, just to close the anxiety trap that controlled his inner, unseen life, he couldn't tell anybody, he had to hide it all the time. He could not tell his drunken mates after the game that no, he wouldn't be chatting up that chick to try and get his leg over because he was scared she would look at him and, with a faint, derisive smile, turn back to the bigger, tougher man who had his hairy arm around her. So he shuffled his feet and made some excuse about going to the toilet but he left the rowdy party and went home, humiliated. Next morning, when his mother said to him: "You came home early last night, dear, what happened, didn't you have a good time?" he smiled agreeably and said he was tired after the game. He was unable to say to her, "No, mummy, I was scared I wouldn't be able to keep it up."

This constitutes a complete explanation of his anxiety, but it is not a matter requiring an explanation in terms of efficient causes. It is a psychological or final explanation but not a biological or efficient explanation because there was no biological failure; we do not need any blood tests to explain this one. I knew, just by looking at him, that there was absolutely nothing wrong with him physically. We cannot start the process once more of trying to find a biological cause for his psychological fear of sexual failure (because chimps don't actually suffer it, *pace* Harry Harlow) or for his reluctance to admit to his mother his fear of sexual failure. Each answer will incorporate yet another psychological explanation, which will then start the cycle again, *ad infinitum*. There is no explanation in terms of efficient (biological) causes that will answer a question phrased in terms of final (psychological) causes. Any attempt to provide such an explanation will inevitably lead to an infinite regress, and infinite regresses lie outside the boundaries of science.

In this young man's case, as in all other mildly anxious young men (it is actually very common), the only reason he would not be able to maintain an erection was fear. The reason his body would not function naturally is because anxiety is powerfully inhibitory of male sexual function (it's not good for female function either). This is true even when the cause of the anxiety is fear of sexual failure itself, as in: He fears sexual failure, but the only time he fails sexually is when he is fearful. The psychological account closes the explanatory gap that biology can never fill. *QED.*

Therefore, the biological program to find "a golden age for neuroscientific discovery in relation to psychiatry... to pursue physical models of the mind and mental disorders" is not a scientific program. It is scientism, the inappropriate application of scientific methods and principles designed to answer questions of an empirical nature to questions of a metaphysical nature or questions with no empirical content. In fact, it is a fantasy, driven by the need to find a single, simple cause for a complex matter so that it can be related to a genetic defect that hasn't yet been found and for which there is not a skerrick of evidence.

What Mr. McK had found was that amphetamines allowed him to function without anxiety. They didn't actually change his performance but they changed his perception of his performance, the bit that counts, because now he remembered: "Hey, I did that PowerPoint presentation like a pro, it went real smooth, the other guys seemed pretty pleased." In all probability, he did perform better as anxiety is a major inhibitor of performance, but he didn't tell his audience anything he didn't already know or make any major discoveries, he just felt better while he was doing it. The drugs "enhanced his lifestyle" in his delicate understatement. Socially, of course, they did make a difference, he felt a lot better walking into parties and was able to talk to people without having to gulp down three or four beers in a hurry. Did it help him get his leg over? I never found that out, but experience of many, many amphetamines abusers says that it doesn't, they just feel better about being failures. Being a failure is no longer a cause of anxiety as the anxiety circuits are blocked. The behavior doesn't change much, only the recollection.

These are explanations at the level of final causes. They are explanations, in the sense that we can now explain why Pres. Bush went to war in Iraq to eliminate weapons of mass destruction. We could offer one level of explanation in terms of his brain circuits and his testosterone levels and hypothalamo-pituitary-adrenal axis and perhaps even his conditioning as a toddler but none of those answers would impinge upon the semantic field in which the question "Why?" is embedded. Imagine if somebody had said to him at the time: "Mr. President, all your talk about preserving peace and bringing freedom to the downtrodden Iraqi people and upholding the dignity of the American flag is a load of tosh. We know that you are only acting as a biological preparation, a festering stew of neurotransmitters with as much insight as a cane toad in the breeding season, because the only explanations that count in human affairs are set at the level of activation of *KoD1* on the third chromosome, so if you'd just take more of the blue tablets which block just that gene, you'll find the fog of what seem like patriotic impulses will fade and you will stop seeing yourself as a Johnny-come-lately messiah."

If anybody had said that (if only), then what would Mr. Bush have said in reply? We know the answer to this question. "My dear Mr. Eliminative Materialist," he would have said, "you know as well as I that an explanation in biological terms does not satisfy a question phrased in terms of human goals and aspirations. Yes, the flow of testosterone as I proclaim the inevitable victory (What, Karl? OK, book a carrier for it) that will be good fun, as good as the old heave-ho but at my age, I get all I want by watching PowerBall on Saturday nights anyway. No, I am doing it because I believe that this country stands for something and dogs like Saddam should not be allowed to cock their legs on the principles in our Declaration of Human Rights (what, Karl? Are you sure?) OK, the US Constitution, just because it is honorable, and any attempt to answer questions of honor with statements of biology will raise another question of values which you will then try to answer in biological terms, and so on until the end of time, but I do not propose to give that slimy wog (what, Karl? Can't I? Why not?) OK, him, until the end of time to back off. I would dearly like the fog of patriotism to fade because it gets in the way of important decisions but your tablets will also stop those important decisions by turning me into an even bigger cabbage so I'll pass on them, thanks."

If we look at that particular UN Declaration, dating from 1948, we see something important. It says:

> "Whereas disregard and contempt for human rights have resulted in barbarous acts which have outraged the conscience of mankind, and the advent of a world in which human beings shall enjoy freedom of speech and belief and freedom from fear and want has been proclaimed as the highest aspiration of the common people..."

Let us try to explain this in biological terms. We can, I believe, readily account for the "disregard and contempt for human rights" in terms of the primate dispositions to territoriality, xenophobia and hierarchical societies. These are crude, unreasoning impulses driven by our genetic heritage but, to our misfortune, they readily take control of our affairs even while we think we are being perfectly rational. The "barbarous acts" I think are directly in line with our origins as foot soldiers in the battle for survival. I don't believe we have to invoke any abstruse mentalist notions to account for those parts of our behavior, any more than we need invoke angels to explain flatus. Where biology does start to seem inadequate is when we try to work out a biological account of the concept of contempt. Do apes hold other tribes of apes in contempt? I don't believe they do. I think the evidence is that they can only be frightened of them, or angry toward them, or indifferent. But move on, let's not stop at the first hurdle. What about human rights? Or just plain conscience? What is that in biological terms? Don't forget that the answer must not confuse the biological mechanism of a belief (that which underwrites the generic class of all beliefs) with the informational content of a particular belief. I think the explanation will not be able to get beyond proposing another value, which will then need explanation, and so on. We cannot write the psychology out of a belief by appealing to biology. All we do is invoke another belief.

However, if we propose a cognitive account of conscience, it will say something like this: "Conscience is a set of rules governing behavior whose purpose is to facilitate groups of people living together in harmony because we know our propensity for intraspecific violence and we believe it needs to be controlled in the interests of our long-term survival, to which end we agree to restrict certain sorts of behavior by an innate sense of guilt and lack of self-worth if those rules are broken, bolstered by the ultimate threat of intraspecific violence." That is, it keeps giving psychological goals until they start to go in circles and we then know there is nothing further to be explained. The circle has been closed, and the final link is just this: This we *believe*. After that psychological endpoint, there is no further discussion because none is needed, unlike the attempted biological explanation in which the discussion never stops. Explanation in psychological terms is brought to an end by a psychological term whereas explanation in biological terms has no end.

My conclusion is that, not only can there be a legitimate explanation of anxiety in psychological terms, but there cannot be a legitimate explanation of anxiety in non-psychological terms. This positively precludes the concept of a biological basis for anxiety disorders. There is now only one step left in this tedious process of drawing a direct causative line between anxiety and a diagnosis of ADHD, the concept of an anxious personality.

16.9 The Concept of an Anxious Personality

We do not have much left to do. The symptoms of ADHD, when they aren't just pseudo-symptoms (i.e. normal but socially undesirable behavior, such as prime ministers picking their noses in public or princes or presidents having affairs), cannot reliably be distinguished from, on the one hand, personality disorder or, on the other, anxiety. Can we meld anxiety and personality disorder to come up with something that will bring joy to the hearts of the splitters of DSM, a new diagnosis? We can and, to this end, I propose a new (actually very old) concept of the Anxious Personality Disorder. This is not a disease so it goes on Axis II, not on Axis I, and it therefore doesn't need to be treated with lots of drugs designed for mental diseases, such as antidepressants and so on, because we all know they don't work on personality. We can start to construct this new diagnosis by answering a series of questions.

Q: What is anxiety?

A: Anxiety is the response of a healthy intact organism to the perception of a threat. It is a normal biological reaction to events in the environment and must never be confused with disease states. The role of anxiety is to prepare us to deal with the threat, either by fighting or by running (or by freezing, or playing dead, or squirting ink or smells or displaying big teeth, etc). It is an immensely complicated, total body reaction strongly mediated by catecholamines, both cerebral and systemic. It is feasible that a flight response is converted into a fight response by the intermediation of the testosterone system.

Q: What is personality?

A: Personality is the totality of the rules that generate our modes of interacting with the environment. Because we want personality to reflect predictive differences (we assign behavioral similarities to the class of cultural imperatives), we narrow this definition to read: The totality of the rules, explicit and implicit, that generate the distinctive, recurrent or habitual patterns in the stable, adult mode of behavior.

Q: What is personality disorder?

A: When the total set of rules, explicit and implicit, that generate the distinctive, recurrent or habitual patterns in the stable, adult mode of behavior are inconsistent with the social rules, thereby bringing the individual into repeated conflict with the social environment, or they are internally contradictory such that they generate discomforting or disabling emotions, then we say this person has a personality disorder. There is no suggestion, real or implied, that the final cause, meaning the individual's set of goals and his rules to achieve them, is insufficient to account for the phenomena of personality disorder in their entirety. This means that no biological explanation of personality disorder is necessary as the brain is entirely normal.

By definition, therefore, an anxious personality just is a set of rules, explicit and implicit, that compels the individual to react to neutral events in the environment as though they were a threat. He sees danger where his peers do not, meaning the danger is private, it exists in his mind only, *but* it is as real to him as a genuine (agreed, primitive) threat would be to his peers.

Next question: How can anybody be so silly as to believe that a frog can be a threat that needs the same (expensive, exhausting) biological response as a crocodile coming straight at you?

Answer: The frog phobic person is not scared of the frog, he is scared of how he will feel if he goes near a frog. He is making a prediction: If I go near a frog, I will feel bad; the thought of feeling bad terrifies me, and terror just is the bad feeling I will experience. So the explanatory loop is closed. The cognitive explanation of a neurosis cannot go into an infinite regress because it automatically closes itself in a vicious circle (a vicious circle is not an infinite regress as vicious circles always end, one unhappy way or another). This is the concept of self-perpetuating and self-reinforcing instability, the same as can bring down a mighty bridge in a breeze [12] or cause an aircraft to shake to bits from trying to go too fast. We need to compare self-maintaining normality (homeostasis) vs. self-perpetuating abnormality. The vicious circle is the crucial intellectual concept that allows us to incorporate the unthinkable. Just as Pythagoras said "give me a fulcrum and I will move the world," so the idea of a tiny error being amplified and magnified by feedback until it brings the whole edifice crashing down is no longer outlandish.

We now have a generic explanation for an anxious personality disorder. An anxious personality is a person whose set of rules consistently sets up vicious circles of anxiety where the act of making a prediction of feeling frightened produces the sense of fear or the physical effects of fear that the person did not want, thereby amplifying his fear. Remember that if the normal anxiety response did not produce somatic effects, then there would be no way for a cognitive loop to be established whereby the prediction produced the feared response. However, because the anxiety response works so fast, the anxious person misses the essential cognitive connection between his mental prediction and his body's response. Why does it act so fast and outside conscious awareness? (1) Silly question: think evolution. (2) The intervening steps are not open to introspection just because that is how the brain works to produce fast responses. This concept is therapeutically vital.

Examples:

Psychogenic male impotence: Rule: I must perform as a man. Consequence of rule: If I am not manly, I will be intensely humiliated. The thought of being intensely humiliated frightens me. Being frightened inhibits my sexual function. Because my sexual performance is being inhibited, I feel even more frightened. Female version: This is going to hurt. I am frightened of being hurt. Fear of being hurt is inhibiting the sexual arousal I need in order not to be hurt.

Hypochondriasis: Rule: I am terrified of death. Consequence of rule: Every variation from physiological normality might mean a dangerous disease. The idea of having a dangerous disease is itself a frightening idea. Having a frightening idea knocking around in my head produces anxiety. Anxiety produces variations in physiological normality. Because my inner normality is being perturbed by a frightening idea, I detect variations in physiological normality and so I feel even more frightened. Because the doctor said there is nothing wrong with me, I do not trust him, he is probably lying to me, which proves he has something to hide, probably a cancer he wants to experiment on so I need to see another doctor for more tests. But I can't afford more tests so the cancer will keep growing and I will die. The thought of impending death terrifies me, and further perturbs my physiology.

Note that the reasoning does not take place in steps as I have set them out, any more than a person running to catch a ball is 'saying' to himself: Take six steps to north-east, then turn and face ball, extend right hand exactly 80cm to 10 o'clock, extend fingers, grasp when ball hits palm... Etc. The mind works quickly. Very often, we don't even know what the intervening steps are, as in: "What was funny about that?" "I don't know, it just was very funny." Every physician has said to a patient: "There's nothing to worry about," only to be told: "Oh, Dr, are you sure? I'm so frightened, I think I need more tests."

Social phobia: Rule: I must appear calm and sensible. Justification for rule: Nobody likes a person who is not calm and sensible. Basis of rule: I want to be liked. Consequence of rule: If I remain calm, I will be liked. Therefore I must always keep myself under control. The thought that I may not be under control frightens me. If I am frightened, I start to lose control. Losing control will lead to ostracism. The very idea of ostracism terrifies me. If I have a terrifying idea in my head, I will start to shake and sweat and stammer. The mere thought that the nice people I have to meet will see I am shaking and sweating and stammering and will not like me frightens me to the point of shaking and sweating etc. At the first sign of shaking and etc., I will know that I have lost this battle and I will have to find an excuse to get out. There are no excuses as my mind goes blank when I am very frightened. I will be left standing there looking a total fool. I wish the floor would open and swallow me. I will never come to anything like this again.

That will have to do. These types of explanations stand opposed to the single "explanation" of biological psychiatry, that an anxiety state represents a chemical imbalance of the brain; since each particular anxiety disorder is different from the next, each one necessarily represents a separate biochemical lesion, and therefore a genetic lesion. But Occam's principle says that the number of explanatory entities must not expand beyond the minimum needed. A single generic cognitive explanation is more parsimonious than a hundred thousand categorical biological explanations and is therefore to be preferred.

Thus, we can give a valid, viable cognitive account of a personality-based anxiety state. It is a personality disorder (an enduring pattern of inner experience and behavior that deviates markedly from cultural expectations in areas involving cognition, affect, social function and impulse control) and it generates endless anxiety. But because orthodox psychiatry doesn't recognize the Anxious Personality Disorder, they have to slot them somewhere else. Because the concept of ADHD is so loose that I could diagnose a ham sandwich with ADHD, then combining the rubbery concept of ADHD with a psychiatrist who is desperate to find a biological disease to treat means that the 15% of the population who are anxious by virtue of their personalities will necessarily end up on a cocktail of drugs which are known to produce serious disturbances of mood in the long term, and by this means they are recruited into the ever-growing ranks of people who form the new epidemic of Bipolar Affective Disorder.

Quod erat demonstrandum.

16.10 Conclusion

On that basis, I am of the view that the biocognitive model of mind passes every test thrown at it thus far with what we might call flying colors. I will therefore terminate this discussion so that it doesn't become endless, on the grounds that anybody who is not yet convinced of the primacy of psychological explanations needs to put up a reasonable counter-argument or vacate the speaker's rostrum (and get his hand out of the honey pot of government research grants and desirable academic posts).

16.11 One Final Shot

I hear the APA has already spent over $35,000,000 on DSM-V, but there is still a huge amount of work still to do before D-Day in 2013. If they had counted all the time paid by universities and government institutions when their staff were away at meetings, I do not doubt the real figure would be five times that amount. However much it may be, it has all been wasted. It should have been spent on articulating a formal model of mental disorder instead.

DSM-V is the wrong project for our time.

In the absence of an agreed model of mental disorder, DSM-V will just be more of the same, then DSM-VR will be rushed out to fill the gaps while they organize the DSM-VI committees, and so it will go on and on. Because they cannot grasp the nettle of a psychological cause, biological accounts of human mental disorder are doomed to endless repetition: isn't there some story about a hog that lives underground and nothing ever changes?

Note:

The "Yellow Peril" was a fear deeply-ingrained in Australians for a hundred years or more, who fretted that this vast, essentially empty continent would be overwhelmed if the swarming masses of Asia just to the north took it into their heads to walk in. In 1949, when China became Red China, the fear morphed into the Orange Peril.

Royal Free Disease. Epidemic hysteria from the hospital of the same name in London, in the 1950s. In fact, it was epidemic anxiety, where excitable people living in close quarters (in this case, nurses) get the idea there is a mysterious disease lurking in dark corners. This too has morphed, into either benign myalgic encephalopathy or chronic fatigue syndrome, depending on who is talking,

Repetitive Strain Injury. A short-lived epidemic of pain and disability of the wrists, mainly affecting young female typists in all-girl settings. In the 1990s, it came from nowhere to be the biggest cause of work health claims, then faded to nothing in a few years. Not to be confused with tenosynovitis.

Conclusion:
The Hungry Dream of Knowledge

"I—a man of thought—the book-worm of great libraries—a man already in decay, having given my best years to feed the hungry dream of knowledge...."

Nathaniel Hawthorne, *The Scarlet Letter*

If depression is purely a psychological frame of mind, of pessimism, then anything at all that produces a more optimistic frame of mind will have the effect of reducing depression (because optimism is the opposite of depression).

As I travel around, reading and talking as I go, it seems to me that psychiatry is in the most serious trouble. Last week, the Australian Federal Government announced a new policy that would see three year old children screened for mental disorders. The screening would be carried out by general practitioners and, if anything were found, the children would be referred to psychologists and pediatricians for further management. Put aside the prodigious difficulties in making decisions about the mental states of such young children and the overwhelming probability that the program won't reach the children who might actually need it, to focus on one point only: psychiatrists aren't involved. Mental disorder in children is no longer regarded as a psychiatric condition.

At the same time, the Western Australian State Government has announced that its new mental health act will contain a section that allows children from the age of twelve to consent to psychosurgery and to sterilization for psychiatric reasons—without their parents' approval. The safeguard will be that the child's psychiatrist certifies that the child is aware of what is involved and has not been subject to undue influence (presumably the same psychiatrist who raised the idea in the first place). The wording of the draft bill is as follows: "11.3.3 : Psychosurgery cannot be performed on a child between the ages of 12 and 18 unless consent is provided on behalf of the patient by a parent or guardian or if they are a competent young person and can provide consent themselves." (Don't worry about the jarring misuse of plural pronouns). This will also apply to ECT: "competent young people" (i.e. from the day they turn twelve) will be able to consent to the procedure. How will they be deemed competent? Presumably because they don't kick and scream when asked to sign the consent form. The same applies to sterilization: "S.12.3.3 Sterilization must not be performed on a child unless authorized by the Family Court. S.12.3.4 The exception to this rule is if the child has sufficient maturity and understanding to make reasonable decisions and therefore has the capacity to provide informed consent. " In addition, a guardian can make the decision regardless of the child's wishes [1].

In the same state, children under sixteen cannot own land, own or drive a car or motorcycle, vote, be in possession of a firearm, obtain a passport, own shares, have a bank account, borrow money, bequeath property, drink, serve in the Defense Forces and so on just because they are considered too young to make those decisions. In particular, a child of fifteen years and eleven months who has sexual contact (of any sort) with an adult, even of sixteen years and one day, is deemed incapable of giving consent and the "adult" involved can be and often is convicted of what amounts to statutory rape. A perfectly normal child of fifteen years and eleven months cannot give informed consent to something that lasts only a few minutes and which, perchance, may even be enjoyable, yet a much younger child with a history of major mental disorder can consent to irreversible, life-altering surgical interventions. Within the psychiatric establishment, there appears to be no awareness of this contradiction. Provisions like that did not get into the draft bill without the full knowledge and consent of the state's most influential psychiatrists.

Within psychiatry itself, training posts are unfilled; the average age of trainees (residents) is rising; the average age of psychiatrists is rising much faster than for the general population; and most western countries have such serious shortages that they have to import foreign psychiatrists to fill their public positions. This shortage comes about because medical students feel psychiatry is not an attractive proposition since it doesn't address people's problems. To students, modern psychiatry is intellectually as inviting as the stairwell in a multi-storey car park on a winter's night. Corruption among senior figures in the psychiatric world is becoming more and more widespread and the cozy relationship between the psychiatric establishment and the overbearing drug companies is drawing increasingly hostile attention from outside the profession.

To a growing proportion of the population, the relentless drive to medicalize what has always been regarded as normality is becoming a source of outrage and contempt. As the consumption of psychotropic drugs rockets skyward, the numbers of people permanently disabled by mental problems keeps pace: if modern treatment is so good, why are all these mentally disordered people in our prisons, on our streets and on welfare? All this is happening despite unprecedented levels of government and drug company publicity aimed at inducing the citizenry to accept that taking pills for every imaginable variation from psychological normality is not just acceptable, but actually represents one's duty to family, employer, fellow students and workers, and self.

Most psychotropic drugs are now prescribed by general practitioners who, increasingly, do not see any point in referring their mentally-disturbed patients for psychiatric assessment before commencing major psychotropic medications. The reason is that they have questionnaires devised by psychiatrists to make the diagnosis and drug company handouts that tell them what drugs to prescribe for each condition, and what to do if the treatment doesn't work (prescribe more). If they feel the patient requires additional management beside the drugs, then they refer to the large numbers of psychologists who are assiduous in establishing and maintaining the closest relationships with general practitioners (Australia has about eight psychologists for each psychiatrist; in France in 2007, there were over 40,000 psychology students who, presumably, would want jobs).

All this was predicted years ago. Psychiatry's determination to "dumb down" the assessment and management of the mentally disturbed has had the result of rendering us irrelevant. These days, every nurse, every schoolteacher and lawyer knows that making a diagnosis is a simple matter of ticking a few boxes. Because of the relentless barrage of drug company propaganda, everybody else knows that drugs are the answer, that drugs are their entitlement, so where does psychiatry fit in? Increasingly, it doesn't.

My case is that this state of affairs has arisen just because psychiatry has no rational or scientific basis. Since it has no declared model of mental disorder, but acts as though biology will explain all even when nobody else still believes this, psychiatry operates in an intellectual vacuum with no points of contact with the larger world. We are busy selling a model of mind that nobody else takes seriously. We wanted to be as biological as the rest of medicine but they still regard us with disdain. We discarded the psychology of being human as it didn't fit with a biological psychiatry, leaving it to other disciplines as though it didn't matter, and now we have no fall-back position, no Plan B. Biological psychiatrists are driving this profession into a position of unassailable irrelevance.

At a conference on biological psychiatry held in Baltimore, Maryland, in 1970, the US psychiatrist Nathan Kline stated:

> "Medicine and science will be *just that much different* because we (Kline's generation of psychiatrists) have lived.... Treatment and understanding of (mental) illness will forever be altered.... and in our way, we will persist for all time in that small contribution we have made toward the Human Venture."

His successors still swear by this but it is a myth, an utterly unsubstantiated ideological claim with no demonstrated basis beyond the dreams of those who hold it. John F Kennedy was aware of the pernicious effects of these stories:

> "The greatest enemy of the truth is very often not the lie—deliberate, contrived, and dishonest—but the myth, persistent, persuasive and unrealistic. Belief in the myth allows the comfort of opinion without the discomfort of thought" (Commencement address, Yale University, 11 June 1962)

Reductionist biological psychiatry is a myth, just as psychoanalysis was a myth, behaviorism was a myth, the biopsychosocial model was a myth, eclecticism was a myth... Myths arise when we try to sidestep the hard work of determining what we mean by "mental." As Thomas Nagel commented in his legendary paper, *What is it like to be a bat?* "Any reductionist program has to be based on an analysis of what is to be reduced" [2]. Most emphatically, that has never been done. No biological psychiatrist in history has sat down to do the hard work of analyzing what it is about the human condition that biology is supposed to explain. No biological psychiatrist in history has offered to show why a final cause in human behavior can be explained in terms of efficient mechanisms. It is assumed that reductionism will work as well in psychiatry as it has in kidneys. No consideration has ever been given to the question of whether it is appropriate.

Biological psychiatry is a tissue of stories illuminated by a roseate promise, a narrative in the worst sense, strung together with the explicit purpose of benefiting drug companies, psychiatrists, nursing unions, psychologists, social workers, general practitioners, builders, cleaners, lawyers, politicians, teachers, parents, prisons and schools... Everybody, that is, but the sufferer himself. And not one of those stories is true. Turing himself noted: "The popular view that scientists proceed inexorably from well-established fact to well-established fact, never being influenced by any unproven conjecture, is quite mistaken" [3].

So here we see the conflict: Man's restless desire to explore and know fenced in by mythology, the hungry dream of knowledge battling the comfort of opinions unburdened by the discomfort of thought. George Orwell had no illusions of the place of myths: "Genuine progress means the continuous destruction of myths." These days, young psychiatrists are not taught to read the classic papers. They are taught to regard anything older than about four years as irrelevant. If the editors can suppress a novel idea for four years, it drops below the event horizon of the new generation of psychiatrists and simply ceases to exist. All our previous mistakes are forgotten, elided from the collective consciousness: "Everything faded into mist. The past was erased, the erasure was forgotten, the lie became truth" (*1984*).

Young psychiatrists are also taught not to question the orthodoxy on which they are force-fed. My own experience is that we were not taught to think at all. When, at the age of thirty-five, a senior specialist in charge of a hospital department, I enrolled in some undergraduate philosophy units, I was shocked to find that students half my age could think with a rigor and discipline I had never seen in my eighteen years in medicine. I had to work hard to catch up but, as I did, I realized that I was taking leave of my psychiatric colleagues. When they were not able to follow something I said in my new language, they dismissed it as not worth their effort. Nothing was allowed to disturb their suave paternalism. They were secure in their myth, mutually self-satisfied by what Chomsky called "...the illusion of a rigorous scientific theory with a very broad scope." Biological psychiatry is an illusion of science, but an illusion that generates vast profits and power for those who surrender to its false promise. It is promissory materialism at its most vapid, it is the easy way out of a difficult problem for people who, quite bluntly, don't know how to think but who can count on their colleagues to reassure them that they are rapier-sharp.

In a genuine science, this would not arise, as criticism of the *status quo* would soon expose the falsity of the claims made for this baseless doctrine.

Carl Sagan saw criticism as the core of the scientific endeavor: "...at the heart of science is an essential balance between two seemingly contradictory attitudes—an openness to new ideas, no matter how bizarre or counter-intuitive, and the most ruthlessly skeptical scrutiny of all ideas, old and new. This is how deep truths are winnowed from deep nonsense." Clearly, that most sane of men had never encountered a profession that now thinks up to half of the population are mentally disordered, the implication being that they all need drugs. For life.

Academic psychiatry is most emphatically *not* open to new ideas. Anything that disturbs the elegant equanimity of the elders of the profession is actively suppressed, anybody with new ideas is shunted aside, and the whole intellectual project in psychiatry becomes a form of brain-washing, of obedience to authority. Does that matter? Stanley Milgram thought it does: "Ordinary people can become agents in a terrible destructive process... Even when the destructive effects of their work becomes patently clear, and they are asked to carry out actions incompatible with fundamental standards of morality, relatively few people have the resources needed to resist authority." For a psychiatrist, with nowhere else to turn, the most frightening sanction is to be excluded from the fraternity. There can be no life after psychiatry.

How does this come about? The radical economist, Joan Robinson, was in no doubt: "Progress is slow partly from mere intellectual inertia. In a subject where there is no agreed procedure for knocking out errors, doctrines have a long life. A professor teaches what he was taught, and his pupils, with a proper respect and reverence for teachers, set up a resistance against his critics for no other reason than that it was he whose pupils they were." But, as that merciless commentator, George Orwell, noted: "If liberty means anything at all, it means the right to tell people what they do not want to hear."

In the case of psychiatry, the intellectual inertia goes much further. It flows from the universal but unstated dread in psychiatrists that if the biological project fails, we are finished. It's all we have, there is nothing else in the barrel. We threw out the humanity in favor of the devastatingly simple idea of reductionism. Carl Sagan again: "One of the saddest lessons of history is this: If we've been bamboozled long enough, we tend to reject any evidence of the bamboozle. We're no longer interested in finding out the truth. The bamboozle has captured us. It is simply too painful to acknowledge—even to ourselves— that we've been so credulous." In this, he echoed Tolstoy: "I know that most men, including those at ease with problems of the greatest complexity, can seldom accept the simplest and most obvious truth if it be such as would oblige them to admit the falsity of conclusions which they have proudly taught to others, and which they have woven, thread by thread, into the fabrics of their lives."

For nearly forty years, orthodox psychiatrists have woven the threads of biologism into the fabric of their minds, starting with the conclusions but never bothering with the premises, and now the fabric is rotten. In a profession whose only source of pride is its glorious tomorrows, there can be no return to the bleak and sterile desert of yesterday's creaking theories. Science, glorious science, is our future salvation. And the future is chemical. Or so the keynote speakers at the endless conferences keep saying.

Granted, the psychiatric publishing industry occasionally prints heart-warming papers on mindfulness or brisk meta-analyses of the efficacy of psychotherapy but these are window dressing, tokenism at its most cynical (see note) as the editors firmly believe that all that counts in psychiatry is biological: "The intellectual basis of this field is shifting from one discipline, based on subjective 'mental' phenomena, to another, neuroscience. Indeed, today's developing science-based understanding of mental illness very likely will revolutionize prevention and treatment and bring real and lasting relief to millions of people worldwide." That is, says the director of NIMH, Thomas Insel, now that the real science of mental disorder is almost within reach, we can dispense with all that silly stuff about trying to understand people or treating them humanely to gain their trust, because it never worked anyway.

In this, Insel speaks with that unruffled certainty granted only to those who are utterly unaware of the complexities of the matter. Henry Mencken knew his type: "The most common of all follies is to believe passionately in the palpably untrue. It is the chief preoccupation of all mankind." But beware, said Chesterton: "The real trouble with this world [is that]... It looks just a little more mathematical and regular than it is; its exactitude is obvious but its inexactitude is hidden; its wildness lies in wait."

We came to psychiatry to satisfy our hungry dreams of knowledge but the establishment fed us pap. Folly, deception, corruption... perhaps we can live with these but their worst crime was that they made psychiatry boring. And that is unforgivable.

Note:

In 2011, the *American Journal of Psychiatry* published 184 original papers. Of these, fifteen were largely or totally irrelevant to the conduct of psychiatry, including obituaries and commentaries on artists (in their *Images in Psychiatry* and *Introspection* series). Three were meta-analyses of the efficacy of psychotherapy and did not address theories or issues of psychotherapy such as values. The remainder, 166 papers in all, including about four editorials per issue, were explicitly biological or epidemiological from a biological perspective.

The same year, the *British Journal of Psychiatry* published 161 original contributions, including three or four editorials a month. Seven were irrelevant (historical notes, obituaries and a debate on whether praying with patients constitutes a 'boundary violation'), one was critical (Dr. J Moncrieff) and one was a meta-analysis of psychotherapy. The rest were epidemiological with a smattering of biological papers.

Two papers in the US journal caught my eye. In May, a paper entitled "Lower ventral striatal activation during reward anticipation in adolescent smokers" required the combined labors of 28 authors. This was eclipsed by one in April which must have meshed perfectly with Dr. Insel's vision of psychiatry's splendid future: "Maternally derived microduplications of 15q11-q13: Implications of imprinted genes in psychotic illness." This opus needed no less than 41 authors to ease its passage to light of day. If nothing else, it seems reductionist biologism will need far more psychiatrists conducting essential research in laboratories which, given our shrinking workforce, means far fewer to treat the explosively increasing numbers of the mentally ill. And why not? For people who think "mental" factors are irrelevant, psychiatry without all those crazy people must be a wonderful career.

References:

Chalmers DJ. (1996) The Conscious Mind: in search of a fundamental theory. Oxford: University Press.

Dennett DC. (1978). Brainstorms: Philosophical essays on mind and psychology. Hassocks, Sussex: Harvester Press.

Dennett DC. (1989) *The intentional stance.* Cambridge, Mass.: Bradford Books.

Dennett DC. (1993) *Consciousness Explained.* London: Penguin Books.

Dennett DC. (2004) *Freedom Evolves.* London: Penguin Books.

Kuhn, T.S. (1970) *The Structure of Scientific Revolutions.* 2nd Edition. Chicago, Ill: University Press (International Encyclopedia of Unified Science, Vol. 2, No. 2).

McLaren N. (2007) Humanizing Madness: Psychiatry and the Cognitive Neurosciences. Ann Arbor, Mi.: Future Psychiatry Press.

McLaren N. (2009) *Humanizing Psychiatry: The Biocognitive Model.* Ann Arbor, Mi.: Future Psychiatry Press.

McLaren N. (2010) *Humanizing Psychiatrists: Toward a Humane Psychiatry.* Ann Arbor, Mi.: Future Psychiatry Press.

Popper KR, Eccles JC. (1981) *The Self and its Brain.* London: Springer.

Whitaker, R. (2002) Mad in America: Bad Science, Bad Medicine, and the Enduring Mistreatment of the Mentally Ill. Revised Edn. New York: Perseus Books.

Whitaker, R. (2009) Anatomy of an Epidemic: Magic Bullets, Psychiatric Drugs, and the Astonishing Rise of Mental Illness in America. New York: Crown.

Introduction:

1. McLaren N. (2007)
2. McLaren N. (2009)
3. McLaren N. (2010)
4. Martinez, M. Institute of Biocognitive Sciences. http://www.biocognitive.com/biocognitive/
5. Chalmers DJ. (1996)

Chapter 1:

1 McLaren N. (2007)

2 Skinner BF. 1978 Why I am not a cognitive psychologist. In: *Reflections of Behaviorism and Society.* New York: Prentice Hall.

3 Whitaker, Robert (2002).

4 Guze SB, 1992. *Why psychiatry is a branch of medicine.* New York: Oxford University Press.

5 Chomsky N. (1959) A Review of B. F. Skinner's Verbal Behavior. *Language*, 35: 26-58.

6 Dennett DC. (1993)

7 Dennett DC. (1989)

8 Dennett DC. (2004)

9 Audi R (Ed.) 1995. *The Cambridge Dictionary of Philosophy.* Cambridge: University Press.

10 Chalmers DJ. (1996)

Chapter 2:

1 Turing AM. (1935). On computable numbers, with an application to the Entscheidungsproblem. *Proceedings of the London Mathematical Society* (1936—37) Series 2; 42:230-65. Available on line: See his author entry in Wikipedia.

2 Shannon CE. (1937). A Symbolic Analysis of Relay and Switching Circuits," unpublished MS Thesis, Massachusetts Institute of Technology, Aug. 10, 1937. Accessed June 24th 2012 at
http://dspace.mit.edu/bitstream/handle/1721.1/11173/34541425.pdf?sequence=1

3 McLaren N. (2007).

4 Eccles JC, in Popper KR, Eccles JC. (1981)

5 Dennett DC. (1993)

6 Dennett DC. (1978)

7 Guze SB. (1992). *Why psychiatry is a branch of medicine.* New York: Oxford University Press.

8 Searle JR (1999). *Mind, Language and Society: Doing philosophy in the real world.* London: Weidenfeld and Nicholson.

9 Searle JR (1993). The problem of consciousness. *Social Research.* 60 (1) Spring.
http://users.ecs.soton.ac.uk/harnad/Papers/Py104/searle.prob.html.
Accessed Dec 30. 2009.

10 Searle JR (1999). The future of philosophy. Paper presented to Royal Society. Available at http://socrates.berkeley.edu/~jsearle/articles.html. Accessed January 4, 2010.

11 Searle JR (2000). Consciousness. *Annual Review of Neuroscience.* 23:557-578.

12 Wiener N (1948, Rev. Ed. 1965). Cybernetics, or control and communication in the animal and the machine. Cambridge, MA: MIT Press.

13 Eisenberg L. (1986). Mindlessness and brainlessness in psychiatry. British Journal of Psychiatry 148: 497-508.

Chapter 3:

1 Shannon CE (1948) A Mathematical Theory of Communication. *Bell System Technical Journal* 27: 379–423, 623–656 (July, October).

2 Shannon CE. (1971). *Scientific American* 225: 180

3 Turing AM. On computable numbers, with an application to the Entscheidungsproblem. *Proceedings of the London Mathematical Society* (1936—37) Series 2; 42:230-65. Available on line: See his author entry in Wikipedia.

4 Chalmers DJ. (1996)

5 Berlinski D. (2001) The Advent of the Algorithm: The Idea that Rules the World. New York: Harcourt.

6 Luria AR. *Higher cortical functions in man.* New York: Basic Books, 1980.

7 Berlinski D. (2004) On the Origin of the Mind. *Commentary* November; 26-36.

Chapter 4:

1 Chalmers DJ. (1996)

2 McLaren N. (2007).

3 Luria AR. *Higher cortical functions in man.* New York: Basic Books, 1980.

4 Popper KR, Eccles JC. (1981).

Chapter 6:

1 Pocock G, Richards CD. *Human Physiology: The basis of medicine.* 3rd Ed. Oxford: University Press, 2006.

2 Bear MF, Connors BW, Paradiso MA. *Neurosciences: Exploring the brain.* 3rd Edn. 2007. Philadelphia: Lippincott.

3 Rhodopsin, in Wikipedia: http://en.wikipedia.org/wiki/Rhodopsin

Chapter 7:

1 Nagel E, Newman JR, Hofstadter D. (2001). Gödel's Proof. Rev. Edn. New York: New York University Press.

Chapter 8:

1 Popper KR (1972a). *Conjectures and refutations: the growth of scientific knowledge.* London: Routledge.

2 Wingfield JC, Hegner RE, Dufty AM, Ball GF (1990). The 'Challenge Hypothesis': Theoretical implications for patterns of testosterone secretion, mating systems and breeding strategies. *Amer. Naturalist* 36: 829-846.

3 Archer J (2004). Testosterone and human aggression: an evaluation of the Challenge Hypothesis. *Neurosci Biobehav Rev* 30: 319–345

4 Liberman SA (2010). Applying the Challenge Hypothesis to wild, adult male Chacma baboons (*Papio ursinus*). Unpublished thesis: University of Michigan, Ann Arbor, MI.

5 McAndrew FT (2009). The interacting roles of testosterone and challenges to status in human male aggression. *Aggression Violent Behav.* 14: 330-335.

6 Klinesmith J, Kasser T, McAndrew FT (2006). Guns, testosterone, and aggression: An experimental test of a mediational hypothesis. *Psychol Sci* 17: 568-571.

7 Liening SH, Josephs RA (2010). It is not just about testosterone: physiological mediators and moderators of testosterone's behavioral effects. *Soc Pers Psych Compass* 3:1–13, 10.1111/j.1751-9004.2010.00316.x

8 Mehta PH, Josephs RA (2006). Testosterone change after losing predicts the decision to compete again. *Horm. Behav.* 50: 684-92. http://www.ncbi.nlm.nih.gov/pubmed/16928375. Accessed Dec 12 2010.

9 Pocock G, Richards CD (2006). *Human Physiology: the basis of medicine.* 3rd Ed. Oxford: University Press.

10 Yin W, Wu D, Noel ML, Gore AC (2009). Gonadotropin-releasing hormone neuroterminals and their microenvironment in the median eminence: effects of aging and estradiol treatment. *Endocrinology* 150:498-508.

11 Shannon CE (1948). A Mathematical theory of communication. Reprinted with corrections from *The Bell System Technical Journal*, 27: 379–423, 623–656 (July, October, 1948).

12 Kessler RC, et al (2006). The prevalence and correlates of DSM-IV intermittent explosive disorder in the National Comorbidity Survey Replication. Arch Gen Psychiat 63:669-678.

13 Möstl E, Palme R (2002). Hormones as indicators of stress. *Domest. Anim. Endocrinol.* 23:67-74.

Chapter 9:

1 Michels, Robert. 1911. *Zur Soziologie des Parteiwesens in der modernen Demokratie. Untersuchungen über die oligarchischen Tendenzen des Gruppenlebens.* Eng. Tr. *Political Parties* Available in PDF at http://socserv2.socsci.mcmaster.ca/~econ/ugcm/3ll3/michels/

2 Bullock, Alan. 1962. *Hitler: A study in tyranny.* London: Fontana.

3 Brown, Donald. 1991 *Human Universals.* Boston, MA: McGraw Hill

4 Doctorow, EL. 2006. *Creationists: Selected Essays, 1993-2006.* New York: Random House.

Chapter 10:

1 Oderberg DS (2005). Hylemorphic Dualism, in Paul EF, Miller FD, Paul J: *Personal Identity.* Cambridge: University Press.

2 Oderberg DS. (2011). Disembodied Communication and Religious Experience: The Online Model. *Philosoph. Tech.* Published on line, October 8 2011. DOI 10.1007/s13347-011-0051-6 Accessed January 24th 2012.

Chapter 11:

1 Insel TR, Cuthbert BN, Garvey M, Heinssen R, Pine DS, Quinn K, Sanislow C., Wang P, (2010) Research Domain Criteria (RDoC): Toward a New Classification Framework for Research on Mental Disorders. Commentary: *American Journal of Psychiatry* 167: 748-751

2 Cuthbert BN, Insel TR, (2010). Toward New Approaches to Psychotic Disorders: The NIMH Research Domain Criteria Project *Schizophrenia Bulletin* (Advance Publication October 7th 2010), at: doi:10.1093/schbul/sbq108 (accessed October 14th 2010).

3 Yan J, (2010). NIMH Builds New Framework for Understanding Mental Illness. *Psychiatric News*; 45:9 (May 21st 2010).

4 Insel TR, (2010) Faulty Circuits. *Scientific American* April 2010, p45

5 Whitaker R. (2009).

6 NIMH Strategic Plan, 3. Strategy 1.4: http://www.nimh.nih.gov/research-funding/rdoc.shtml,

7 McLaren N (2007).

8 McLaren N (2009).

9 McLaren N (2010).

10 McLaren N, 1992. Is mental disease just brain disease? The limits to biological psychiatry. *Australian and New Zealand Journal of Psychiatry*; 26: 270-276. Revised version: Brain disease, mental disease, and the limits to biological psychiatry. Chapter 2 in ref. 7.

11 Kuhn TS. 1970. *The Structure of Scientific Revolutions.* 2nd Edition, Chicago, Ill: University Press (International Encyclopedia of Unified Science, Vol. 2, No. 2

12 Guze SB, 1992. *Why psychiatry is a branch of medicine.* New York: Oxford University Press.

13 Kandel ER. 2005. *Psychiatry, psychoanalysis and the new biology of mind.* Washington, DC: American Psychiatric Publishing.

14 Hawkins RD, Kandel ER, Bailey CH. 2006. Molecular mechanisms of memory in *Aplysia. Biological Bulletin* 210:174-191.

15 Bear MF, Connors BW, Paradiso MA. 2007. *Neurosciences: Exploring the brain.* 3rd Edn. Philadelphia: Lippincott.

16 Benjamin PR, Kemenes G, Kemenes I. 2008. Non-synaptic neuronal mechanisms of learning and memory in gastropod mollusks. *Frontiers in Bioscience* 13:4051-4057.

17 Wiener N. (1948) *Cybernetics: Or Control and Communication in the Animal and the Machine.* Cambridge, MA: MIT Press 2nd revised ed. 1965.

Chapter 12:

1 Szasz, T.S. (1974). *The Myth of Mental Illness: Foundations of a Theory of Personal Conduct.* Revised Edition. New York: Harper and Row (Perennial Library). Page numbers refer to the revised edition, 1974.

2 Szasz, T.S. (1970). *The Manufacture of Madness: a Comparative Study of the Inquisition and the Mental Health Movement.* New York: Harper and Row (Harper Colophon Books). Page numbers refer to the reprint, 1977)

3 Szasz, T.S. (1977). *The Theology of Medicine: the Political-Philosophical Foundations of Medical Ethics.* Baton Rouge: Louisiana State University Press.

4 Szasz, T.S. (1979), *The Myth of Psychotherapy.* New York: Anchor Press/Doubleday.

5 Szasz, T.S. (1987). *Insanity: the Idea and its Consequences.* New York: Wiley.

6 Ryle G (1949). *The Concept of Mind.* London: Hutchinson. Reprinted Penguin University Books, 1973.

7 Dennett DC. *Consciousness Explained.* London: Penguin Books, 1993.

8 Skinner BF. *Beyond Freedom and Dignity.* New York: Knopf, 1971.

9 McLaren N. (2007).

Chapter 13:

1 McLaren N. (2007)

2 McLaren, N. (2009)

3 McLaren, N. (2010)

4 Szasz, T.S. (2004) An autobiographical sketch, in Schaler J (Ed.) *Szasz Under Fire: the psychiatric abolitionist faces his critics.* Peru, Illinois: Open Court Press.

5 Ryle, G. (1949) *The Concept of Mind.* London: Hutchinson. Reprinted Penguin University Books, 1973.

6. Szasz, T.S. (1974) *The Myth of Mental Illness: Foundations of a Theory of Personal Conduct.* Revised Edition. New York: Harper and Row (Perennial Library).

7. Kandel, E.R. (2006) In search of memory: the emergence of a new science of mind. New York: Norton.

8. Kuhn, T.S. (1970) *The Structure of Scientific Revolutions.* 2nd Edition. Chicago, Ill: University Press (International Encyclopedia of Unified Science, Vol. 2, No. 2).

9. Whitaker, R. (2009) Anatomy of an Epidemic: Magic Bullets, Psychiatric Drugs, and the Astonishing Rise of Mental Illness in America. New York: Crown.

10. Whitaker, R. (2002)

Chapter 14:

1 Turner EH et al. (2008) Selective Publication of Antidepressant Trials and Its Influence on Apparent Efficacy *New England Journal of Medicine* 358:252-260.

2 Healy D (2003) ABC debate on antidepressants.
http://www.abc.net.au/radionational/programs/allinthemind/part-a---the-antidepressants-debate-depressed/3455258

3 Whitaker, Robert (2002).

4 Whitaker, Robert (2009).

5 Torrey EF A review of Mad in America: How Robert Whitaker got it wrong.
http://www.treatmentadvocacycenter.org/index.php?option=com_content&task=view&id=2085 Accessed June 21st 2012.

6 Beyond blue at http://www.beyondblue.org.au. Accessed June 2nd 2012.

7 Horwitz AV, Wakefield JC. (2007) *The Loss of Sadness: how psychiatry transformed normal sorrow into Depressive Disorder.* New York: Oxford University Press.

8 WebMD at http://www.webmd.com/depression/features/antidepressants. Accessed June 2nd 2012

9 Lynn J, Jay A (1989) *The Complete 'Yes, Minister.'* London: BBC

10 Autism risk and antidepressants in pregnancy (CNN): http://edition.cnn.com/2011/HEALTH/07/04/antidepressant.pregnancy.autism.risk/index.html.
Accessed June 2nd 2012.

11 Autism risk and antidepressants in pregnancy (WSJ): http://online.wsj.com/article/SB100014240527023044506045764197 61141034324.html

12 Autism Support Network (TM) http://www.autismsupportnetwork.com/news/study-links-anti-depressants-use-during-pregnancy-increased-autism-risk-39829332. Accessed June 2nd 2012.

13 Incidence of autism http://www.autismaus.com.au/uploads/pdfs/PrevalenceReport.pdf. Accessed June 2nd 2012

14 Labrie, V., Pai, S. & Petronis, A. (2012) 'Epigenetics of major psychosis: Progress, problems and perspectives'. *Trends in Genetics*. Article in press. DOI: 10.1016/j.tig.2012.1004.1002. Accessed May 30th 2012.

Dean ET. "Shook over hell: Post-Traumatic Stress, Vietnam and the Civil War." 1997; Harvard University Press: Cambridge, Mass. P200.

Chapter 15:

1 Road trains. I'd really like you to watch these, this has been my life for the past twenty-five years (it has nothing to do with psychiatry). http://www.youtube.com/watch?v=QObGu_WQIts
http://www.youtube.com/watch?v=RRNRbfiyHWA&feature=related
http://www.youtube.com/watch?v=dbNtwSHJe1Q&feature=related.
If they aren't available, just search "road trains in Australia" in Youtube.

2 The implausible antics of Silvio Berlusconi: a Must See.
http://www.youtube.com/watch?v=81vQje8bWmo

3   BCCI
http://en.wikipedia.org/wiki/Bank_of_Credit_and_Commerce_International. June 4th 2012

4 Nugan Hand http://en.wikipedia.org/wiki/Nugan_Hand_Bank. Essential reading for anybody who wants to know what the psychopaths in government get up to. June 4th 2012

5 Zimmerman M et al (2010). Psychiatric diagnoses in patients previously over-diagnosed with Bipolar Disorder. *J. Clin. Psychiat.* 71: 26-31.

6 WebMD: http://www.webmd.com/bipolar-disorder/guide/cyclothymia-cyclothymic-disorder. June 16th 2012

7 Dreyfus, J: http://en.wikipedia.org/wiki/Jack_Dreyfus June 4th 2012

8 Kirsch, I. (2009). The Emperor's New Drugs: Exploding the Antidepressant Myth. London: The Bodley Head

9 Gibbons RD et al. Benefits from antidepressants: Synthesis of 6-week patient-level outcomes from double-blind placebo-controlled randomized trials of fluoxetine and venlafaxine. Arch Gen Psychiat [e-pub]. (http://archpsyc.ama-assn.org/cgi/content/full/archgenpsychiatry.2011.2044)

Chapter 16:

1 Whitely M (2010). Speed Up and Sit Still: the controversies of ADHD diagnosis and treatment. University of Western Australia Press: Perth, WA.

2 Whitely M (2012). The rise and fall of ADHD child prescribing in Western Australia: Lessons and implications. Australian and New Zealand Journal of Psychiatry 46: 400-403.

3 Freeman, Walter: "The Lobotomist" Documentary on PBS Frontline.
http://www.pbs.org/wgbh/americanexperience/films/lobotomist/

4 Dean ET. "Shook over hell: Post-Traumatic Stress, Vietnam and the Civil War." 1997; Harvard University Press: Cambridge, Mass.

5 Morrow RL (et al), Influence of relative age on diagnosis and treatment of attention-deficit/hyperactivity disorder in children. CMAJ, March 5, 2012,
http://www.cmaj.ca/content/early/2012/03/05/cmaj.111619.full.pdf+html

6 Valle, M. ADHD: Biological Disease or Psychosocial Disorder? Accounting for the French-American divergence in Ritalin consumption.
http://www.irle.berkeley.edu/culture/papers/vallee09.pdf

7 Adult ADHD http://www.webmd.com/add-adhd/10-symptoms-adult-adhd June 5th 2012

8 Helpguide http://www.helpguide.org/about.htm Accessed June 6th 2012. See page "About us"

9 Youngson R: "Scientific Blunders" Robinson: London, 1998.

10 Bullmore E, Fletcher P, Jones PB (2009) Why psychiatry can't afford to be neurophobic. Brit. J. Psychiat. 194, 293–295. doi: 10.1192/bjp.bp.108.058479 T

11 Broad, Wm and Wade, N. "Betrayers of the Truth: Fraud and deceit in the halls of science." London: Century, 1983. p212

12 Tacoma Bridge collapse, 1940. http://www.youtube.com/watch?v=j-zczJXSxnw
http://en.wikipedia.org/wiki/Tacoma_Bridge

Conclusion:

1.
http://www.mentalhealth.wa.gov.au/mentalhealth_changes/mh_legislation.aspx. Accessed June 23rd 2102.

2. Nagel, T: What is it like to be a bat? *The Philosophical Review*, Vol. 83, No. 4. (Oct., 1974); pp. 435-450.

3. Turing AM (1950). Computing machinery and intelligence, *Mind* 59: 236: 433-460,; p442

Index

www.ingramcontent.com/pod-product-compliance
Lightning Source LLC
Chambersburg PA
CBHW080228270326
41926CB00020B/4186